Presumed Crazy

A Fisherman Gets Entangled in the Mental Health Gulag

Gerald D. Otis, PhD

DEDICATION

This book is dedicated to all those who have suffered or died as the result of arrogant, inept, ill-informed and unethical practices in the courts and care facilities that oversee individuals who are presumed to be mentally ill.

CONTENTS

PREFACE AND ACKNOWLEDGMENTS

Deprivation of liberty on grounds of mental illness is unjustified....I believe that the severity of the mental illness cannot justify detention nor can it be justified by a motivation to protect the safety of the person or others. Furthermore, deprivation of liberty that is based on grounds of a disability and that inflicts severe pain or suffering falls under the scope of the Convention against Torture.
Juan E. Mendez, UN Special Rapporteur on Torture
Statement to the UN Human Rights Council, 04 March 2013

I had not planned on writing this book. I would have been quite content to continue writing historical books about the interesting characters associated with the early years of my home town of Northfield, Minnesota, even though I had not lived there for half a century. At first, I thought the crisis would just blow over, the mistake would quickly be found and my old friend would be back in his usual habitat. When that didn't happen, I thought that surely I would be able to talk with someone who had some common sense and understanding of mental phenomena and would get the situation straightened out. But a cursory evaluation by a court-contracted psychologist, guided more by a desire to avoid a snow storm than to comply with ethical standards, produced a report with totally absurd diagnoses that could not be supported by the data obtained. Meeting over the phone with a court that was resistant to reason and determined to draw blood - to make my friend pay for his misdeeds as if he were a criminal even though he had committed no crime - I began to get desperate. I called numerous state agencies that were supposed to help in such situations and was met with indifference and no help, if I even got so far as to explain the situation. Most of the time, I didn't get that far.

Disbelief changed to outrage at the inadequacies of a state that I used to proudly consider progressive. My friend was beginning to panic too because his physical problems were being ignored while he was at the same time being psychologically abused - disparaged by hospital staff as "paranoid," "delusional," "grandiose," and, when they could provide no evidence to support any of those attributions, they reasoned he must be "in denial." The court forced him to take a neuroleptic medication, despite evidence of its dangers and warnings about its use in patients of his history and physical conditions, to which he subsequently had multiple adverse reactions. His physical condition deteriorated and he

i

began to lose hope, a necessity (along with courage) to be able to continue on when locked up in an insane asylum.

By a stroke of luck, a competent doctor discovered the travesty and my friend was freed, only to be cast into the clutches of a new set of state certified wardens who had no interest or incentive in correcting the situation. Health care workers were, with a few exceptions, largely incompetent and uncaring. The legal profession was, at best (again, with a few exceptions), contemptible in all of these proceedings, ignoring the laws regarding human rights that they had sworn to uphold. Even an appeal to the office of the governor, by way of a signed petition, was totally ignored.

This book recounts the story of Bill Tollefson, a pseudonym for a real person, who was caught up in the net of Minnesota's mental health jurisprudence system and the web of "practitioners" who live off the suffering of the poor, infirm, elderly and downtrodden. While Minnesota has what seems to be a decent set of laws on the books, including reasonably prudent statutes for civil commitment, a *Patient Bill of Rights* and a *Bill of Rights for Wards and Protected Persons*, they are routinely ignored. There does not appear to be anyone in state government actually taking responsibility for monitoring the legal proceedings to see that they are implemented. It may be that the recession and consequent reduction in court budgets has led to neglect of these laws, but there is nothing in the statutes themselves that indicate that these rights can be suspended due to a shortage of money.

Because these laws and rights are not honored, erroneous information gets placed in a defendant's file, which accompanies him from place to place in the "system" and is never corrected. The "carry-over diagnosis" is accepted as if it were a fact. Poorly trained, poorly paid, and poorly motivated health care workers (including doctors) simply accept what has gone on before, never questioning the quality of the data, never exercising independent judgment, and they do a perfunctory job of "processing" the patient (or, in this case, the poor sap who was misidentified as a psychotic mental patient). Nursing homes, group homes and other residences for individuals who get caught up in what I refer to as the "mental health gulag," add to the problem. The corporations who control most nursing homes develop policies that stretch staff too thin and they deliberately cut corners on quality of care in order to extract as much profit as possible from government programs. Those few nurses and nurses aides who are ethical and conscientious are soon driven to seek employment elsewhere or succumb to the prevailing nursing home culture and do as little work as possible, neglecting patients in the process. By requiring a legal hold on their clients in order for them to be admitted, the nursing homes have spawned growth in the "guardianship industry" while at the same time discriminating against potential residents who are competent and denying them the rights that they are due. Of course, some guardians exploit their positions for personal gain and get away with it because there is inadequate oversight.

Bill's story offers a glimpse into a bizarre world of paradoxes, one that would do less harm if it did not exist. I hope that telling his story will spur concerned citizens to make the necessary corrections to this shameful system. I thank him for providing, as much as possible, a blow-by-blow account of what was happening to him and for his endurance in the face of unbelievable degradations by a heartless system.

One other note about this book: it is not written as an academic tome with proper footnotes, references and the like. It is written to be read quickly, with the least number of impediments to comprehension and appreciation of the plight of those who get caught up in this web of despair. I tried to tell the story more or less as it unfolded before me. I hope I have provided enough description in the text for those who want to get more information to be able to find it using the many Internet search engines that are available.

I wish especially to thank my comrade-in-arms and boots on the ground in Minnesota during this whole dreadful affair, the character in the story named "Jake Heckler." Jake was a constant encouragement to go on when things looked really dim. He was always there and would not hesitate to make trips to gather important information, check claims made by involved persons, and visit Bill as often as possible. He contributed valuable ideas and insights as to the dynamics of what was going on behind the scenes and the deceptions presented by others. He also has a delightful sense of humor that helped keep us grounded when we were the most aggravated.

Jake and "Gloria" helped to increase our numbers and get signatures on our petition to governor Dayton. The members of the *Free the Fisherman Network* also provided useful criticism and ideas and an emotional boost to try to solve this vexing problem. Members of my writers group – Barbara Villemez, Koro Myers, Sonia Segura and John Duncklee – all did their best to help make this manuscript interesting and readable. Penny Dunklee deserves a special thanks for catching most of my spelling and grammatical errors.

Encouragement as well as leads to research and thoughtful documents on the many aspects of the problem were provided by Jim Gottstein of Psychrights.org and Bonnie Nelson of Mindfreedom.org. Cindi Fisher of M.O.M.S in Washington State contributed her first and second hand knowledge of the foibles of mental health jurisprudence problems and made helpful suggestions regarding this book. Susan Freiman, a former federal attorney now practicing in Israel, used her experience to provide direction and insights as to legal matters. Dr. Janet Parker helped me to navigate the pathways of government agencies, national and international law regarding persons with disabilities and file the appropriate complaint forms.

Most names in the book are pseudonyms except for those individuals who are in the public eye and those who actually tried to do something positive for Bill and others in similar circumstances.

Finally, I wish to thank my wife Connie for putting up with my endless hours at the computer, near daily talks on the phone with Bill, and frequent ravings at the sources of my frustration.

1 <u>FAST TRACK TO THE CACKLE FACTORY</u>

"Hey, Bud. Guess what?"

I recognized the voice on the phone immediately. "Hi, Bill. What's happening?"

"They locked me up!"

"Holy shit! Locked you up? What on earth for?"

"I don't understand it," said Bill. "They think I'm nuts. I was in my wheelchair and slid down on the seat pad and couldn't reposition myself because of the pain in my leg. I asked for some help from the staff but they decided to call the police."

I could believe there might be difficulty moving Bill - he was 6' 6" and weighed 350 pounds. A year ago my wife and I had been in town and Bill was going to prepare a spaghetti dinner for eight of us at a friend's house. I had helped him get from the car to the house steps and warned him that I wouldn't be able to catch him if he started falling. I could picture myself being accidentally squashed by this gentle giant.

"Don't worry, Bud. I've got this thing down. Just steady me a little bit as I get up these stairs. If I lose my balance, get out of the way and I'll make a controlled descent, cushioning myself with my big fat ass."

"What happened after the police got there?"

"Well, they wanted me to go to the hospital. They said they were concerned about the looks of my legs."

The previous time we had been there Bill had been wrapped up in some kind of leggings that applied pressure to help reduce fluid retention and swelling in his legs. He said his legs weren't any different than they had been for several years.

"Yeah, so....?"

"I told them I didn't want to go because it would cost me $150 if I got admitted and I could use that money for something important rather than just getting told for the umpteenth time that I had a problem with my legs. But those assholes thought they knew better and insisted I go. When I resisted, they gave me three shots of Haldol until I didn't give a shit any more and they hauled me off."

"Where did they take you?"

"To the Northfield Hospital. I got in a fight with the doctor there. He didn't like my religious beliefs."

I shuddered. Northfield Hospital was the place where a long-time personal friend and Bill's campaign manager when he had run for mayor back in 2004, had died after coming into the ER several times within a week complaining of chest pains. He was told he had "indigestion" or "stress," or, on the day of his death, that he had pneumonia. Actually it was the patient in the examining room next door to him who had tested positive for pneumonia.

After consulting a passel of lawyers my wife and I learned that it is virtually impossible to institute a malpractice suit in Minnesota because, just to get things started, it is required that you have a doctor testify that one of his peers did something wrong. While her doctor suggested that the wife sue, he was too frightened of retribution from his peers to voice his suggestion publicly. A small town physician could expect to be ostracized if he did so.

Ninety-five percent of all malpractice incidents were never prosecuted in the state, according to one lawyer. In the meantime, the CEO of the insurance company that insured doctors for malpractice received more money in compensation than was paid out in all the malpractice actions in the whole state combined.

The young man left a wife and two children with an outstanding loan on a partially completed home and office building and no income. The bank convinced her to spend half her insurance payment on completing the home so it could be sold, and then foreclosed on her. Yeah, I thought, those good old small town values – help your neighbor and all that. Guess those have vanished into a fond memory with the town doubling in size since I grew up there.

I knew Bill had very fundamentalist kinds of religious beliefs but couldn't imagine how the topic would have come up in a physical examination. "What do you mean, Bill? What do your religious beliefs have to do with your doctor?"

"He didn't like the fact that I had stopped taking some of my medications. He asked me who had told me to do so and I told him that I

2

had consulted with God, meaning that I had prayed about it. He was mad as hell and said, 'Well I've got something here that will over-ride your instructions from God.' and he pulled out this paper, filled it out with a flourish and shoved it in my face. 'You're going to a mental hospital on a 72-hour hold.' And then he stormed off. Oh, Oh! They're coming to get me now. I'll call you the next chance I get."

I hung up the phone. It had been only two months since we had seen Bill at his apartment in Minnesota. He had been looking forward to going out to a lake with us, seeing some of his old haunts and maybe we'd go out to eat. But he was not feeling well. When we saw him, he just sat in his wheelchair and struggled to make conversation, excusing himself for his uncharacteristic lapse in social skills. He didn't know what was wrong and wondered if his lethargy and difficulty in thinking could be the result of depression.

"I don't think so," I said. Having been a clinical psychologist for over 40 years, and knowing Bill for nearly 60 years, the symptoms - lightheadedness, photosensitivity, drooling, "nodding off," and weakness – aren't what you usually associate with depression and appeared to me to suggest some kind of organic problem. Either he was having an adverse drug reaction (which is the most likely suspect in elderly patients) or the negative interaction of two or more drugs, or possibly a stroke. Bill had had unusual reactions to certain drugs in the past and my hunch was that this was another instance. He was able to respond to specific questions and we managed to get the telephone number of his local physician.

Over the phone, I related Bill's appearance to the nurse who relayed the information to the doctor. She came back and said the doctor thought he was suffering from "thyroid toxicity" and should come in to see the physician at the hospital since he was pulling ER duty for the next few days. Bill refused, saying that he would have to pay $50 just to see the doctor in the ER and $150 if he was admitted. He was saving to get a phone from his meager Social Security funds. Finding it hard to believe that there would be such expensive co-pays for someone on Medicare and SSI, we called the insurance carrier and found that it was indeed true. We offered to pay the fee but, apparently out of pride, Bill refused. He promised to see the doctor at his office the next week. Surveying the disarray in Bill's apartment, we inquired if he could get homemaker service from the county and he indicated that he could but they didn't seem to want to do what he thought was needed.

We had been back in our home in New Mexico for about a week and hadn't heard from Bill. I contacted his county social worker to see if she could arrange housekeeping assistance for Bill while he was ill. She said workers from the home care agency had been there and Bill had turned them away. She complained that he "doctor hopped," was "non-compliant" and was "verbally abusive" to the home health care workers. I could visualize her puffing out her chest when she huffed that, "Contrary to what Mr. Tollefson seems to think, agencies have the right to pick up or decline a case." Nevertheless, she agreed to send out a Vulnerable Adult Worker to do a health and safety report on Bill. I had never heard of such a thing as a "vulnerable adult worker" but the name sounded like someone who would attend to the welfare and interests of an impaired individual. It was only later that I learned my assumption was inaccurate.

Damn, he must have really pissed somebody off, I said to myself. I began to wonder if he was really depressed and being cantankerous with others, like depressed people often are. At seventy years of age he had little control over his life and was at the mercy of the state and county, and dependent on "the kindness of strangers." I thought that was bound to make him depressed and angry as he approached the end of his life. Was he sitting in his apartment alone, moping and waiting to die? His father had suffered from depression in his later years. I remembered his father, the once proud and robust businessman, sadly saying during a visit, "You know Bud, I've had a lot of disappointments." I suspected that what he was referring to was the fact that his dream of having his sons take over the business that he had worked so hard to create, did not work out.

Bill certainly had lots of recent reasons to be depressed. He had been unable to work for several years after having a hip and knee replacement and he continued to have difficulty with that leg. The orthopedic surgeon wanted to replace both the hip and the knee, a procedure that would have Bill laid-up for nearly a year. Not knowing how much time he had left to live, given his age and health problems, Bill did not want to be out of commission for that long and sought a more conservative approach. He found a physician who agreed to try an antibiotic treatment that seemed to be effective. Of course, the parties who lost out on the hundreds of thousands of dollars the operation would have generated labeled Bill as "non-compliant" and a "doctor shopper." I thought he was using good judgment.

Bill had to use a wheelchair to get around but managed fairly well: he could hand-paddle himself about three quarters of a mile downtown and back, he could go into the local pub and have a beer with his friends, and he could sit on the river bank in his chair and fish. He had some cardiac problems but had good medical care at the Mayo Clinic in Rochester when he could get there.

About a year earlier Bill had made a trip to Florida to see if he could resurrect his career as a fishing guide. He had worked the waters of northern Minnesota during the summers and the rivers and lakes in Florida during the winters for several years, had participated in fresh-water fishing competitions and had worked with others to develop a professional fishing guides association (until the treasurer ran off with all of their funds).

A physically able 50 year-old man wanted to apprentice himself to Bill to learn the fishing guide business from the master fisherman. He was a recently divorced ordained minister and wanted to make a new start. Bill thought he could trust this man because they shared a religious outlook. A bonus was that the man, Terry, had auto-mechanic skills and was eager to help Bill get his old motor home running. That vehicle was to be their transportation to Florida and their base of operations once they got there.

For a couple of years, Bill had been in contact with a woman who owned a fishing resort in the Gainesville area. She encouraged Bill and his partner to come to Florida and implied that she would employ them to repair her boats and motors and act as fishing guides for tourists once they got there. Bill set about planning the kind of equipment and accommodations he would need to adapt to his physical limitations. He and Terry were to work as a team: Bill had the knowledge and skills associated with the fishing guide business while Terry could do the mechanical and physical things Bill could no longer perform.

Because their vehicle was over thirty years old, it was quite a task to get parts for it and get it running after being immobile for several years. But Terry did a yeoman's job and finally they were ready to start off on their adventure. They filled the motor home with Bill's fishing gear and tied a seventy year old aluminum boat – "the best trolling boat I've ever had" - on the top. Bill planned to give the boat to his grandson who lived in Florida. They attached his partner's SUV to the back and took off while there was still snow on the ground.

Unfortunately, the trip met with one disaster after another. They ran into bad weather and the motor home broke down several times on the way so that what would ordinarily be a 3-4 day trip ended up taking a month. When they went to the resort, they learned the owner had sold it because the resort business had dried up due to the recession. She was just managing it in a "holding" mode for the new owners. They checked other resorts and learned they had either gone bankrupt or had been sold to real estate investors. They depleted their financial reserves, Terry had to sell his SUV, and tempers were short. Terry threatened Bill with physical harm and demanded that Bill turn over title to the motor home with the proviso that Bill be paid back a certain portion of the proceeds if it was sold. It was sold but Bill never received his share of the proceeds. Bill left his boat in the tourist park where they were staying and it disappeared, although the sheriff later returned the boat to Bill and he arranged for it to be stored at an old friend's place.

Shortly after they arrived in Florida, Bill contacted his daughter's boss and the boss told him where he might find her. He and Terry went to that place and Terry went into the restaurant to see if she would talk with Bill. The two of them had been estranged for a time even though, a few years prior to that, she had told Bill that he could come live with her family if he moved to Florida. Now she refused to see him and, through Terry, said she would call the police if he pursued the matter any further. His daughter told Bill's sister that she loved her father but "I just can't have any more chaos in my life right now." It later turned out that she was having marital problems and Bill's presence would have complicated her plans.

Bill was dejected after that and went to the hospital that had saved his daughter's life shortly after she was born, to see if he could get some psychological help in accepting this rejection from his daughter. In order to get insurance coverage, he had to admit himself on a voluntary 72-hour hold. Within a day or two the hospital decided they did not want Bill to be there and forcibly evicted him. He was physically abused in the process and called the sheriff who took photos of the injuries and wrote down the allegations from Bill for a report.

I received nearly daily updates over the phone from Bill as he went from one place to another trying to find shelter and get some help. For a time, he was staying at a trailer camp and would roll himself several blocks in his wheelchair to get to a phone. He managed to gain admission at another hospital but was again discharged. He then thought he might get some help with his medical problems at Mayo Clinic in Jacksonville, since he had been a long-term patient at Mayo in Rochester. They too discharged him after a short stay and no help. Although he was wearing down during these multiple frustrations and disappointments, I was amazed that he remained remarkably resilient through it all. It warmed his heart when a compassionate "woman of the night" let him use her cell phone to make a call while all the official "helpers" treated him like a pariah.

Obviously, the hospitals did not consider him a danger to himself or others and didn't feel it an ethical violation to discharge a wheelchair-bound 70 year-old man to the streets. Perhaps their motives are not so pure, I thought. His Medicaid may have been discontinued because he hadn't returned to Minnesota in time to fill out papers for his annual review. In these hard economic times, all that counts to these government agencies and health care institutions is the bottom line, not the viability of their patients.

Bill made it back to Gainesville but was not admitted by a shelter that had earlier, over the phone, offered to do so. Finally, a friend of his brother-in-law came to the rescue and found Bill a motel room, made arrangements for storage of some of his belongings and got him on a plane back to Minnesota. Prior to his return, he talked to his financial worker in Rice County to see if she could get his Medicare/Medicaid continued until he got back. She refused, apparently happy to be rid of the fat man who complained too much. Now there's a woman with a heart of gold, I thought. She needs a little experience living on the streets. Maybe she'd learn a little humility from the ladies she would meet there.

Bill had been back at his Northfield apartment for five or six months before he became ill. I looked up "toxic thyroid" on the Internet and learned that it is a possible side effect from the use of amioderone, a medication used for atrial fibrillation, and may have some interactions with warfarin too, both medications that Bill had been taking. Sometimes the amioderone causes high toxic levels of thyroid hormones, which apparently was the case for Bill.

At some point after we had left town in October, Bill decided to halt his amioderone as well as his blood pressure medications. The result was that his level of functioning returned to normal: he was lucid, full of energy and could think logically. And he had no adverse effects from not taking the medication – his heart beat was regular and his blood pressure was normal. But stopping his medications was interpreted as "medical non-compliance" by his doctor and when Bill said he had stopped taking them after praying (consulting with God), the physician decided he was crazy.

So, according to the doctor, discontinuing a drug that is making you ill and possibly killing you without consulting him is madness, in spite of the fact that there are at least 106,000 fatalities due to medication errors every year and despite the fact that medical care errors are now considered the third greatest cause of death in the U.S. When Michele Bachmann says that God told her to run for office, she wasn't hauled off to the funny farm. And when George Bush went to war in Iraq after his consultation with God and thousands of people were killed, there was no such declaration of mental instability raised. Therefore, one would have to conclude that imperviousness to accusations of madness is one of the perks to being president or running for the office.

"Doctor shopping" is a concept invented by doctors and their defenders to disparage those patients who are dissatisfied with incompetent medical care and/or arrogant physicians and persist in trying to find that healer with a conscience who doesn't try to baffle them with bullshit and genuinely tries to solve their medical problem. It is a concept that helps to soothe over-inflated egos bruised by rejection from mere patients that those doctors think are so inferior to them in every way.

Is it a sign of mental illness to seek a competent doctor who approaches his task with a manner compatible with one's expectations? Considering the number of errors made by physicians that result in death or injury and the fact that 80% of research findings that physicians rely upon in their practice ultimately turn out to be in error (according to studies reported in the online science journal PLoS One), everyone should be skeptical about their physician's pronouncements and seek other opinions if the doctor's beliefs conflict with their bodily experience or with common sense.

According to Dr. Marcia Angell, former Editor in Chief of the *New England Journal of Medicine*, "It is simply no longer possible to believe much of the clinical research that is published, or to rely on the judgment of trusted physicians or authoritative medical guidelines. I take no pleasure in this conclusion, which I reached slowly and reluctantly over my two decades as an editor of *The New England Journal of Medicine*."

Unfortunately, when you are on Social Security, like Bill, you do not have the option to "doctor shop" like other people with good insurance, transportation and availability of resources to find appropriate health care. And most judges have not read either PloS-One or Dr. Angell's comments and do not wish to broaden their horizons by doing so. Instead, they defer to the nearest doctor who currently has their ear. If what he says turns out to be bullshit, the judge can always blame the bad outcome on the doctor.

A hospital social worker called me to say that Bill was being transferred to United Health Care Hospital in St. Paul for a mental evaluation. This hospital was owned by the same corporation that owned the clinic in which Bill had been treated in Northfield. Since his "72-hour hold" did not include weekends, he would actually be detained for at least five days.

Expressing my disbelief, I said "There is no way in hell this thing will go through, is there?"

The evasive answer, "Well, you never know about these things" told me that Bill might be in real trouble.

On the day Bill was hauled off to the hospital, his county nurse wrote to me in an email:

"Bill was removed from his apartment today via 2 cops and 2 Ambulance personal. He was given 3 shots of Haldol, and was still yelling. His apartment was full of alcohol bottles and bottles of urine. He will be taken to NFLD hospital, and probably transferred to Mayo in Rochester. That is all I know at this time. VA [vulnerable adult] worker was involved and several VA reports came to the county via the hospital/clinic regarding recent visits."

I got a call from Bill a couple of days later and he sounded quite lucid and his account of what happened was markedly different than the report from the social worker. He denied there were any empty booze bottles or jars of urine sitting around. He admitted that he had some wine stored up for the Christmas holidays.

I have seen many people in minor positions of power in hospitals and other "total institutions" concoct stories to get rid of or cause trouble for someone they didn't like, so I was a bit hesitant to accept their accounts without verification. Less than a month earlier when the nurse and vulnerable adult worker visited Bill, they made no mention of seeing empty booze bottles or jars of urine and my wife and I saw no such evidence when we were there in October. A set of pictures of his apartment taken by Jake after Bill was hauled off revealed no jars or bottles of anything. His apartment was cluttered and messy, primarily because he had no shelves and cabinets to organize his stuff. On the other hand, I knew Bill sometimes tried to paint a rosy picture of his innocence too. Oh how I wished for the testimony of a disinterested witness!

About a week later I sent Bill's court-appointed lawyer an email in which I informed him that I was a retired psychologist and that I had known Mr. Tollefson for a long time. I said that if he had access to competent medical care, I thought the proposed commitment action would be neither necessary nor advisable and might actually have adverse consequences. He replied by sending the Pre-petition Screening Report and the Independent Examiner's Report.

He wrote, "The Rice County Attorney's Office usually places great stock in the examiner's recommendations so it is a vital piece to this puzzle. I want you to answer the following questions: Have you had sufficient contact with Bill over the past month so that you can address the issues relating to the proposed commitment, and if so, are you willing to testify to what you think is appropriate for Bill. If you can, I will move the Court to allow you to testify by phone as his next court date which is set for Monday, December 27th at 10:15 am. I will probably be seeing Bill again at the hospital on Sunday, the 26th."

The prepetition report was written by the Rice County Vulnerable Adult worker, although it looked like it had been written by a grade-schooler turned loose with a psychiatric dictionary. I decided to pay attention to the psychologist's report. Quickly reading through it, I started muttering to myself, What is this shit? Crap! More crap! Idiots! Why don't they check their facts! They even missed his weight by 100 pounds! It was replete with errors, innuendo, and unjustified conclusions. I showed it to my wife.

"That doesn't sound like the Bill I know," she said.

Relying on statements in the report created by the Vulnerable Adult Worker without bothering to check its veracity, the psychologist asserted that the patient's statement that he had graduated from the University of Minnesota School of Mortuary Sciences to be a "confabulation," "grandiose" and a "delusion" even though he did, in fact, have a diploma from that institution and practiced as a mortician in his father's mortuary and furniture business for a few years.

Another "delusion" that the psychologist claimed Bill manifested, was when he talked about a taxicab war in Northfield. Back in the 1950's there were "wars" between two of the three competing taxicab companies in town. My father, who started one of the companies with his two brothers in 1927, was involved in them. I observed some of the physical skirmishes and had talked with Bill about writing a book called *The Great Northfield Taxicab War* as a parody of *The Great Northfield Bank Robbery* (about the Jesse James Gang raid). Both Bill and I drove cab for one of these companies in later years. A subsequent owner, now deceased, was apparently swindled by someone who bought the company and told Bill about the "war" he fought to recover his lost funds. In line with this history, Bill deemed his difficulties with the current cab company - their refusal to provide him transportation, presumably because of liability issues – as another "taxicab war." The interviewer's lack of knowledge of Northfield history and her failure to appreciate Bill's account of it, apparently lead her to think it was just another delusion.

Bill made comments about the governor that the psychologist characterized as part of some paranoid delusion. To her it was like claiming a connection with royalty and must be the result of a sick mind.

10

Actually, his comments were right on target because the soon to be unemployed governor denied to the citizens of the state federal funding that could have been used for maintaining the excellent health care insurance that Bill had had previously. Had it not been for the governor's actions, Bill would not have had to pay $150 if he were admitted to the hospital through the ER and $50 just for an examination by his primary care physician there. Bill did not trust any assurances that the county would pay the fee since he had been burned before, accumulating a huge health care debt on paper. While it was probably not collectible, he feared that it might prevent him from getting hospital care when he really needed it and he may have been right.

The examiner claimed Bill had a "manic spell" and bought 21 pizzas for residents of his apartment complex. In fact, he did treat the residents to a different, less expensive, kind of specialty from a pizza shop, one that cost $60 in total, a price he could afford at the time. It was meant to be a Thanksgiving celebration with his friends in the apartment complex. So, spending $60 for a party is a manic spell? Yeah, his friends would really think he had gone off his gourd to splurge that much on a bunch of old farts who could die any day. If you want to be considered sane, you better save your money for a rainy day and say to hell with your old friends.

Bill is a colorful character and has many a story to tell about his life, and he will do so in great detail to anyone willing to listen. Some people find his loquaciousness to be obnoxious while others find his stories entertaining. The examiner pathologized this personality trait as "tangential thinking" and inferred that he must have a thought disorder. Oh, for Christ's sake, I thought! Yeah, it is true that Bill often doesn't get directly to the point when communicating, but many people operate under the same assumption as he does - that, in order to adequately describe an event, it is necessary to fill in the total context. And yeah, he may think, as he is telling his story and is reminded of another anecdote, 'Oh, and you'll be interested in this digression.' This may make him aggravating and a little unusual but it doesn't make him insane.

The examiner gave him a diagnosis of Cognitive Disorder, NOS or organic brain disorder. But there was no psychological test data in the psychologist's report and there was no MRI or EEG performed. Bill was probably anxious, scared and overwhelmed by the procedure he was forced into so it is not surprising that he did not finish the one psychological test that was attempted. Results would have been invalid anyway because of his distracted mental state. What a dipstick this psychologist must be, I thought. A competent examiner would have established rapport and calmed him down before attempting any assessment of intellectual functioning.

Rhetoric is speech uttered in order to persuade rather than simply to communicate information. One rhetorical device is what Aristotle called "pathos" or an appeal to the listener's emotions. Thus, a disgust reaction, for example to other people's bodily fluids, can be used as a rationalization for persecution, sometimes called the "yuck factor." Even though there is no evidence to support it, the "natural" repugnance itself is claimed as evidence for the harmful nature of the object. References to Bill's urine seemed to be aimed at eliciting this yuck reaction.

The "scare tactic" is another method to create support for a proposition by exploiting the listener's existing fears. Thus, it was claimed that Bill had Methicillin-resistant Staphylococcus aureus or MRSA, the drug resistant infection that is often found in hospitals and high density living facilities. Bill had been tested for MRSA on more than one occasion but never had a positive result. This unverified claim was, presumably, the justification for claiming he was "dangerous" to others. However, if that were true, he should have been placed in quarantine and health care workers would have attended him clothed in disposable full-body suits and gloves, like my neighbor was when he actually contracted MRSA in a hospital during surgery. If a hospital or health care worker did not follow that protocol, he or she would be guilty of endangering the public.

But this was not done in Bill's case. In fact, he had been told he had cellulitis in the legs, an infection of the subdural layers of the skin that is not ordinarily contagious. The only purpose in labeling his condition as MRSA was to manipulate people's fears of having someone running around spreading a contagious disease. In criminal law, such use of this form of scare tactic is considered defamation while in civil law it is considered libel or slander.

In a similar vein, the examiner claimed Bill was diabetic. Health care workers frequently let their implicit assumptions run away with them, assuming that everyone who is fat has diabetes. Although Bill's blood sugar levels had been consistently normal, it was nearly impossible for him to get this entry erased from his medical records even though he had tried several times. Later, his care givers didn't even believe the results of their own tests that showed Bill's blood sugar level and A1C test to be in the normal range.

By pairing reports of Bill's excessive alcohol use and a single positive test for THC at the hospital, the examiner implied that his Hepatitis C was from use of shared needles in drug abuse. Again, unfounded rumors were accepted as fact without any attempts at verification. He contracted Hepatitis C during a hospitalization for surgery for a pyloric valve problem associated with development of gall stones. I remember him telling me about it at the time. He thought the place where the surgery was done was unsanitary and voiced his concerns but was ignored. When he found out that he had contracted Hepatitis C, he wanted to sue the hospital but never followed through on it.

Bill grew up in a very religious family and has some strongly held religious views. Those beliefs were important to him when trying to comfort the families of deceased loved ones when he was working in the mortuary. It is one of the factors that allows him to keep a positive attitude when in dire circumstances, such as this coerced hospitalization. When first hospitalized, he tried to construe it as a test of faith or a situation God had designed for him that he might learn a lesson. Construing traumatic events in such a manner is considered one of the positive ways of coping with Post-traumatic Stress Disorder. I recalled a recent article in a psychological journal that pointed out the many ways in which religious beliefs support social organization and fulfill the human need for finding meaning in otherwise unfathomable events.

I have always distinguished ordinary "religious talk" used by preachers and religious folks from true hallucinations and delusions which make reference to religious concepts. Ordinary religious talk understands much of human experience through the metaphorical language of spirituality. God is the ultimate cause of everything in this language so when Bill was asked "Who told you to stop your medication?" it was like asking "Who makes your impulses?" His response to the "who" question was cast in the format of ultimate religious explanation. That is not the same as hearing acoustical signals from some disembodied figure, which would indeed be an hallucination. Similarly, like many other religious individuals, Bill uses the concept of "devil" to explain the complex of forces that make life painful and difficult. It is a *personified* concept which makes it more comprehensible to our human minds than, say, talking of an array of abstract multiple regression equations comprising huge numbers of variables. It is not like the user of this concept actually visually perceives a red, human-like figure with horns and a tail. It is a metaphor, for crying out loud!

Is there any justification for "pathologizing" religious beliefs and concepts when 80% of the world's population thinks in such terms? If so, a point of view held by the minority becomes redefined as "the norm" and the majority become defined as mentally ill. Welcome to the Topsy-Turvy world of modern psychiatry. With the advent of DSM 5, psychiatry does, indeed, appear to diagnose the majority of the population as mentally ill, a ludicrous position fueled by greed and lots of money from Big Pharma.

For a number of years Bill had wanted to write a book, tentatively titled *I Digress,* a title which is a joke on himself and his penchant to go off on tangents while telling a story. The examiner did not "get" the joke and thought wanting to write a book about his life was a sign of Mr. Tollefson's "grandiosity." Bill certainly had a varied and interesting life with a large number of set-backs and disappointments but also numerous life-affirming experiences and he wanted to share them with others. I had considered writing a short story about his Florida trip and how he had been able to persist in spite of all the obstacles that would have taken down a less resilient person. All the members of my writers group thought it was a great idea. It's a good thing that a psychiatrist was not in earshot of that conversation. We all would have been considered grandiose and carted off to the asylum. I guess it is beyond the limits of a mental health worker's vision nowadays to think that anyone who wants to write an autobiography could be anything except screwy. Conform! Stop that imagination! Stop that creativity or we'll send you off to the cackle factory!

I had to admit that, as a literary creation, the psychologist's report was pretty slick in making Bill sound like a lunatic. Unless, of course, you asked the embarrassing questions like who said what, who observed the alleged auditory hallucination and how did you know he was hearing something that, by definition, others couldn't hear; where is the evidence to support the assertion that he has MRSA; how did you ascertain that he was drunk when all you observed was that he was sleeping – where is the breathalyzer results; why didn't he receive treatment for his legs when he got into the hospital, since that was the reason for taking him there in the first place; why didn't he have DT's if he was an alcoholic rapidly withdrawn from his addictive substance, etc.

This couldn't be considered to be an acceptable psychological assessment - no way- I thought. I went online and looked up the ethical standards for psychologists put out by the American Psychological Association. Under article 9.01 *Bases for Assessments*, I found:

a) Psychologists base the opinions contained in their recommendations, reports, and diagnostic or evaluative statements, including forensic testimony, on information and techniques sufficient to substantiate their findings. (See also Standard 2.04, Bases for Scientific and Professional Judgments.)

b) Except as noted in 9.01c, psychologists provide opinions of the

14

psychological characteristics of individuals only after they have conducted an examination of the individuals adequate to support their statements or conclusions. When, despite reasonable efforts, such an examination is not practical, psychologists document the efforts they made and the result of those efforts, clarify the probable impact of their limited information on the reliability and validity of their opinions, and appropriately limit the nature and extent of their conclusions or recommendations. (See also Standards 2.01, Boundaries of Competence, and 9.06, Interpreting Assessment Results.)

c) When psychologists conduct a record review or provide consultation or supervision and an individual examination is not warranted or necessary for the opinion, psychologists explain this and the sources of information on which they based their conclusions and recommendations.

And, under article 9.06 *Interpreting Assessment Results*, I found:

When interpreting assessment results, including automated interpretations, psychologists take into account the purpose of the assessment as well as the various test factors, test-taking abilities, and other characteristics of the person being assessed, such as situational, personal, linguistic, and cultural differences, that might affect psychologists' judgments or reduce the accuracy of their interpretations. They indicate any significant limitations of their interpretations.

Yeah, that's it, I said to myself! You can't just make shit up. You have to have some data to back up what you claim or else make cautionary statements about the inadequacy of the data and place limits on your interpretations. I didn't see any of that in this psychologist's report.

I sent the lawyer an email with over thirty points of contention about the psychologist's report. On Monday, December 27, I received a call from the court which was in session. The judge started out by saying, in a very hostile manner, "You will *not* say anything about the psychologist's report and you will *not* say anything psychological about Mr. Tollefson."

Caught off guard, I stammered, "But I can't just stop thinking the way I usually think. I am a psychologist and I think like a psychologist. What can I say then?"

"You will *not* say anything about the psychologist's report or make any comments of a psychological nature about Mr. Tollefson."

At that point the defense attorney stepped in and began to ask some innocuous questions I could answer, e. g., about how long I had known Bill, when was the last time I had seen him, and so on. Eventually he asked if I had ever known Mr. Tollefson to hallucinate, be out of contact with reality and the like, all of which I answered in the negative. The subject of Bill's use of amioderone came up and I explained the effect it had on him. In the background I could hear the prosecutor saying, "There's no evidence he ever took that medication." Before I had a chance to say that it was the generic term for Corderone, which was on the drug list they had before them, the telephone line went dead. About ten minutes later they called again and I resumed my testimony, such as it was.

Two days later I heard from the lawyer who defended Bill. He said that since I was not Bill's treating psychologist and "just his friend," the judge would not let me comment on the other psychologist's report, no matter what my credentials. The judge ruled that Bill be committed to the old state hospital at Anoka for a period of six months.

What about the requirement in the *American's with Disabilities Act* about placement in the least restrictive environment? Minnesota didn't seem to believe in it until they were sued on that basis but by the time they finally developed their *Olmstad Plan*, it was too late for Bill. I remembered two "town characters" in Northfield, Squint and Lonnie, who used to do odd jobs between bouts of heavy drinking. Much more dysfunctional than Bill, there was never any thought about carting them off to a state hospital in the days before the town had lost its sense of humaneness. When they got too old to work, the city bought them a pair of chairs in which to sit on the sidewalk and watch the traffic go by. Another image that came to mind was the two main characters in *Grumpy Old Men* (played by Jack Lemmon and Walter Matthau) , the movie about the friendship/rivalry between two elderly Minnesota ice fishermen, both interested in a new woman in town (played by Ann Margaret). Would the court have committed these two lovable old men to the loony bin for the hostile pranks they played on each other? Probably so in 21st Century Rice County.

I imagined the newspaper headlines in my mind's eye: *Insane Rice County Court incarcerates man of sound mind on the basis of erroneous evidence! Hanging judge prefers fiction rather than fact! Assessment said to violate Ethical Principles of Psychologists, ignores Practice Guidelines for Psychological Practice with Older Adults, Guidelines for Evaluation of Dementia and Age-related Cognitive Deficit. Judge silences defendant and disallows testimony that would correct errors! Panic in the Streets! Anyone living in Rice County could be next! Read all about it!*

2 <u>HELP IS JUST A PHONE CALL AWAY</u>

I sent an email to one of Bill's old friends, Jake Heckler, a man who was to become a major player in what was about to unfold. Jake's sister was in my high school class and we soon discovered that about a half century earlier we had been on an overnight scout camping trip together in Nerstrand Woods, outside of town. I remembered the trip because we had been camped near a creek below a small bluff and had come under attack from another scout troop who rained clods of dirt down on us from above. I led a group of volunteers up the hill under cover of darkness. We crouched down and allowed the "enemy" to pass us by, and then jumped out, made a big commotion and surprised our adversaries who ran off screaming.

I told Jake what had happened to Bill and he gladly volunteered to go to St. Paul, get Bill's keys and retrieve some essentials from Bill's apartment as soon as the ice storm was over and the roads were passable. Bill's thoughtless kidnappers had failed to consider that he might need shoes and a change of clothes as well as a toothbrush and other personal care items. Jake had talked with Bill earlier and commented, "He sounded very logical, calm, and lucid over the phone. I know his apartment manager doesn't like him and hasn't for a long time. His apartment is a little messy, but I've lived in worse myself." To be sure Bill's apartment manager did not like him – she had heartlessly sent an eviction notice along with him to be served while he was in the Northfield hospital. Jake carried out his task and also took some pictures of Bill's apartment to document what was there in case pilferers decided to take advantage of the situation.

Both Bill and I expected there would be an appeal of the judge's ruling. Bill had called his public defender several times to talk about it but never got a response. On New Year's Day I sent an email to Bill's lawyer asking if he was going to be on board for the next stage of the process, meaning an appeal. He did not respond to me either.

In the meantime, I wrote up a sarcastic editorial in which I expressed my outrage at what had happened to Bill and sent it in to the *Northfield News*. I waited for a response for some time but never did get so much as an acknowledgment.

I started browsing around the Internet to see what resources might exist in Minnesota to provide Bill with some legal assistance. I tried the Minnesota Disability Law Center and listened as the phone rang for about an hour. When I finally did get through, the intake woman who answered didn't even allow me to get the question out of my mouth before she was saying they didn't deal with commitment matters and didn't know anyone who did. Sounding incredulous at my question, she responded "You mean you want legal help *for free?*"

Figuring I must have missed something, I again looked at the web site for this organization. The proud self-promotion jumped out at me:

"At Legal Aid, we specialize in providing professional civil legal help to Minnesotans who traditionally lack access to the American justice system and cannot afford the services of a private civil attorney...Minnesotans with mental and physical disabilities face a variety of day-to-day civil legal challenges. Legal Aid assists citizens with disabilities primarily through our state-wide protection and advocacy organization, the Minnesota Disability Law Center (MDLC)."

Wow! And I had thought that a wheelchair-bound 70 year old with multiple physical problems living on welfare who is accused of being crazy would be a candidate for their services. How could I have been so stupid!

It was slowly dawning on me that this might not be over quickly and that I had better get organized so I had a record of what happened, when, and who was involved. I reconstructed a "time line" for what had happened so far from my scattered notes and emails. I had yellow pads available at the dinning table and next to my computer so I could jot down events as Bill related them in our many telephone conversations. I established a separate folder of emails to and from Jake and others regarding Bill which ended up being nine folders containing hundreds of email messages. I made notes about people to contact and things to do in my search for help. I did a lot of Internet searches using Google. Every now and then I would write up summaries so I wouldn't get completely buried in details.

I talked with Bill over the phone several times. He would go from being mad as hell at the imperious manner in which he was jerked out of his apartment and railroaded into the nut house, to being astonished and saddened to find himself in such a situation at this stage in his life, to trying to put a positive spin on his plight - "God is giving me a lesson to be learned and if I keep my faith and get through it, maybe there is something I am supposed to do with what I learn."

"Yeah, Bill. That might be a good way to look at it," I said. That was one of the things I had learned from working with hundreds of veterans who suffered from post-traumatic stress: any kind of positive spin you can put on the dreadful experience helps you to put it into a context you can at least live with enough so that you can go on.

Bill asked me if I could find him a cheap tape recorder to use to keep a record of what was done to him and also to record things he needed to remember, since his arthritis made it difficult for him to write. In the past he had used a tape recorder for taking notes and recording conversations over the phone. He knew the legal requirements for recording other people's conversations and said he adhered to them. Long before the advent of digital recording, Bill had toyed with the idea of collecting personal recollections of people washed ashore from the economic mainstream by life's vicissitudes, the kind of thing that had happened to him. His plan was to give informants free low-tech tape recorders, have them tell their story at their leisure and then transcribe the results into a book, like Studs Terkel did in his book *Working*. It was one of the techniques I had used to follow a medical student through his educational experiences day by day for four years back in the 1970s.

Scrolling through Amazon.com, I found a tape recorder that used mini-cassettes with a phone attachment and a set of three 90 minute tapes. It arrived at the hospital the following week. However, the machine was confiscated immediately. They told Bill it was against policy but never did give him a reason for the policy. However, I suspect the real concern was that one or more of the staff might be caught doing or saying something they shouldn't and that could lead to legal difficulties. For the ethically challenged, a witness-free environment is the only safe environment in which to work.

Bill thought the eviction would be final during the week of January 16th. He had learned from Jake that after 60 days from when someone is evicted, if the tenant hasn't picked up his belongings, paid for the movers, and paid the storage bill, the landlord can either trash everything or sell it to collect money due for the removal and storage. He had been warned about the mess in his apartment several times over the last few years, but even then he never cleaned up the place.

"Bill sounds a little depressed," said Jake, "because he now knows that five years of not cleaning up his mess has done him in and he'll lose everything he owns. Nothing can stop what's about to happen."

I said, "I know Bill is a pack-rat but he's not as bad as those hoarder stories you see on TV. Why, I had to build an 8 x 16 foot shed to store all the extra crap that my wife and I collected over the years. He's got all this stuff that he has picked up along the way that he thinks he might find a use for at some time in the future. When you have all that stuff and it's in such a disorganized mess, it's hard to work up the enthusiasm to even start cleaning it out, so I bet he has let it go for years. He probably needs some help but, knowing Bill, I suspect he would be bull-headed about wanting to make all the decisions himself to keep it or throw it out.

"I would think the law would take into account Bill's situation. Since he's legally committed, how can he be expected to clean out his apartment in the prescribed time period? They should extend his grace period until after he gets out of the hospital. Of course, it would probably take a court order to stop the removal of his property. At any rate, if the apartment manager has to hold the stuff for 60 days, she would have to get it moved and stored or leave the apartment vacant until he can move it. I would think she would expect to be left holding the bag on any moving or rental expenses since she doesn't know Bill could or would pay her for it."

At the time, I was operating under the assumption that Bill's "sentence" was 6 weeks and that he would be out of the hospital within 60 days which would give him a couple of weeks to recover his stuff. When I learned that his term of commitment was for six *months*, I gulped and said out loud, "Oh, shit! This could cost some real money and Bill may never be able to recover financially."

Bill was worried that things were being taken from his apartment and, indeed, some clothing items that he knew were there were not present when Jake entered the apartment to recover them. When appraised of the new dimensions of the situation, one of Bill's sisters, Jane, asked her wealthy brother, Gary, if they could store Bill's stuff in one of the storage units he owned. He said he would consider it. However Bill resisted agreeing to that arrangement.

There was bad blood between Bill and Gary. After he had become disabled, Bill moved in with his widowed mother, who suffered from severe osteoporosis that caused her to be quite bent over as she walked. Bill lived in the basement while his mother lived in the ground floor of the home situated directly across the street from the local hospital. My wife and I had visited them several times over the years and noted they seemed to get along quite well. Bill's mother was always very gracious, making lunch for us all and engaging in intelligent conversation. She was especially interested in solving the problem of obesity, which had plagued most members of her family.

When Bill's mother had to go into the hospital, Gary decided to sell the house to pay for her care. Bill refused to move and Gary had him evicted and had his belongings hauled to the dump. So placing his belongings in Gary's care did not appeal to Bill. His sister was not strongly inclined to help her brother either. She thought his feet should be held to the fire until he took more responsibility for his actions. She thought he had a problem with alcohol but wouldn't go so far as to say it was an addiction and she thought that he didn't keep his leg elevated often enough when he was up and about in his wheelchair.

I responded to her in an email that, "Bill may have a problem with excessive alcohol use but I can't say that I have seen it from my own direct observations, since he has either drank moderately or not at all when I have seen him over the last 20 years. Of course there has been a lot of that time when I have not observed him. In any event, he was apparently committed for 'Cognitive Disorder, Not Otherwise Specified' presumably due to 'organic brain disorder.' I don't believe there is any evidence that Bill has either of those conditions or that he is psychotic, delusional or has hallucinations (all of which the prosecution claimed). Usually, commitment requires that the person be "imminently" (in the next few days) dangerous to himself or others and I do not see that being the case here either.

"Treatment standards usually require that treatment be in the 'least restrictive' environment possible. Anoka was not a "least restrictive" environment since it is a locked facility. So, while Bill may have psychological problems and bad habits, none of them required that he be incarcerated. Besides, forced treatment has been shown to be ineffective and the stigma of having been committed (or even treated for psychological problems) has negative consequences that stick with you for life (including, the likelihood that physicians will disregard your real physical problems). Yes, Bill is difficult to persuade on any matter that he thinks he should be in control of, but what has happened to him now is likely to make matters worse and reduce the quality of life he has for however many years he may have left."

She too didn't think he should be committed to a mental hospital and she volunteered to pay for a storage unit. His youngest brother, Pat, and some friends offered to help move Bill's stuff out of his apartment when it appeared imminent that the apartment manager was going to do something.

Since his apartment was supported by Housing and Urban Development, Bill had contacted them to see what his rights were. The person he talked with told him his contract was with the corporation that owned the facility and not with HUD and, therefore, they would not get involved. Unsatisfied with that kiss-off response, Bill managed to get an attorney from a non-profit legal aide group to represent him on the housing problem. I talked with the lawyer, who sounded like a very ethical and reasonable man, and told him that I had looked up tenant rights on the HUD website and it did not sound right to me that a person could be evicted while he was in the hospital. The rules were quite clear that a disabled person could not be evicted because of his disability and that special considerations applied if the person were in the hospital.

The lawyer agreed to look into it and found that not only could she not evict him without specific cause and that time in the hospital was excluded from the required notice period, but she had to bring an "Eviction Action" against the tenant in district court. He found that she had not, in fact, filed the required action and attempted to notify her of what she must do and the consequences of taking any action to dispose of Bill's property. She ignored several phone calls from him and he finally sent her a letter, to which she never responded. With the situation in a stalemate, no rapid decisions had to be made and Bill's possessions remained in his apartment.

I had not heard from Bill for a couple of days and decided to call. He was discouraged and losing hope after meeting with his treatment team the day before.

"There was no empathy from any of them. They don't care about my physical problems. They are trying to convince me that I'm an addict. If I try to explain my behavior, they say I'm 'in denial'. How can you win when they play that kind of game? "

From what I understood, he may have had times when he drank too much but his drinking behavior did not hold a candle to the kind of alcoholics I had seen when working in the VA. And no one in any of the hospitals noted that Bill had any signs or symptoms of withdrawal from an addictive substance. Even the breathalyzer test result of .07 obtained at the Northfield Hospital proved that he was legally sober at time of admission.

"Bud, you've got to see these people here! Some of them have been in lock-up for long periods, like years. That could happen to me. I'm getting really scared."

Bill knew from people he had met before he was hospitalized about the cascade of events that get inmates trapped in the mental hospital system, starting with the commitment, the subsequent confiscation of Social Security or SSI by so-called "guardians," the loss of possessions and the inability to have the resources to get back into independent living. It then becomes overwhelming to figure out how to escape since the agents of the system don't provide any information to the patients about options and plans. So quite naturally the victims anxiety and depression levels increase, the manifestations of which are taken as proof of their mental disturbance, and a lot of patients simply give up.

God, I thought, I hope this wont be the course for Bill. There are standards for appropriate discharge planning in most decent hospitals, but unless you have a lawyer in tow, they can probably get away without following them.

Bill was still worrying about his stuff and how much of it was being stolen from his apartment. He was trying to realistically appraise what should just be tossed because it was of little value and what he really wanted to keep and might actually be able to use some day. He expressed his anxiety and depression to Jake about the deconstruction of his household after he received a box of "clothes and other junk" in the mail, which obviously meant that someone had been in his apartment going through his belongings without his permission.

Jake said, "Bill seemed so upset that he could hardly talk. He thinks the apartment manager might just toss most of his stuff in the trash. I think I'll head down there today or tomorrow after she has gone for the day and look around. If she hasn't changed the lock, I can look around the apartment and see if most of it has been tossed. If it has, I'll hold off telling Bill until he feels better and can accept what's happened. I'll check the trash dumpster to see if I notice any of Bill's stuff in there. I double checked with my lawyer who's done a lot of evictions. Legally, she can toss absolutely nothing for 60 days. If she does, she could be in big trouble."

A few days later Jake reported on his trip to "The Field," as he called our home town. "The stuff on Bill's door was still there and the key let me in. Everything looked the same as about two weeks ago. I didn't notice anything missing except the T-shirts which weren't there today but were there a couple weeks ago. I'd say about 4 were missing including a bright yellow one and a red one. Also, his wheelchair was gone. It needed new bearings, but Bill had been using it every day - it was just harder to push. I will give him a call tomorrow to let him know what I saw. I did find his check book and a bunch of checks on the bed under a bunch of stuff. He'll be glad to hear that."

Bill received a notice from the CEO of Minnesota Department of Human Services saying he was being charged $910/day for his hospitalization but that his ability to pay was zero. What that meant was that they could then charge Medicare or Medicaid $910/day for his hospitalization. For this price he was getting room and board but, as far as I could tell, no treatment for any of his physical problems. The much ballyhooed "dangerous-looking" legs (for which the police decided he needed to be taken to the hospital) were not being treated, just as they hadn't been treated at the Northfield Hospital or United Hospital in St. Paul. It was simply a lie they told to suck him into the mental health gulag. The state institution had no facilities for hydrotherapy and did not make any other kind of exercise available to him.

Bill was unable to provide a urine specimen because of an unusual condition that he had for some time – hypogonadism. This problem caused his penis to shrivel up and that, in turn, made it difficult to access himself and control his urination. Use of testosterone would ameliorate the problem to some degree but he had been deprived of this medication for some time, probably because of cost to the county, and he had not been provided assistance by his doctor in obtaining a more effective means to contain his urine. The problem was exacerbated when he took Lasix, a diuretic, to control the swelling in his legs. And the swelling in his legs was exacerbated by not being able to exercise, such as in hydrotherapy. So the process fed on itself, aided by the practices of his care givers.

Bill commented, "This might not be just a six month sentence, it may be a death sentence. I told the judge that when he sentenced me."

Pondering the situation, I thought since they don't appear to know what they are doing, it might not be so bad that he is not getting any medical care. At least they are not making matters worse by implementing the wrong interventions!

I called the *Minnesota Innocence Project*, which works on cases of people falsely accused of criminal behavior, to see if they knew any similar group or agency for people wrongly committed to a mental institution. The response of the managing attorney was, "I really don't have any suggestions for a referral for someone who might handle that kind of case for free. Sorry I cannot be of more assistance." Hmm. One more confirmation of my growing belief that one is much better off being accused of a crime than of being accused of being mentally ill.

I looked up the Minnesota statutes regarding civil commitment online and learned that Bill's legal rights were violated when they did not inform him that he had the right to be examined by a second doctor of his own choice. In addition, they violated his rights by not informing him he had the right to appeal the hearing decision. In fact, Bill had called his court appointed lawyer two times to ask about an appeal but the lawyer never responded. I also contacted the lawyer by email and gave him a deadline by which to respond regarding an appeal and he never did. It was only later that I found out that these were just the most glaring violations of Bill's legal rights.

Bill's sister, a former psychiatric nurse, wrote to me. "I worked in psychiatric facilities for years but never experienced the kind of fraudulent practices that you are attributing to the people taking care of / evaluating Bill. My experience was that everyone respected the laws and were concerned about the licensing requirements." She said she couldn't talk with Bill when he started using terms like "the devil" to explain goings-on in the world.

I replied, sarcastically, "Yeah, I must be paranoid too."

Then I listed some of the incompetent, unethical and fraudulent practices I had seen in the mental health industry over 40 years without even being in the work settings most prone to such abuses. And I lectured her on the nature of religious language, noting that even the American Psychological Association no longer sniffs their noses at fundamentalist religious beliefs.

"Although I'm a non-believer, I do not think it makes Bill crazy to think of the world in spiritual terms," I said. "Eighty percent of the people in the world think like that." After that, communications with Bill's sister were rather chilly.

I contacted one of Bill's old friends to see if he might be able to generate some support for Bill in his time of need from some of his Northfield buddies. He did not respond. When I told Bill of his friend's diffidence, he quickly came to his defense. He explained that his friend had recently received a lot of competition from a new business in town and he did not want to stick his neck out for fear of alienating his clientele. Maybe that was true, but I still thought the guy was a coward and fair weather friend.

I called the Ombudsman for Mental Health in Minnesota, whose office is in the same town as the hospital. Their web site proclaims:

"The Office of Ombudsman for Mental Health and Developmental Disabilities is charged under Minnesota Statutes 245.91 – 245.97 with promoting the highest attainable standards of treatment, competency, efficiency and justice for persons receiving services for mental illness, developmental disabilities, chemical dependency and emotional disturbance in children."

I explained to the person I talked to that Bill's sister and I, both professionals in the mental health field, and a number of his friends who had known him for decades did not consider Bill to be psychotic, dangerous or in need of hospitalization. I described the court procedure and the spokesman seemed to be particularly interested in the fact that Rice County did not give Bill the opportunity for being evaluated by a doctor of his own choice nor did they give him an opportunity for an appeal (both requirements, according to state law). I asked if he could do anything to help get a fresh evaluation of Bill. He said he was going to take the matter to his board and get back to me.

After more than a week, I called back and left a message for them to call me. No response. I called again. This time, the person said, "We don't give legal advice."

"Well, what can you do besides that?"

"I'll get back to you on that."

Another week went by and no one called. I called back and asked what the man I first spoke with was doing about my inquiry.

"I can have someone from his treatment team call you."

"Fine," I said, and I gave him my telephone number.

Of course no one ever called. I was beginning to develop an attitude about state agencies in Minnesota. What the hell! They are supposed to work for the rights of patients with psychiatric labels attached to them. But they don't give legal advice and they can't get off their fat asses to walk across the street and find out what's going on. I haven't seen that they do anything but make excuses for why they can't do any real work!

I learned about Jim Gottstein's organization in Alaska, The Law Project for Psychiatric Rights, a public interest law firm devoted to the defense of people facing the horrors of forced psychiatric treatment. His www.psychrights.org website is filled with information about the many facets of the problem. I wrote him an email letter about Bill's plight. He quickly responded.

"Finding good representation is always a huge problem in these situations. I wish I knew someone in Minnesota for you and your friend. As a general matter and without speaking to Minnesota law, your position as a substitute decision maker should give you the right to say no to the drugs if they say your friend is incompetent to decline them. However, being able to enforce that right is the problem."

Being a Harvard trained attorney and with a decade of fighting for legal, human and civil rights for people labeled with psychiatric diagnoses, I figured he must know what he was talking about. He was right as far as enforcing the law with regard to Power of Attorney. In fact, almost all agents of the court and state agencies ignored my status as Bill's attorney-in-fact. And he anticipated the next abomination to appear on Bill's horizon: forced drugging.

Forced commitment and forced medication have been shown in several studies, including one funded by the MacArthur Foundation, to be ineffective and, in many cases, to make matters worse. A number of well-known mental health professionals have voiced their opposition to it. Lawrence Stevens, JD has argued that it violates due process of law. Even the American Psychological Association has come out with a report that discredits the practice of indiscriminately restricting psychiatric patient rights. They concluded that "there is no consistent psychological profile or set of warning signs that can be used reliably to identify such individuals in the general population" and called for primary violence prevention and behavioral threat assessment which tries to identify and intervene with individuals who have communicated threats or engaged in behavior that indicates planning or preparation to commit a violent act.

But rational analysis of the problem appears to have had little effect on the practice in the states. The shootings of congresswoman Gifford and others in Tucson and the mass shootings in Colorado and Sandy Hook will probably result in the states ceding yet more authority to psychiatrists, even though it is not justified. Not only can psychiatrists not predict dangerousness but a person has only one chance in 14.3 million of being killed by a mentally ill person; his/her chances of getting killed by lightning is three times greater. Yet legislators and presidential commissions, trying to make themselves look like they are doing something to halt the carnage in our violent society, are attempting to rush bills through legislatures to limit the rights of individuals more likely to be victims than to be perpetrators of violent crime.

I decided to give the attorney general of the state of Minnesota a try. I drafted a letter in which I voiced two different types of complaints: formal and substantive. In the former, I complained of the failure to provide Bill with the opportunity to have a second opinion by a doctor of his own choice, the failure to allow him to appeal the commitment decision, and the failure to prove that he was dangerous.

Under the substantive complaints I identified some 20 instances of defective or false information used to commit Bill to the hospital. I didn't know it at the time but Minnesota law requires that such information meet certain standards in order to be allowed into evidence, and this information did not meet those standards. I included copies of ten articles on how involuntary commitment violates due process of law and basic human rights, on the unreliability of psychiatric diagnosis, the lack of effectiveness of coerced psychiatric treatment, the lack of evidence to support use of anti-psychotic medication, and a statement against use of coerced psychiatric treatment made by about 20 leaders in the field of mental health.

About a month later I received a reply signed by the attorney general, Lori Swanson. She expressed sympathy but explained that her office had limited jurisdiction. Specifically, she said, they did not have any authority over the courts. She suggested the patient appeal, which option I had already told her in my letter had been denied. Finally, she referred me to the same state offices that I had found unresponsive and inadequate. It wasn't until much later that I realized that her office would be the one defending any state agencies, including the state hospital, if they were accused of wrong doing.

However, I was interested in one of the attachments regarding Minnesota Statutes 2010, 253B.23 General Provisions, Subd. 3. False Reports. This section states:

"Any person who willfully makes, joins in, or advises the making of any false petition or report, or knowingly or willfully makes any false representation for the purpose of causing the petition or report to be made or for the purpose of causing an individual to be improperly committed under this chapter, is guilty of a gross misdemeanor. The attorney general or the attorney general's designee shall prosecute violations of this section."

I had previously concluded that the only way to clear up this miscarriage of justice was to prosecute in criminal court those people responsible for making false statements on the prepetition report and all those subsequent reports in the case that carried forward the initial false statements without any attempts at independent verification. The AG's office was the place to file the criminal charges.

I called Bill, enthusiastic that we might finally be able to get things going in the right direction. I laid out the situation and said we had to go over each assertion in the prepetition report to identify all those that were false or misleading.

"I can't do it now, Bud. I am just barely hanging onto my life. Besides, they lost all my papers, my 'office,' and I can't remember all that happened right now."

Bill had a morning nurse that was waking him up and harassing him for not being up in time for breakfast. "Well, I guess you'll just have to not eat then," she said. "You're too fat anyway." Bill missed three breakfasts in a row.

"How do they expect me to get up on time? My wristwatch was stolen at United Hospital and they lost my alarm clock here. There is no clock in my room and she comes in at the last minute and tells me I'm late and I'll have to go without breakfast."

The treatment team refused to believe what he said about his past life, made fun of what he said, accused him of being paranoid and grandiose when he made some factual statement about his past life, and did not give him any credibility in the so-called "meetings" with the team. There was no give and take, no planning to get him out of the institution, and no therapy. In addition, his medical problems were being ignored. This sounded to me like the place was being run by a bunch of incompetents.

I wrote back to the attorney general. "At this point Bill is just struggling to survive his captivity and is not up to the emotional demands of filing charges and being involved in even more litigation. Once he is free of the punishment and increased stress of forced incarceration as well as deprivation of treatment for his physical conditions, I think he will recover his emotional reserves and be able to initiate criminal proceedings."

I found a reference to The Citizens Commission on Human Rights (CCHR) on the Internet and looked up their web site. Although co-founded in 1969 by the Church of Scientology and Thomas Szasz, MD, a well-known psychiatrist and author of *The Myth of Mental Illness*, it claimed to now be a non-political, non-religious, non-profit organization. Its objectives sounded reasonable enough: to protect individuals from abusive or coercive mental health practices and to foster informed consent regarding psychiatric diagnosis, proposed treatments and alternatives to those treatments. Although I had a few doubts about just how independent the organization was, I thought if it had a chance of helping Bill, it was worth a try.

I wrote a one page letter briefly explaining the case and sent it via their online submission site. A short time later, I received a reply from their "Director of Litigation," who said they might be able to help. I then sent copies of the prepetition report, the psychologist's report and my letter to the attorney general, expecting that he would have additional questions. After a couple weeks with no response, I sent another email asking if he was still considering the case. I received not even the courtesy of a rejection letter. What I later suspected was that, after reading the prepetition report and without any critical thinking, he became just as biased as the rest of the legal people involved in the case. Or perhaps he just didn't think the case was winnable or that it would not garner the kind of favorable publicity his organization desired. To my mind, his was just another useless organization pumping itself up with rhetoric but doing nothing for those suffering from injustices wrought by the mental health system.

After talking with Bill, who was at that point kept totally in the dark as to any aspect of his treatment, I called the hospital to find where to send my credentials as Power of Attorney, so that I could talk with them about the case. I was redirected to someone in the social services section. She made an appointment to talk with me on the phone but did not call at the appointed time, instead sending an email that she had gotten busy doing something else. She made two more appointments but did not follow up on either of those, again sending emails to excuse herself. I could understand there being one holdup but not more than that. Something wasn't right and they seemed to be trying to buy time for some unknown reason.

I didn't know what this person wanted to discuss but thought it might have something to do with the fact that I was Bill's Power of Attorney and was his health care representative in his Advanced Directives. At the time I thought that there were certain matters that legally would require my permission, such as the coerced use of medications, electroshock treatment (ECT) or psychosurgery. If so, I expected to deny the use of any anti-psychotic medications and, of course, ECT and surgery, all of which are known to have permanent deleterious effects on the brain. I hoped I could find out what they had in mind for Bill in terms of length of stay, discharge planning and so on.

Finally, she called and I told her that I thought Bill did not meet the criteria for involuntary commitment and that his legal rights were violated in the process. She said she thought Bill's psychiatrist would like to talk with me. She said that the psychiatrist had a speech impediment. I knew that from Bill, who said that the man had surgery on his jaw. Bill had urged me to be patient and give him a chance to articulate what he was trying to say.

On February 1st I talked with Bill's psychiatrist. He told me he was an assistant professor at the University of Minnesota and liked to do research on schizophrenia but had difficulty getting funding and was working at Anoka part time. (At the time I did not know of the Dan Markingson death case or that a university ethicist was calling for an investigation of that case and of university research practices, especially in the Department of Psychiatry). He was quite difficult to understand but I talked with him for about an hour and was able to correct or counter some of his misconceptions, although he was not completely convinced. He requested that I send him a copy of my letter to the Attorney General's Office. I talked with Bill and told him what I planned to send and he was all right with that. The doctor said that he would give Bill a copy of the email I sent.

I asked him what kind of time line he was thinking of and he indicated possibly a month but he couldn't be positive. Bill had not been a problem there, he said. They had talked about casual things but Bill hadn't really trusted him enough to open up so as to convince the doctor that he was safe to go out. He was unclear about Bill's living arrangements and I told him what Bill's lawyer in Rochester said about HUD regulations and the fact that his apartment manager could not evict him without a proper court hearing. I told him that if she did not have adequate reason for eviction, according to HUD rules, she could lose her status as a HUD housing facility or be taken into court to explain why.

The psychiatrist did not seem to know what a social worker's job was or was supposed to be. But I knew that finding housing is usually one of their tasks. So, if Bill was unable to go back to his apartment, it would be up to the social worker to find a place in Northfield for Bill. I did not trust his previous Rice County case worker to find the best place. I knew that Bill had an eye on some place near the Retirement Center that would make it convenient for his ongoing hydrotherapy.

After talking with Bill's doctor, I was optimistic that his ordeal would soon be over. At least he was thinking in terms of a short stay and was considering the need for post hospital placement. I received an email from the hospital social worker expressing her concern about Bill's property and whether it should be disposed of or should be stored and, if the latter, who would pay for it. I explained that the eviction was being contested and that, if it was necessary to move his belongings, a plan for doing so was in place.

After reading my letter to the attorney general, Bill's doctor responded, "I read this letter with interest as a source of information about Bill Tollefson and as a very well-written narrative that makes a number of valid and well-argued points." We set an appointment for another phone call.

When the doctor called, his speech was especially distorted and I continually had to ask him to restate his comments. Even the restatements were difficult if not impossible to understand. However, I was able to recognize when he said that even though Bill showed no evidence of psychosis on the ward, he was going to diagnose him as paranoid schizophrenic on the basis of information in the reports used against him in court.

I said that to call Bill schizophrenic of any stripe was totally absurd. He would not listen and said he had filed for authority to force Bill to take anti-psychotic drugs. I said I could not allow that. The hearing was to be in the same court with the same cast of characters as in the previous hearing. I supposed the outcome would be the same since none of the arrogant bastards would ever admit that they could be wrong. But I had to at least try to derail this additional abomination of the legal process.

Bill had referred to the doctor who had placed him on a 72 hour hold in Northfield Hospital as "Dr. Flakey" and he laughed when one of his interviewers duly transcribed that name into her notes. We soon began to refer to his doctor at Anoka as "Dr. Quack" in our phone conversations.

Expressing my outrage in an email to Jake, I said, "By the way, schizophrenia usually first makes it's appearance in a person's late teen's and early 20's. It is virtually unheard of to first make it's debut in a 70 year old! I'm afraid the wrong person is locked up! The drugs have not been shown to have any positive effect and are not really safe when used for a long period of time. Both the psychiatrist and the psychologist that Bill talked with yesterday have threatened him that the only way he will get out of the hospital is if he takes the meds. The folks at CCHR say that this should be grounds for charging them with assault - a criminal charge. I agree with them on that."

Jake emailed back, "Bud, it's been many moons since I thought about the words "paranoid schizophrenia" so I picked up an old college text book, *Abnormal Psychology And Modern Life*. It is about 50 years old but still a great text and as relevant today as it was 50 years ago. I read about 20-30 pages in various sections about many of the paranoid and schizophrenia syndromes. If Bill is anywhere close to being paranoid schizophrenic, then I must state with great certainty that I am the King of France. The head psych guy with the speech problem hasn't got a clue about Bill. There must be some easy money to be had by keeping their hands on him as long as they can. I feel like renting a kangaroo costume somewhere and attending the February 11 court hearing in Faribault. If the judge asked me what I was up to I'd have to tell him that I was just dressing for the occasion and trying to accurately reflect the ethos of the court!"

I sent an email to the Minnesota Psychiatric Society to see if there was any requirement for licensure of a psychiatrist that he be able to communicate with his patients. They did not respond. Apparently, communication with anyone who is not a member of their club is not high on their list of important things.

A number of people suggested I contact the American Civil Liberties Union. On the organization's web site I found the email address for the Minnesota branch and sent them an inquiry. When I didn't get a response after a few weeks, I went to the Minnesota ACLU web site and found that they did not respond to emails that were not submitted using the form on their web site. So I went to their submissions page and found that one had to have a residential address in Minnesota in order to submit anything on their form. In other words, if you were not a Minnesota resident, you could not submit an inquiry on their site, even though that would be the appropriate place to take up the matter. Frustrated, I went back to the national ACLU web site and submitted my inquiry to them. They did not deem my question - whether or not they would be interested in a case like Bill's - worthy of a response. So much for the ACLU.

GERALD D. OTIS

3 <u>BETTER LIVING THROUGH CHEMISTRY</u>

By now I knew it would be an uphill battle to get Bill out of the hospital and Bill was not helping matters by some of his behavior. When angry about some mistreatment or insult delivered by staff, Bill would yell that he was going to sue them all, but that was interpreted as being "paranoid." From the staff's point of view, any angry display could not be a consequence of something they did but had to be a result of his craziness, exactly the same erroneous interpretation placed on patient behavior that had happened in a well-known study where "pseudo-patients" gained admission to several mental hospitals back in the 1970s. And the more Bill talked about religion, the more evidence they had that he was "grandiose," even though a rash of TV pundits and politicians could spout the same kind of verbiage with impunity.

Bill was not taking his blood pressure medications and they interpreted that as "noncompliance" due to his madness. He was likely correct that being treated rudely was what made his blood pressure go up when they measured it; I had observed the same effect in my doctor's office due to aggravating political broadcasters on the waiting room TV. I knew that most nurses did not measure blood pressure correctly and their method was grossly different from the British standard of taking three measures and averaging the results. I had tried it myself three times per day for three months using three different machines. The variability of results could be analyzed statistically for machine effects, time of day effects and order of administration effects and they were substantial. A single measure did not allow canceling out of these spurious effects. When Bill did manage to get his blood pressure measured at a time when he was not aggravated, it was normal.

At this time I was still waiting to hear from the attorney general's office. I encouraged Bill's sister to send a complaint letter to the attorney general also, thinking that the more complaints they received, the more likely they would take the matter seriously. Although she agreed that the diagnosis of paranoid schizophrenia did not fit her brother at all, she balked at writing a letter. She still wanted to hold Bill's feet to the fire until he admitted that he was part of the problem.

I responded, "Yes, Bill has problems and he has probably hurt you in some way I don't know about. I guess you cannot get past that at this time."

She then explained that she had grown up in Bill's shadow and resented how their mother always favored Bill and let him have his way, a treatment that she felt caused him to not learn to take responsibility for the consequences of his actions. Some time later, I mentioned this to Bill and he was incredulous. He had always thought that his sister was just more reticent and studious than he, not that she was harboring resentments toward him for the way his mother treated him.

I emailed back to his sister, "You may be right about Bill being overindulged as a child, I don't know as I never saw that side of him. I did know your parents and thought they were very kind. Your mom was a very interesting, bright and understanding woman and my wife and I enjoyed talking with her when we stopped by to see Bill. When we were kids, I always liked to go to your house during Christmas time because she would have a couple of counters filled with Swedish delicacies, which she would urge us to sample. Like many parents who lived through the depression, they may have been too eager to give their kids things they never had growing up (although I can't say that my parents were like that!). Unfortunately, it is too late to go back and correct things.

"Considering all the physical problems that Bill has, the odds are against him for having a long life. In fact, I am surprised that he has made it this far. Thus, I would prefer that he live in a situation that provides him some sources of enjoyment, such as fishing, and a certain degree of autonomy. The psychiatrist and someone Bill talked with yesterday are threatening him with continued incarceration if he doesn't take anti-psychotic medications. These drugs are not as safe as they like to claim and research indicates that they don't really work anyway. I was never greatly impressed with them when they were used on patients I saw in the VA.

"What is likely to happen is that they will hold this position until he gives in, then discharge him to some group home or, if he is lucky, to an assisted living facility, where he will be allowed $75/mo. for spending on personal needs and all his other income will go to the facility and his guardians. They will receive any government benefits that are due Bill (his Social Security) and have authority to administer psychotropic medications (without having any liability for the consequences). Since these places are usually without any storage facilities, all his property might be turned over to them and they can do with it what they want. About all he will be left with is the right to vote. Some of these places are reasonably good, given their tight budgets, and they take patients on outings every now and then and provide some entertainment. But some are hell-holes with minimal concern about patient welfare (and sometimes even worse). Hopefully, Bill will get placed in one of the better residences."

On February 7th Bill was jerked out of bed in the early hours of the morning and taken to Rice County for a guardianship hearing. Bill tried to defend himself, in spite of his lawyer's urgings to keep quiet, but to no avail. He learned there was to be another hearing on the 11th with respect to forcible use of anti-psychotic medications. His sister wrote a "To whom it may concern" letter and sent three copies to Bill to use as he pleased. She stated that she thought it inappropriate and futile to treat Bill as a schizophrenic and suggested that a Christian mental health provider would be more appropriate treatment than drugs.

I learned that Jim Gottstein, the attorney CEO of Psychrights.org had made up a legal defense package for forced medication issues and made it available through Mindfreedom.org, an advocacy organization with patients, ex-patients and supporters as members. The package can easily be modified for the specific state and includes 50 years of research that show these drugs actually make recipients into chronic patients and can be very harmful physically in many cases (i. e., cause weight gain, precipitate heart attacks, cause Parkinsonian symptoms, etc.). It includes all the forms for "pleadings" and other actions that lawyers do to make things official. I sent the package to Bill's lawyer and he obtained a continuance in order to get certified copies of the affidavits referred to in the legal defense package.

I also sent him descriptive information about a conference being put on by two New York attorneys. It was designed to help defense lawyers counter the tactics used by hospital forensic experts, such as using scare rhetoric to convince judges and juries that "otherwise preposterous big lies and Catch 22's are not only plausible but compelling." One such tactic was to claim that a patient who showed demonstrable signs of improvement was feigning sanity! Another was to claim, with no evidence whatsoever to support it, that a patient was stable only in the protected environment of the hospital and that he would fall apart if released.

In order to provide to the court a "less-restrictive alternative" to drug treatment, I contacted Lutheran Social Services in Rice County to see if Bill qualified for counseling there and how it could be set up in advance so that the court would believe it was legitimate. They were quite understanding and agreeable and indicated how Bill could become one of their clients. Their office was in the same building in which Bill had been receiving his hydrotherapy.

At the same time, the two women proposed as Bill's "guardians," were pushing to have his belongings removed from his apartment. I told them that Bill's apartment manager had to call Bill's attorney since she had been non-responsive with regard to his phone calls. She had still not filed a formal eviction notice and would have to comply with HUD rules regarding evictions when she did, something Bill's attorney and I figured she could not do. According to state law, she had to safeguard Bill's belongings for 60 days after she filed an official eviction notice. Later I was to learn that the time period was 180 days if the person was in the hospital.

In the event that Bill's case was not settled in his favor, his sister, brother and friends worked out logistical plans for moving his belongings. Jake went over to Bill's apartment and made estimates of what kind of containers would be needed and Jane rented a storage unit just outside of town. She tried to talk with Bill about moving his stuff but he became overwhelmed and stressed out just trying to think about what he would need in a new place, what things could be left in long term storage, what papers he wanted with him, and what could just be abandoned.

Bill tried to get me to travel to Minnesota at his expense for the upcoming hearings on Friday, February 25 for temporary guardianship (which was supposed to last only 2 months) and for the forced use of anti-psychotic drugs. I agreed with Jake that it probably wouldn't do any good for me to be there. I wouldn't be able to testify as an expert witness because I was not treating him and I was not licensed in Minnesota anyway. They wouldn't let me testify about the drugs because I am not an MD and I can't prescribe medications, even if I know from reading the research they aren't any damn good! His lawyer should have the certified copies of the expert testimony about the uselessness and potential harm of the drugs and could present that himself. The forced drugging defense package I had sent him told him how to do it and the lines of argument to take. The guardianship was thought to be not much of an issue since it was to be short term (60 days) and would be over before the commitment order was over.

I thought Bill could better use his money to hire a psychologist of his own choosing to examine him. He probably couldn't afford to pay for court testimony (since with the inevitable delays it might run into several hours) but he should be able to get someone to come talk with him for an hour or two, give him some short mental status tests and write up a report and submit it to the court or to Bill's lawyer. Actually, the court should pay for it since they didn't allow him to get a second opinion the first time around, which is written in the Minnesota law regarding commitment. The trick, of course, would be to get a psychologist who wasn't a jerk and keep him from being adversely influenced by Bill's current captors or the spin doctors from Rice County Social Services. What was desired was a "pristine" report based solely on his own observations. I located a Lutheran Social Services office in Minneapolis that might have someone who could do that.

I received a phone call and email from a young woman, Lucy, who had known Bill for several years and wanted him to become a distributor for her nutritional products. She was a bright, energetic graduate of Carleton College and visited Bill when he was in the hospital. However, she was bothered by doubts about Bill raised by her friends.

"I was so upset by the whole situation. I can't understand how someone's rights can be taken away like Bill's have. I was informed by many that there must be information that I don't know, that Bill hasn't told me. When I last saw him he was pretty down and out and talking to him yesterday he sounded better. Speaking with his sister Jane this week also helped. He made it sound like they were going to keep him there for $1000 a day indefinitely and that he couldn't do anything about it. Is there a way you could give me more information so that I can explain the situation better to others so that I might find some other resources."

I wrote back that I knew of no deep black secrets about Bill. I allowed that he is a unique and colorful character and maybe had more than his share of adversity, but I didn't think he ever had been psychotic in the 60 years I had known him. I said that he had participated in community life in his home town and had a varied career which included working for Goodyear Tire and Rubber, being a mortician, running a furniture store and being an outstanding fishing guide in both Minnesota and Florida. I said he had always been ready to lend a helping hand to those less fortunate and tried to live his life according to Christian principles.

I told her about the thyroid toxicity and his cellulitis, the imperious actions of the police and other parties on the scene, and the anti-religious bias of the doctor who saw him at Northfield Hospital. I sent her some articles about the sad state of present-day psychiatry, the arguments for forced psychiatric treatment being unconstitutional and a violation of the international code of human rights, and the research evidence that it did not help patients and, in many cases, made matters worse. I sent the same articles to Jane but she said she didn't have time to read them.

About this time, Mindfreedom.org was having a letter writing protest in the case of a woman from Moorhead, Minnesota. She had been court-ordered to have a series of involuntary outpatient electroshock treatments. When the results were adverse, she and her husband decided to refuse to leave her home for any more such treatments, which an FDA panel had called "hazardous and untested." The county sheriff then picked her up and hauled her off to Anoka, the same place where Bill was being housed. I wrote email letters of protest to the two senators from Minnesota and to the representative from her district. Eventually, the campaign met with success but not until after she was forced to undergo more indignities at the hands of a legal-mental health system that is out of control.

Dr. Quack had requested authority to use involuntary electroshock or ECT on Bill at the same time that he requested authority to use involuntarily administered drugs and I soon learned from Mindfreedom that 49 people in Hennepin County alone were being forced by the courts to have involuntary electroshock. Both Bill and I dreaded the possibility that Quack would resort to this barbaric form of "therapy." Bill had previous experience with ECT when his father, in his later years, was subjected to the procedure. His father had pleaded with Bill to get them to stop shocking his brain, but the doctors in charge did not provide Bill with the required facts about this form of psychiatric abuse in order for him to decide against it.

As the day approached for the Jarvis Hearing to determine if anti-psychotic medication could be forced upon him, Bill learned from one of his attorneys that letters of support for him could be sent by email to the court. I alerted Pat, Jane, Lucy, Jake and another long time friend, Big Jim, to this fact and sent them all a sample letter and some guidelines about what to write. Jane thought the letter she had given to Bill would suffice to express her sentiments. The judge provided no indication that he had ever read any of these messages.

Lucy, Jake and Bill's cousin, a retired minister, attended the hearing. Dr. Quack appeared on an Internet TV arrangement, to the use of which Bill objected. The court went ahead with it anyway and it soon broke down. Lucy interpreted the breakdown as a divine intervention and commented, "Bill has a strong connection with God. He got what he wanted!" The judge was someone that Bill had known for 40 years – they were both on a local committee when Bill was running the furniture store and mortuary and they both were campaigning for elective office back in 2004. He probably should have recused himself from the case but he did not.

Jake said he was able to pick up about 60% of what Dr. Quack said. That was about two or three times the amount I could understand on the phone. However, he didn't know how the court reporter could understand very much when Dr. Quack talked about the various drugs.

"Quack mentioned that having 'treated' Bill for once a week at first then twice a week lately, he could observe nothing that suggested a mental health issue. All of Quack's opinions and drug treatment plans have come from Bill's first court appearance records which Quack had in his files. Bill's lawyer objected at that point that everything Quack had on Bill was basically hearsay from previous records. The judge allowed Quack's testimony anyway. A good lawyer would have made chopped liver out of everything Quack said!"

So Dr. Quack didn't even believe his own eyes when he said he saw no evidence of mental illness himself. He was just diagnosing on the basis of all the preceding reports, all of which depended upon the prepetition report concocted by the so-called Vulnerable Adult Worker. I was, at that point, convinced that what was needed in order to get Bill's situation straightened out was to establish what was true and what was false in that prepetition report. Unfortunately, filing criminal charges and waiting for the results of an investigation and trial would be a lengthy process and Bill didn't want to wait to get his freedom, thinking that he would die if he didn't get out of Anoka soon. I feared he might be right.

The judge said he would research the drugs Dr. Quack wanted to use and make a ruling the following week. Bill instructed his lawyer that he wanted to be present when the decision was announced but his wish was ignored. Whether the judge read the summary of 50 years of research in the affidavits obtained by Bill's lawyer is not known. However, it was clear, in his ruling to allow forced drugging, that he did not listen to the drug manufacturer's own warning on their TV adds that Abilify was not recommended in elderly patients with dementia (which his examiners claimed Bill had) and that it could increase blood sugar levels to such an extent that it could cause death (and they claimed that Bill had diabetes too). Other studies showed that it can cause weight gain and increase blood pressure and results of drug trials showed that 4.5% of patients in

41

Bill's age group died within 10 weeks of ingesting the drug. Yet another study showed that the drug worsens psychotic symptoms in schizophrenia, a second psychiatric label that Quack bestowed on Bill. I thought that was an outrageous risk to take when it was not necessary and that it could not be justified by Quack's own reasoning.

Bill didn't hear about the ruling until some two weeks after it had been made and then through "a little bird," a friendly attendant in the asylum, who told him. He did not hear it from his lawyer or the judge or even his doctor. The first "official" notice he received was when a large group of staff members captured him in the hallway and forcibly held him down while he was twice injected with Abilify in his shoulder. The second time he was overpowered by what he estimated to be about a dozen staff members, even after he had consented to take the pill form. I thought to myself, "Now get it through your head, Bill. 'Involuntary' means they get to beat the shit out of you while injecting you with a harmful substance!"

Jane, a former psychiatric nurse and devotee of traditional medicine, talked with a psychiatrist friend who thought Abilify would be just fine for Bill. I sent her seven references to studies that indicated otherwise but she just glanced at a couple of them. She really didn't want to hear about adverse reactions and seemed to wish for a bit of chemical magic that would make her brother less of a problem.

Both Jake and I ran across an article on how psychiatrists have gone out of the "talking cure" business because it doesn't pay as well as 20 minute sessions devoted to deciding on a drug to be used as "treatment." I sent Jake another article written by Nathaniel Lehrman, a traditionally trained psychiatrist, called *Psychiatry: 60 years in an increasingly corrupt specialty* in which the author decries the changes that have occurred in his profession over the last 30-40 years.

I commented to Jake, "I saw the article and downloaded it to my file of articles related to Bill's plight. I think it is time to do away with the specialty of psychiatry all together. They are being trained without any emphasis on learning what makes people tick, on how to understand their patients, on how to tell the difference between a normal personality trait and a mental disorder, on how to help patients learn how to change their thinking and behavior. Then they give them an arsenal of dangerous drugs and turn them loose on the public - size up a patient in 12 minutes and give him a pill! The psychiatrists have all sold their souls to the fucking drug companies! Anyone who goes to one should have his head examined!"

A member of the Twin Cities branch of Mindfreedom referred me to a professor at the Mitchell School of Law at Hamlin University. He had been director of the Mental Patient Law Project at Berkeley and served on the Minnesota Supreme Court Study Commission on the Mentally Disabled and the Courts. The school itself had a selected topic area of mental health law.

I wrote an email letter to the professor to see if he could help get me oriented in the right direction on the legal matters. After two weeks and no response, I called and learned that he no longer actively practiced law. The secretary, trying to be helpful, referred me to the school's law clinic. After briefly talking with a representative, she told me their law clinic didn't handle matters like that.

Hmm. Too complicated for law students? Maybe they just get practicum experience in filling out legal forms - the kind any educated person can download from the Internet and fill out? Oh, god. I am really getting cynical, I thought.

Big Jim, a long-time friend who is about the same size and weight as Bill wrote to complain that many of the adverse side-effects of Abilify "could have a tendency to really screw-up a guys weekend." He thought the lawyer had dropped the ball in Bill's case and he observed that depriving Bill of his normal medical regimen was taking a toll on his body. In 1995 after Bill had his hip and two knees replaced, he received physical therapy in heated pools at the Courage Center in Golden Valley. It was instrumental in making him relatively mobile and he credited it with saving his life. Bill continued working out in a therapeutic pool at Faribault and for years in a pool at the Northfield Retirement Center.

Bill did, indeed, want to draw up charges against his lawyer for the Minnesota Bar Association. I knew that the attorney disregarded state law in not informing Bill that he had the right to a second opinion from a doctor of his own choosing and not responding to either Bill's request for an appeal or my request that he state if he were going to represent Bill or not in the next stage of the process.

I looked up on the Internet the Minnesota law regarding commitment and found that state law also requires that statements to be used against the defendant must meet certain requirements in order to be considered evidence. MN Statute 253B.07 Subdivision 1(6)d requires that the facts contained in the written report must meet the requirements of subdivision 2, paragraph (b)." And Subdivision 2, paragraph b. states:

"The petition shall set forth the name and address of the proposed patient, the name and address of the patient's nearest relatives, and the reasons for the petition. The petition must contain factual descriptions of the proposed patient's recent behavior, including a description of the behavior, where it occurred, and the time period over which it occurred. Each factual allegation must be supported by observations of witnesses named in the petition. Petitions shall be stated in behavioral terms and shall not contain judgmental or conclusory statements."

Nearly all of the statements in the prepetition report were disembodied assertions, such as "Bill is paranoid" – no witnesses were specified, no time periods were noted, no behavior was described and judgmental and conclusory remarks were included. As far as I could see, the judge should not have allowed such a document into evidence and the defense attorney should have questioned the author of the document to force her to name names, specify times, and provide objective evidence to support her claims. One glaring error was that she claimed Bill had a drug-resistant infection (MRSA) when, in fact he was never diagnosed with it and had at least two lab tests which showed that he did not have it. Even Dr. Quack testified in court that he was keeping Mr. Tollefson's MRSA under control when he knew very well that Bill did not have the infection.

Online I found the Minnesota Rules of Professional Conduct which outlines the responsibilities of lawyers to their clients and to the law. After going through the 115 page document, I was able to pull out a number of rules where Bill's lawyer seemed to fall short. I abstracted a set of complaints to submit to the the Minnesota Bar Association.

Although the brochure distributed to those making a complaint to the Minnesota Bar states that they do not deal with matters of incompetence or malpractice, their first rule of professional conduct, that they call "Competence," requires that a lawyer possess the legal knowledge, skill, thoroughness, and preparation necessary to adequately represent their clients. Bill's lawyer did not, as far as Bill could remember, cross-examine the author of the prepetition report to establish the factual nature of each allegation contained therein by observations of witnesses named in the petition, as required by state law. Was this a lack of knowledge of the law, a lack of skill, or a willful disregard of his client's welfare?

I asked Jake, who was present at the second hearing, what he thought of the performance of Bill's lawyer. "He could have objected several times, but only did so once that I recall. He objected to the fact that Dr. Quack was reporting nothing but hearsay from the first hearing. And that was rejected. He should have objected when Quack kept calling Bill 'Mr. Johnson.' He should have objected to the fact that Quack was impossible to understand. He should have objected to the whole thing when they lost the TV picture from Anoka."

The lawyer did not contest the allegation that Mr. Tollefson was dangerous to himself or others, in spite of the fact that Mr. Tollefson has no history of violence or indications of suicidal intent. The element of "dangerousness" must be present, according to state law, for any commitment to occur. If the prosecution was arguing that Bill was dangerous because he was running around with an infectious disease, his lawyer should have required them to provide evidence that he in fact had the infection.

The second rule where Bill's lawyer was deficient requires that a lawyer abide by a client's decisions concerning the objectives of representation and consult with the client as to the means by which the objectives are to be pursued. A lawyer is supposed to abide by a client's decision whether or not to settle a matter.

Bill's lawyer did not allow his client to appeal the results of the initial hearing and disregarded his requests to be heard at the final Jarvis hearing. He prevented his client from objecting when the psychiatrist testifying against him called him by the wrong name, "Mr. Johnson," on *five* different occasions.

Rule 1.3 requires that a lawyer act with reasonable diligence and promptness in representing a client. Bill's lawyer did not act with commitment and dedication to the interests of his client and with zeal in advocacy upon the client's behalf. He did not advise Bill that he had the right to have a second opinion rendered by a doctor of his own choice, as specified in Minnesota Law. He overlooked the statute of limitations for appeal so that Bill's legal position was destroyed. He allowed doubt to grow about whether a client-lawyer relationship still existed and did not clarify it either in writing or verbally, so that Bill supposed his lawyer had ceased to look after his legal affairs. His lawyer handled a judicial or administrative proceeding that produced a result adverse to the client and he did not respond to the client's request, or the inquiry of his power of attorney, to have him handle the matter on appeal. He did not consult with the client about the possibility of appeal before relinquishing responsibility for the matter. All of these things are required by the Rules of Professional Conduct.

According to Rule 1.4, a lawyer is supposed to communicate and consult with his client. He is supposed to keep him reasonably informed about the status of the matter; consult with him about the means by which the client's objectives are to be accomplished; and promptly comply with reasonable requests for information.

Bill's lawyer did not keep Bill reasonably informed about the status of his case; he did not inform him at all about the result of his Jarvis hearing so that the first Bill knew of it was when he was being forced by a gaggle of hospital staff to submit to injection of a potentially harmful substance in his veins. This caused considerable pain and distress for Bill and, as the UN special rapporteur has decided, constitutes torture.

His lawyer did not promptly comply with reasonable requests for information. According to this standard, when a client makes a reasonable request for information, a prompt compliance with the request is expected, or if a prompt response is not feasible, the lawyer, or a member of the lawyer's staff, is expected to acknowledge receipt of the request and advise the client when a response may be expected. Client telephone calls are supposed to be promptly returned or acknowledged. Bill's lawyer ignored all phone calls and emails sent by me, Bill's durable power of attorney. He also did not explain matters to the extent reasonably necessary to permit Bill to make informed decisions regarding continued representation by the lawyer.

The final standard that seemed applicable was that dealing with professional misconduct. The first statement in this rule is a recursive one: it is misconduct to violate or attempt to violate this set of rules. The lawyer can also be faulted for engaging in conduct that is prejudicial to the administration of justice and knowingly assisting a judge or judicial officer in conduct that is a violation of applicable rules of judicial conduct or other law. Bill's lawyer and the other officers of the court, by their silence, failed to uphold the laws regarding civil commitment in the State of Minnesota.

I wanted to get other examples from Bill to include in the document but he was in a strange mood. Big Jim noticed it first.

"Everyone that has any idea what's been going on with this travesty should get on the band wagon, as it were, and pile into these bastards as hard as we can. The other thing we need to do is convince Bill that this "Fools" bullshit is wholly inappropriate at this time. While we are all trying our damnedest to get him out of the muck, he is off on another one of his pipe-dreams wanting to do this and the timing is all wrong. It just seems counter productive. But then you know how he gets when he gets a hair-brained idea in his head, thinking that its all a big joke. We must remind him that the past 110 days haven't been a joke of any sort, then perhaps he will see the light."

A few years earlier, Bill had been a member of an informal friendship group called "The Fraternal Order of Fools." They got together for fun and merriment, which included drinking, feasting and entertainment of various types. The more outrageous their antics, the more fun they had. But after a while the more prominent members, concerned about their economic welfare, began receiving shaming reactions from some of the stuffy town elders and decided to end their involvement. Bill wanted to resurrect the organization using modern communication technology and had been talking about it with his new found friends in the hospital. In my mind's eye I could see Bill regaling his audience with tales of roasting a whole pig in a pit in the ground while drinking and cavorting around as a band played um-pah music. He would have been the center of attention as he entertained those gathered around, something that would have raised his spirits greatly.

Bill always liked to think about the possibilities, whether in terms of developing some new type of fishing tackle or how to develop a new business enterprise or how to get himself out of some jam he had gotten himself into. He liked the problem-solving process, at least in fleshing out the big picture. He relied on his ability to generate a lot of different ideas quickly. It would not be uncommon for him to be expanding the implications of several alternative ideas all at once, knowing that 90% of them would turn out to be unworkable, but "someplace in there" would be the gem that would solve the problem. In other kinds of circumstance, both Big Jim and Jake would have liked to watch Bill's mind operate when he was working on a problem, but this didn't seem to be the right time. On the other hand, this kind of "daydreaming" allowed Bill to escape, at least for a time, the horrors of his current situation.

I thought maybe the Abilify was making Bill giddy. Jake commented, "I just hope they don't turn him into a 'veg' with no personality left over." Bill did seem to be off on cloud nine recently, somewhat oblivious of his surroundings and more accepting of the hospital staff than he had been previously. I had some fears that he was beginning to show signs of the "Stockholm Syndrome," the tendency of captives to identify with their captors (like Patty Hurst). My major fear was that they would kill him through neglect of his physical problems - his legs were swelling up pretty bad and nobody there was paying any attention, even when Bill would plead for help. He was not getting any exercise and his hydrotherapy had been crucial to keeping him alive and moving for several years.

Jake said he had talked to Bill. "He had to have eight people hold him down the other day as they hit him with the needle after he told them he wouldn't take the Abilify anymore. He has gained weight and his legs keep getting worse. He said the drugs make him extremely confused and disorganized."

I talked with Bill the next day. "One of the nurses helped me measure my legs on two different occasions. One leg increased in circumference by 1.25 inches and the other by 2.75 inches in just one day! I'm drooling all the time and my muscles are killing me. I've been swearing a lot more and you know I don't like to swear. They gave me a double shot of Abilify on Saturday and I'm totally spent today and I can't get organized."

Crap! If Bill loses the integrity of his skin because his legs are expanding so much, I thought, he will then be subject to any number of infections lurking in hospitals and then we will be talking about a wrongful death claim rather than a complaint about simple incompetence.

Jake had made the 100 mile round trip to see Bill and give him $40 to feed the vending machines in the building. "He does not sound good and said that the meds are killing him and he feels like he might die at any time. Sounds like every bad side effect from Abilify is hitting him all at once. Sounds like they're going to keep hitting him with that drug until he is dead or completely agrees with everything they tell him: who he is, what he is, what's best for him, and that every thing he did was because he was nuts and needed confinement. It just boggles my mind that they can treat him with a dangerous drug for a disease which he does not have!"

After his sister Jane talked with him she said, "He really sounded frightened but his vitals were holding good. I truly do not see how he's going to get out of this if he stays in his "war" [with the hospital staff]. I expressed my opinion at first but then stopped because it was clear he just wanted to be listened to and wasn't getting that--couldn't reach you. I did call my favorite prayer line again this morning to continue prayers for him. I had a dream about him this morning. In my dream, he did not live through his war but there were redeeming circumstances and, all in all, it was not a bad dream, but very colorful in the way that Bill is colorful."

Oh, oh! The question hit me, "Is that a prophetic dream or a *wish* to have Bill out of the way?"

Bill told Jake that he had this constant urge to move that was driving him bonkers. Jake looked up the side-effects of Abilify in his *Physicians Desk Reference* and found that 15 % of patients on Abilify had this experience. The closest common language term would probably be "restlessness" but that sounds more benign than it really is - it is more like a compulsion to move, "ants in your pants," "gotta move" type experience.

Jake said, "It seems to be one of the main reasons why patients run away if they can from the hospital when they are being treated with antipsychotics. I can't imagine what it must be like to be stuck in a wheelchair and yet have an almost uncontrollable need to get up and move around. It would for sure cause me to flip out."

I remembered running across on the Internet some kind of organization that accepted complaints regarding hospitals and other institutions. It turned out to be the Office of Health Facility Complaints and their web site had a place where you could file your complaint on line.

I looked up several web sites that listed the side effects of Abilify and made a list of all those Bill confirmed were present. They included side-effects affecting 11%-27% of users - anxiety, sedation, agitation, fatigue, drowsiness, nausea, and constipation; those side-effects affecting 2%-10% of users - weight gain, dry mouth, joint pain, blurred vision, overall pain, increased salivation, swelling or water retention in chest, armpits, legs, and feet; those side-effects with implications for development of diabetes - frequent urination, extreme hunger, large or rapid weight gain; those side-effects with implications for neuroleptic malignant syndrome (which can be fatal) - stiff muscles, confusion; and those side effects suggesting an allergic reaction - unexplained rash, unexplained swelling.

I included in my complaint letter that Bill also reported (and demonstrated to several outside observers who had known him most of his life) the symptoms of forgetfulness, difficulty concentrating, loss of motivation and interest in the usual things he was interested in before he started the drug, excitability, agitation and an increased propensity for expression of anger and use of swear words.

"Mr. Tollefson has made the staff aware that he is suffering from these side-effects and they have continued to disregard them. Besides causing discomfort for Mr. Tollefson and defeating the purported purpose for which the drug was prescribed, these symptoms may be precursors to debilitating and irreversible physical conditions. It should also be remembered that this drug has a fatality rate of 4.5% within 10 weeks of use in Mr. Tollefson's age group. I ask that you investigate this situation and take appropriate corrective action before this turns into another medical tragedy."

A few days later, after talking with Bill, I told his siblings and three friends that Bill was very depressed, lacking energy and dispirited.

"He was in a lot of pain and no one at the facility would help. Either last night or this morning they tried to move him using a rolled-up blanket rather than the appropriate transfer equipment and screwed up his shoulders. Then his right ankle went out and apparently is now 'numb.' He was very angry that no one would help him and that a doctor was not available. I expect that the anger will turn into another round of depression. Ever since they forced him to take Abilify his mood has worsened and his ability to cope with the situation he is in has been more impaired. Prior to the Abilify, his mental coping mechanisms or "tricks" to keep a positive outlook and keep going were working reasonably well. Now that is gone. I don't know what to do. I have received no answer from the Office of Health Facility Complaints and suspect that they are just as inadequate as all the other Minnesota agencies I have contacted."

4 <u>PRESUMPTIVE BLINDNESS</u>

It was amazing to me how so many people (with a few exceptions) were blinded by their presuppositions about Bill. All of his behavior and expressions were pushed into the concepts and labels someone earlier in the course of his travels through the mental health gulag had applied to him, just as Procrustes had his arms and legs "resized" by the inn-keeper so he would fit into the bed that was available. That is to say, they presumed to "see" evidence in his behavior or his verbal expressions of the concepts that they already had of him without ever questioning the nature or appropriateness of those concepts. He must be "schizophrenic" or "paranoid" or "demented" because someone applied those labels to him and recorded them in his chart, which document followed him where ever he went, like the ball and chain attached to a runaway slave.

No thought was given to the idea that concepts are not an intrinsic aspect of nature but are *invented* by human users of concepts in order to "explain" things (relate one aspect of nature to another) or for practical purposes. The degree to which concepts can be made to be "operational," so that they can be consistently applied by different observers, varies a great deal. Psychiatric diagnostic concepts are some of the poorest concepts in existence, lacking sufficient operational definition so that they can be consistently applied by different observers, their inter-rater reliability being only slightly better than chance and their coefficients of validity being virtually non-existent. Sometimes they are no more than lists of symptoms that are supposed to cohere with each other in a given condition, but research evidence fails to support their coherence and psychiatric theory provides no explanation for why they should cohere in the first place.

Sometimes psychiatric diagnostic concepts seem to be made up out of whole cloth and for economic purposes, such as the concept of "Somatic Symptom Disorder," which includes all those individuals who are "overly concerned" about some physical condition, such as a malignancy, heart condition, paralysis, etc. It's scope is so broad as to include nearly all persons with some physical condition that it would be absurd for a person to be unconcerned about. The diagnosis was applied to the recent internationally known case of Justina Pelletier, the teenager with mitochondrial disease who was "kidnapped" from her parents by psychiatrists at Boston Children's Hospital. It's only "virtue" (for psychiatrists, not patients) is that it expands the range of potential clients for whom services can be offered and drugs can be developed.

What all of these individuals seemed to be lacking was a knowledge of *normal* personality and how it is different from perturbations in normal personality that require some kind of assistance (help that is not necessarily psychiatric or even psychological in nature). Concepts in the field of personality have their own ambiguities but the ones to be discussed below have a respectable degree of reliability and numerous studies have been done to support their validity.

Although there are a number of different ways to conceptualize personality (or "relative uniqueness"), two approaches have a lot of empirical support: the Five Factor Theory and the Theory of Psychological Type proposed by Jung (1923) and later operationalized and clarified by Isabel Briggs Myers and others. The Five Factor Theory is largely an empirically derived set of five dimensions of "source" variation that appear to run through the population of humans and their primate cousins and ancestors. Some people have either more or less of this source feature than do other individuals. The source feature is thought of as "causing" the observable behaviors that are probabilistically associated with it. Because it does not yet have much theoretical elaboration other than to say that the dimensions exist, I prefer the more theoretically rich Jungian approach which includes four of the dimensions in the Five Factor Theory (although they are not called "dimensions" but rather "bi-polar contrasts" in the Jungian approach). The dimension that is left out in the Jungian scheme is "Neuroticism" or "Emotionality." Jung, quite correctly, considered these manifestations as deviations from a person's normal operation that occurred under different circumstances for different kinds of individuals.

Jung distinguished two different ways of perceiving (taking in information), *Sensing* (S) and *Intuition* (N), and two different ways of judging (making decisions), *Thinking* (T) and *Feeling* (F). He called

52

these four methods of operation "functions," and each function could be used in two different "orientations," *Introversion* (I) and *Extraversion E)*. So we actually have eight function-orientation pairs available to us (the four functions in each orientation). Everyone is capable of using all four functions in each orientation, but they differ in their natural preference for one member of a pair rather than the other. Research indicates that these preferences are, to a great degree, genetically determined but people also tend to develop and become good at their preferred functions through practice, leading them to acquire specialized skills, abilities and knowledge.

As a person grows, one function comes to dominate the conscious personality and the others are forced into serving the dominant, or are neglected or remain largely unconscious. (This one-sided development is necessary for crystallizing an identity but it is also limiting in a number of ways). The *Dominant* function is the one that is most highly developed, most conscious and most easily controlled and directed. We enjoy using it and use it as much as possible.

The *Auxiliary* function is the second best developed function and serves the interests of the Dominant, complementing and balancing it by being the opposite *kind* of process from the dominant. If the dominant is S or N, then the auxiliary is T or F. If the dominant is T or F, then the auxiliary is S or N. In Introverts the Auxiliary indicates which function is used when dealing with the "outside" world while in Extraverts the Auxiliary indicates which process is used when dealing with the "inner life."

The *Tertiary* function is the opposite of the Auxiliary but the same kind of process (either perceiving or judging). It may be uncomfortable to use and is not easily controlled or directed by conscious effort.

The *Inferior* function is quiet and lies dormant while the Dominant function is in control but may erupt and take over if the Dominant is depleted of energy. We can't consciously control or direct it. When operational, the Inferior may make the person look like a caricature of a person who has that function as the Dominant, i. e., the person's performance may be characterized as exaggerated or extreme, undifferentiated or categorical, and immature or inexperienced.

According to this theory, in order to have a "balance" in adaptation, one must have one reliable method of dealing with the outside world (an extraverted function), one reliable method of dealing with the inner life (an introverted function), conscious access to one kind of differentiated perception (either Sensing or Intuition), and conscious access to one kind of differentiated judgment (Thinking or Feeling). Thus, an Introverted-

Thinking (IT) type's Dominant function is balanced by Extraverted Intuition (EN) (Auxiliary function). And an Extraverted-Sensing (ES) type's Dominant function is balanced by Introverted Feeling (IF) (Auxiliary function).

The objective questionnaire that Isabel Myers developed to assess individuals' psychological type, the *Myers-Briggs Type Indicator* (MBTI), is the most used test of its type in the world, having been translated into several different languages and used on every continent. It identifies the respondent's relative preference for each of the basic functions, orientations and attitudes (Sensing/Intuition, Thinking/Feeling, Introversion/Extraversion, and Judging/Perceiving) and which one of the 16 *Psychological Types* (created by bifurcating these contrasts) a person is most like in terms of expressed preferences. Newer versions of the test allow assessment of *facets* of each of the four major preferences as well.

The MBTI is the preferred way to measure psychological type but, if test results are not available, one can get a pretty good idea of a person's psychological type by looking at the definitions and associated characteristics of the function preferences in relation to the manifest behavior of the person you are trying to identify (providing you know him or her fairly well). I have known Bill Tollefson for over 60 years, have observed him in many different kinds of situations, and have talked with him for hundreds if not thousands of hours, so I think I qualify in terms of knowing him fairly well. I have also counseled thousands of people using the MBTI and have used it in many empirical research studies, so I am acquainted with the nature of other psychological types as well as that of Bill Tollefson.

Let's start with the distinction between Extraversion and Introversion. Since the population is about evenly divided between these two camps, establishing Bill's preference distinguishes him from half of the people in the world.

When we are using Extraversion *as a process*, we scan the environment for stimulation, affirm the importance of the environment and try to increase it, want to be involved and want to get into action to effect the environment. We may use trial and error procedures to do so. Individuals with a *preference* for Extraversion tend to create a life with lots of action, are sociable and outspoken, find it easy to communicate, think out loud by talking, rely on the environment for guidance, prefer "extensive" rather than "intensive" experience and may be impulsive.

Extraverts may be seen by others as charming, outgoing, sociable, enthusiastic, and energetic. However, if they overdo their Dominant function, or if the observer is someone with a quite different set of preferences, they may be seen as boastful, bossy, loud, intrusive and rude.

In contrast, Introversion is a process whereby we dampen the immediate effect of the environment and direct attention inward to get a clearer appreciation for the significance of what is "out there." When we use Introversion as a process we look inward for guidance from ideas, concepts and inner impressions, are reflective, and consider carefully before taking action. Individuals with a preference for Introversion create a life with time for contemplation and reflective thought, socialize mainly with close friends and intimates, prefer "intensive" as opposed to "extensive" experience, and are interested in the clear conceptualization of ideas. They may be unaware of changes in the environment and would discount its importance in any major decision.

Introverts may be seen by others as deep, detached, calm, reserved and discreet. If they are overdoing their dominant orientation or if the observer is much different than the object of observation, the Introvert may be seen as aloof, inhibited, withdrawn, timid or shy.

One of the clichés about the distinction between these two orientations is: An Extravert cannot begin to understand life until after he has lived it while an Introvert can't begin to live life until after he understands it. Another is: If you don't know what an Extravert thinks, you haven't been listening but if you don't know what an Introvert thinks, you haven't asked him.

When we consider Bill in terms of this distinction, it is quite clear that he is an Extravert. As a youngster, he associated with a variety of people, from kids with a similar socioeconomic status, to the poor and the old. He often played with older kids, had many adult mentors and respected his elders, figuring there was always something to learn from them. He loved interacting with and entertaining people. He was an accomplished story teller and often referred to himself as "the phone monster" for his extensive use of the telephone. He often related long, elaborate stories about his exploits and would often go off on tangents during the telling. He was a Boy Scout leader. He loved to party and took great delight in preparing meals for others and organizing the elaborate bashes of the Fraternal Order of Fools. His youngest sister described him as an outgoing, sociable person who needed to have others around. He would become quite enthusiastic about whatever new idea struck his fancy and, as shown above, he could act impulsively. Prior to his physical impairment, he was very active in numerous different kinds of activities and, even after his impairment, he still managed to get around town quite well in his wheelchair. One time, when his wheelchair could not navigate a flight of stairs at a local pub, he got down on his enormous behind and lifted himself up the stairs one at a time in order to get to a party he wanted to attend.

The next distinction we want to consider is that between the two perceptive processes – Sensing and Intuition. Sensing is defined as perception of the physically observable by means of the senses. When we are using Sensing as a process we attend to facts and practical details, the present moment, and what is said and done. We are seeing the "little things" in everyday life and "letting the eyes tell the mind." We are using established skills and paying attention to step-by-step experience. Individuals with a strong preference for Sensing tend to develop acute powers of observation and have a good memory for facts and details, trust conventional ways of doing things and rely on experience rather than theory. They consider "real intelligence" to be sound and accurate common sense. Persons with a Sensing preference like to work with tangibles and use well-learned knowledge and skills rather than develop new solutions.

When viewed in a positive light, Sensing types might be described by others as patient, steady, thorough, and pragmatic. If they are overdoing it, or if the observer is quite different from the subject, they might be described as dull, fussy, overly literal, and obsessive.

Intuition is defined as the perception of meanings, relationships and possibilities by way of insight. When we are using Intuition as a process we are seeing patterns and meanings and projecting possibilities for the future. Our perception is influenced by memory and associations more than physical details. "The mind is telling the eyes." We read between the lines, have hunches, try to see the big picture, have ideas come to us "out of the blue." We rely on inspiration more than past experience and are interested in the new and unproven.

Individuals with a preference for Intuition are often said to have insight into complexity and to be capable of seeing abstract, symbolic or theoretical relationships. They are more interested in creating new knowledge than in applying existing knowledge.

When viewed in a positive light, Intuitives might be described as insightful, curious, imaginative, ingenious and quick-witted. If they overindulge their intuition, or if they are being described by a strong Sensing type, however, they may be described as absent-minded, disorderly, eccentric, erratic, and unrealistic.

There are differences between introverted and extraverted forms of both Sensing and Intuition but they will not be considered here. The interested reader is referred to the fine book by Isabel Briggs Myers and

Peter Myers called *Gifts Differing* (1980, Consulting Psychologists Press).

Bill's ideational productivity was one of the things that fascinated and drew Jake to him. He was always coming up with new ways of doing things, new solutions to problems, new business opportunities, new ways of getting around his physical limitations, new possibilities in general. When he took over responsibility for his father's furniture store, he went to Minneapolis to attend a class in interior design so he might be more creative when serving his customers. Unfortunately, the "modern" ideas he learned in the big city may have been too advanced for his customers - small town residents and farmers - as I learned from some of the people who lived there at the time.

Bill trusted and relied on his intuition to make his way in the world. When he went to Florida in an attempt to resurrect his career as a fishing guide, he had a vision of the possibilities and had worked out in his mind how to overcome most of the obstacles in his way.

Unfortunately, he did not count on the economy going bad at that particular time and changing the whole opportunity structure he had pictured. When Lucy suggested he work with her in selling health food products, he could see the possibilities that awaited in multi-level marketing and the new electronic technology and he imagined how he might be able to use his established contacts to carve out a niche for himself among outdoors men. When he learned of a new manufacturer of wheelchairs for use in the out of doors, Bill immediately traced down the owner in Mexico and discussed with him the possibility of becoming the North American representative for the company. A similar arrangement seemed a possibility with the manufacturer of a specialized boat that Bill thought he could sell. Even when he was in his first nursing home, he fantasized about buying the place and spent time thinking about what it would take to pull it off (financing) and what was required to actually make it an effective nursing home serving the needs of its patients (training and organization). It was not that he actually thought he would do it; what he liked was the mental exercise of figuring it all out. He had previously done the same kind of "mapping out the possibilities" for the old Northfield Hospital and the old high school and tried to sell the ideas when he ran for mayor in 2004.

The examples could be multiplied over and over but it appears certain that Bill was an Intuitive type and not a Sensing type. He was a "big picture" kind of person and would leave it to the Sensing types to work out all the details. The likelihood that he relied too much on his Intuition will be discussed once we identify all the other parts of his personality and put them together into Bill's psychological type.

The distinction between the two kinds of decision-making – Thinking and Feeling – is next to be considered. In this framework, Thinking is defined as a logical decision-making process aimed at bringing back a true or false answer resulting in impersonal findings. When we use Thinking as a process we are engaging in logical analysis using objective and impersonal criteria. We want to be firm-minded and skeptical, draw cause and effect relationships and value the logical ordering of things. Individuals with a preference for Thinking are impartial and weigh facts objectively. They try to be fair, just and work best in settings where technical skills are more important than interpersonal skills, where truth is valued above tact, and where tough-mindedness may be required.

When Thinking types are viewed in a positive light, they may be thought of as rational, lucid, objective, sound and succinct. If they overdo this function, or if they are being described by someone with a strong preference for Feeling, they may be described as argumentative, dominant, intolerant or defensive.

Feeling is defined as a process whereby judgments are made in terms of a set of personal subjective values, a weighing of relative merits of the issue. Feeling judgment depends on an understanding of personal and group values. When we use Feeling we are applying personal priorities, weighing human values and motives, and *appreciating* people, things or activities. We are being trusting, prizing harmony and valuing warmth in relationships.

Feeling types are said to possess a highly developed set of values, to know what matters most to themselves and others, to tend toward being warm, compassionate, and empathic. Feeling types understand others and wish to affiliate, and are bothered by lack of harmony or conflict. They like to work in settings where understanding and communicating are more important than technical skills, where it is possible to treat others as unique individuals, and where "tender-heartedness" is seen as a virtue.

When viewed in a positive light, Feeling types are considered appreciative, congenial, loyal, considerate, and tactful. When viewed in a negative light, they may be thought of as evasive, high-strung, moody, hypersensitive and spineless.

As with the perceptive functions, there are important distinctions between Introverted and Extraverted forms of the Judging functions that will not be developed here. See *Gifts Differing* for an explanation of these differences.

Bill appears to have had a preference for Feeling rather than Thinking. His tenderheartedness led him to "take in strays" that needed temporary lodging and was revealed in his proposals for the old unused buildings in town – to use them for the elderly, those down on their luck and for disadvantaged youth. He had, at one time, considered Social Work as a profession. The part of the mortuary business he liked the most was in helping families grieve and work through the loss of their loved one while he had little interest in the technical aspects of the business. He liked to be of service to others, whether it be helping them catch fish or improving their health through the products he sold. Even when he worked as a bouncer, he was regarded as a "gentle giant" who would subdue unruly patrons by sitting on them rather than handling them roughly. He was quick to come to the defense of someone who slighted him because he could understand the motivation and constraints they were operating under that had caused them to do what they did. While in hospitals, he was an understanding ear for many other patients and would try to help them work out or understand their problems. The lack of compassion shown to him and other patients in both hospitals and nursing homes was particular galling to him but he was constantly trying to reach out for some common ground that could be built upon so that everyone could move forward. He kept giving unethical staff members or disappointing friends "one more chance" until he was so frustrated he would explode in anger – then he would apologize and give them yet another chance. Unfortunately, his experience over the last three years was mostly disappointing in that respect.

Isabel Myers added a fourth bi-polar contrast (and a scale to measure it) to Jung's original theory in order to clarify the nature of the dominant function. It is said to measure which function is preferred when the subject is extraverting, i. e., when dealing with the outside world.

Perceiving is a process whereby we are open to input from the environment, are curious and want to see more. When we are operating in Perceiving mode, decision making is put off and data is collected. We are using Sensing or Intuition outwardly, taking in information, adapting and changing and resisting closure. We are open-minded, curious and interested in what is out there.

People who have a strong preference for Perceiving might be described as receptive, flexible, adaptive and understanding. They feel little pressure to control events and may not decide within the appropriate time frame.

When viewed in a positive light, the Perceiving person might be called flexible, easy-going, adaptable, and self-determined. When overdoing it or when being viewed in a negative light, the person may be seen as unreliable, scatter-brained, and procrastinating.

Judging is a process whereby input from the environment is closed off so that a decision can be made. Judging refers to Thinking and Feeling which are both considered "rational" functions in contrast to the Perceptive functions (Sensing and Intuition) which are thought of as "irrational" functions because they are "just there" in experience without any effortful evaluation of them. When we are in Judging mode, we are using Thinking or Feeling judgment outwardly, trying to decide or plan, organize or schedule, control or regulate. We are goal directed and want closure even if the data are not all in.

People who prefer the Judging process tend to be called responsible and dependable, They are inclined to stay in the Perceptive mode only long enough to get the basic information necessary to make a decision and then they want to get going, get organized and get things under control. They may make decisions too quickly, without all the necessary facts.

Viewed in a positive light, Judging types may be regarded as planful, efficient, methodical and persevering. If they rely too much on Judging, or are being evaluated by a strong Perceptive type, however, they may be seen as opinionated, rigid, compulsive and impatient.

Bill appears to have operated mostly in a Perceptive mode. He was extremely adaptive, even in adverse circumstances. His ability to roll with the punches during his years of confinement without going completely mad or becoming violent was a marvel to behold. I know that I would not be able to adjust to the kind of torture and maltreatment he received without becoming totally despondent or being consumed with murderous rage and striking out against my oppressors. He could "make do" with what was at hand when camping or fishing, even when he was confined to a wheelchair. He liked to keep his options open and put off decision-making until that one bright idea would come to him that would make a solution to the current difficulties possible. Much to my consternation when I thought it was time to file complaints against his inept lawyers and guardians, he would put it all on hold, waiting for what he considered the opportune moment.

Putting all of these preferences together, Bill's psychological type turns out to be Extraverted Intuitive Feeling Perceiving or ENFP in the shorthand of the Myers-Briggs Type Indicator. This means that his Dominant function was Extraverted Intuition and therefore he would prefer to use his Intuitive perception in the outer world of people, things and activities. He would like the possibilities more than concrete realities and attack his environment with trust and optimism. He could be expected to take risks that others would not and find new enterprises more desirable than the tried and true, often with an extraordinary aptitude for discovering future trends. ENFPs are inclined to leave no option or possibility unexamined and are bored by mere facts, details and repetitive activities. They like to travel because it provides opportunities to experience different kinds of people and cultures. To concentrate on just one possibility would seem to Bill to be too narrow a focus and he would feel boxed in by it. The ENFP's desire to be open to new developments outstrips his desire to be organized and consequently he may find himself living and working in cluttered surroundings. ENFPs find it especially difficult to estimate time requirements for an activity because ideas cannot usually be implemented as fast as they can be generated, especially for an ENFP. If a new project needs a visionary spokesperson, the ENFP may step up and take charge

ENFPs constitute 4.1% of males in the United States. They are adaptable innovators – unconventional, spontaneous, innovative and independent. They scan the environment for anything new and try to change or reshape it. More frequently than other types, they are attracted to counseling as a profession, work in religious settings, the arts and education, teamwork, and cooking. They rate relationships and friendships as being "very important" and use "talking with someone close" as their preferred method of coping when stressed (which is often over financial matters).

The goal of the ENFP's *Auxiliary* function, Introverted Feeling, is to achieve an ideal of inner harmony and serve as a guide to acceptance or rejection of different aspects of one's emotional life. ENFPs try to adapt themselves to the objective environment by simply excluding from awareness that which is unacceptable or pretending it just doesn't exist. The latter may cause a problem in intimate relationships because the ENFP tends to romanticize their partners, overlooking some obvious fact that would make other types suspicious and on guard for signs of deception and artifice. They tend to focus on their partner's best characteristic and shower them with affection, gifts and promises of undying love and to proclaim themselves in love with their true soul mate, thereby making apparent their youthful spirit and zest for life (which certain other types may cynically view as "immaturity"). When the disagreeable fact about his partner that he has been trying to exclude from awareness finally can no longer be avoided, the relationship might dissolve quite rapidly. This seems to have been the case in both of Bill's marriages, although I will refrain from discussing the details here.

A person is said to "fall into the grip of their *inferior* function" when an aspect of himself emerges in a startling "Jeckyl and Hyde" fashion as atypical or out-of-character thoughts, feelings and behaviors. Although the experience may be unsettling to the one it happens to, it may have long-term beneficial and adaptive effects. The experience does not mean that one is falling apart or going crazy (unless, of course, some poorly trained mental health or social service worker gets involved and starts insisting on medication and hospitalization).

The inferior function for ENFPs is Introverted Sensing. In the person who has this function as the dominant, it is likely to be manifested as solitude and reflection but when this function is used by an ENFP it is likely to be manifested as withdrawal, sadness and despair. This is a result of the decrease of energy flowing in the extraverted direction and its redirection inwardly, an unfamiliar and uncomfortable condition for Extraverted Intuitives. Normally enthusiastic and fun-loving, the person begins to feel isolated, unloved and trapped.

ENFPs who are "in the grip" may also become obsessively fixated on one fact or detail, whereas in the person who has Introverted Sensing as a dominant function the process would be manifested as attention to facts and details and a well differentiated awareness of internal experience. In contrast, the ENFP in the grip of his inferior function loses his trusted everyday companion, the sense of new fantastic possibilities. He may become picky, irritable and peevish and make mountains out of mole hills, particularly when it involves personal comfort.

Unlike the person who has Introverted Sensing as his dominant function, the Extraverted Intuitive who has fallen into the grip is not able to recognize the nuances of his internal sensory experiences in fine detail. Instead he may have exaggerated concerns about physical symptoms and think the sensations he is experiencing are signs of a major disease.

What kind of factors are likely to cause an ENFP to use his inferior function, i. e., to be thrown into "the grip?" Extraverted Intuitives are prone, for one thing, to overextend themselves, leading to physical and mental exhaustion. Prompted by their enthusiasm and ideational productivity, they get themselves involved in too many projects and disregard their needs for food, rest, and sleep. They may also overextend themselves by overeating and partying too much - "Let the good times roll!".

Another cause is when they are required to deal with practicalities or have to learn or pay attention to details for an extended period of time. They may be "driven up the wall" by what seem to them to be nonsensical corporate, bureaucratic, or simply practical requirements in order to implement one of their pet projects.

Another trigger is when some value that is important to them is desecrated. In her manual, *In the Grip,* my former colleague, Naomi Quenk, related how one ENFP thought his experience of being thrown into his inferior function was precipitated: "It happens when I feel the pain of others who are the victims of someone's extreme aggressiveness." Bill frequently spoke of experiencing this kind of pain when he saw other patients in the hospitals or nursing homes (as well as himself) being treated in an abusive, degrading and inhumane fashion.

Sandra Hirsh and Jean Kummerow, in their book *Life Types* (1989), wrote that "...if ENFPs become disabled or experience a lack of resources, such as money, they may become despondent because this restricts their ability to quest after new experiences. A worst-case scenario for ENFPs is to live alone and be incapacitated, with few resources and little contact with the outside world....Because they focus on possibilities, rather than the realities, retired ENFPs often do interesting things that may not be thought possible by other, more 'realistic' types."

Well, this "worst-case scenario" was what Bill's life had turned into and it only got worse when his care givers violated his basic values and principles. Quenk writes, "Extraverted Intuitive types need time to reflect, fully experience themselves, even 'wallow' in their inferior state. Meditating is particularly appealing to them. Others need to back off and to avoid patronizing them, but they can help by relieving them of some of the burden of overwhelming details. Attempts to assist by taking over and solving the problem for them, however, are not appreciated. Talking to trusted friends helps, as long as the friends don't offer advice, make judgments, of try to talk them out of their negative state...ENFPs, who may be communicating uncharacteristic coldness and indifference, respond with their auxiliary Feeling to others' warmth, kindness, and approval." In other words, Bill's so-called care givers not only failed to do the kinds of things that would improve his functioning but they did just about all the wrong things that would make him worse.

Bill did have some problems, of course. Most of them had to do with his life circumstances (physical disability and lack of financial resources) and his over-reliance on his Intuition to get along in the world. He also failed to develop aspects of his personality, such as the practically oriented Extraverted Thinking process, to help balance his Extraverted Intuition and assist with the harsh facts in his life.

It seems likely that some of the people who badgered Bill into the state hospital knew quite well what they were doing and were consciously and deliberately getting even with Bill for what they considered his insolent treatment of them. But most of the legal and agency people that Bill encountered on his journey in the mental health gulag were blinded by the poor quality concepts they used to characterize him, construing traits and behaviors that are quite normal in a person of Bill's psychological type into pathologizing psychiatric concepts. His production of "possibilities" was seen as grandiosity, his dislike of details and practicalities was seen as being "in denial," his extensive range of acquaintances and experiences was construed as "delusional," his criticism of their lack of humane treatment of patients and abusiveness was construed as "paranoia," his religious values were transformed into "hallucinations."

If they weren't blinded by the inadequate psychiatric diagnostic concepts that someone else had placed "in the chart" before they received it, they were blinded by their own type bias. Most of the people in the world are different from Bill Tollefson and those people who work in state agencies are often types that are extremely different from Bill. Being untrained in what constitutes the normal range of behavior and experience, and unaware of their own predilections, they were unable to separate out themselves from the situation. They decided that anyone who experienced the world differently from the way they experienced it must be crazy.

So what did they miss by their presumptive blindness? They missed the essence of Bill Tollefson, the kind of person he really was.

5 THE PRICE OF JUSTICE

On April 12th when I talked with Bill, he was fit to be tied. "I've never been so mad that I just wanted to start breaking things, but yesterday I felt that way. Those fuckers are trying to screw me every way they can. They don't give a shit that I'm in pain. They don't give a shit if I croak!"

The following day he was just plain depressed and couldn't do or say much of anything except to curse out the staff for not paying attention to his physical problems.

I gave Jake an update on Bill's mental status and he wrote back, "He hasn't called me for a week or so and then he was so sick he couldn't talk. Now I just hope his legs improve and they don't decide he needs to have them amputated. That's what they did to my wife's aunt in Brainerd.

"And then to get Bill out of his depression (which they caused) they might start to think that he needs some shock therapy. Hope they never got permission to do that, although I see they tried to do so when I looked up the list of proceedings in Bill's case.

"I am going to head to Faribault on Wednesday or Friday and see if I can pick up a copy of the court reporters transcript for Bill's two hearings. If they tell me I can't have or buy copies I'll just tell them that they are for Bill and should be mailed to him or me. Will see what they say. "

After Jake's trip to the county seat, he reported, "The court reporters are on the 3rd floor, but you can't get in. So I went to the information desk on the 2nd floor. I gave them the file numbers and was told that Sharron was the reporter for the first hearing and Alice for the Jarvis. They gave me their phone numbers so I called Sharron. She said she couldn't talk as she was just heading into court. Then I talked to Alice. I gave her the file number and she said yes, she could remember that one. She told me that I could get a copy but that they were about a month or more behind in their printing of the transcriptions. She didn't know what it would cost but would let me know by phone. She called later today but left no message."

When he called back, he learned that the cost for the records of the forced drugging hearing alone would be $650. This was the shortest of the two hearings and would place getting transcripts out of sight financially.

I responded, "That is absolutely disgraceful! Talk about putting up barriers to justice! The whole system is insane! I just talked with Bill and he is really down. His ankles and shoulders are causing him 'killer pain' and they tell him, 'Well, if you can't get up to make the meals, you'll just have to go hungry.' So he has missed 4 meals. But he did manage to get up and get some fluids in him so he can maintain his electrolytes and not get dehydrated. He says he is just trying to keep on breathing!"

Bill's apartment manager had sent a letter to Bill saying she was going to treat his belongings as abandoned property on April 15 . That would leave no time to move anything if she actually did it. I thought she might gamble that Bill wouldn't sue her if she acted. I would have loved to see his apartment manager get sued but I didn't think that it was worth losing Bill's possessions.

I talked with Bill and he was unable to even think about it. I told Jane "My best guess is to move it into storage until Bill gets out of the hospital. He had another visit by his court-appointed guardian today who told him they are trying to find a place for him to reside, so it probably won't be too long from now. The place they had lined up on Greenvale Avenue is now filled up."

I talked with the partner of the lawyer who was handling Bill's eviction problem and she gave me a brief version of the contents of the letter they sent to Laura Biggs, Bill's apartment manager. She said what Biggs was proposing was illegal and that it did not comply with the rules for subsidized housing, that it was "ineffective." Biggs had to give specific reasons why she was evicting Bill. The lawyer said that the property was not abandoned and that if Biggs disposed of it she would have to respond to legal remedies for having done so. Also, Bill had 180 days after receiving notice of eviction, not the 30 days that Biggs claimed.

The attorneys had received no response from Biggs or her attorney. The partner said that Biggs might still dispose of the property but they could do nothing about it until after it happened Then someone representing Bill could take legal action. So, she said, if you are willing to take the chance of losing the property, then do nothing. If the property itself is worth something to Bill and you do not want to risk losing it, then get it moved into a storage locker.

I told the partner, "If things continue to go the way they are going in Anoka, the question of the property may all be moot and that the family could then file a wrongful death suit."

In the end, Jane reneged on her agreement to provide storage. "At this point, since he is not evicted, I would rather not be paying that money until it's needed and God only knows when that might be. The unfortunate reality for us is that we really can't afford to save Bill's 'stuff' at this point. "

I told Jake, "I just got off the phone with Bill for over an hour and we discussed the pros and cons of letting it go to court or moving the stuff out. Jane has reneged on her deal to provide storage, so we decided to let it go to court. Jane said that Laura Biggs told Gary Tollefson that the city of Northfield had declared the place unfit for habitation and threatened Laura's license if she didn't clean it up. I doubt that that is true but it really doesn't make any difference. I think she will have to provide storage for Bill's stuff for 180 days even if she has to move it out of the apartment or risk getting in trouble with HUD. So, we'll let the court decide. If Bill loses his stuff, so be it. But I think any judge with a heart would let him keep some mementos. He is really low on energy and strength now, but he got mad enough to get a little fight back in his system during our conversation. He believes his blood pressure and pulse are low, which is probably true and not a good sign. They may kill him yet!"

Jake talked with Gary who said he was let into Bill's apartment and made the assessment that the only things worth saving would be the electric lift chair, hospital bed, TV set, roll-top desk, some kitchen items and family photos. He thought everything else should be dumped. Gary confirmed to Jake that some kind of inspector looked at the place and decided it needed to be cleaned up.

But something did not sit right with Jake and he began to doubt the building inspector story. "Next time I'm in The Field, I'll stop and see the building inspector. They probably only have one person doing it. He can tell me what's going on and if a re-inspection is scheduled."

It was about ten days before he got around to visiting the building inspectors. "My lawyer friend in Albert Lea told me that when an apartment is condemned by an inspector, a notice has to be stuck on the door giving the reasons why and state when a re-inspection would take place. This notice may not be removed under penalty of law. So today I just got back from The Field. Bill's apartment door had no notice on it. The lock had been changed, and all of the stuff Bill had on the door was gone including his name plate. I went around to the outside and looked in the windows. Bad news. The place had been completely cleaned out. Nothing left in the bed room and only a TV and small box in the main room. I bet you-know-who will try to sell the TV to whomever might move in.

"I then went to the city hall inspection office. Three guys were sitting there. They told me they were the only inspection people in town. They said no one from that office had looked at anything at that facility for at least 10 years or longer. I guess Biggs made up another good story."

I talked with Bill's attorney, Bill Zimbledon, who handled the guardianship matter and he informed me that Laura Biggs was attempting to get around the HUD regulations to force Bill out of his apartment and get rid of his property. The attorney was aware that Bill was being represented by Brian Landers in the eviction action and said that he thought Brian had put forth a very good argument and statement of the HUD regulations regarding Bill's apartment (e. g., He cannot be evicted in the middle of a month. He has 180 days before he can be evicted when he is sent to the hospital. They have to list specific reasons why he is being evicted. They have to make an inventory of all the items in the apartment, etc.). He said he thought that Laura was just trying to get around the law and have someone else do the dirty work.

Biggs claimed it was an emergency to get Bill's stuff out of his apartment because building inspectors might shut her down otherwise. Bill's lawyer argued that there was no emergency and that she should follow the law and regulations. Unfortunately, he did not have the information at that time that city inspectors had not been out to inspect the place for any violations. If he had, he might have been able to nail her for perjury. He lost the case but the court required that Bill's temporary guardians store the stuff someplace rather than destroy it.

In theory, Biggs should not have been able to re-rent the apartment until the issues regarding HUD rules were resolved and it was uncertain when that would go to court. Then there was the matter of guardianship coming up on May 9th. The prosecution was now going for "permanent" guardianship rather than the six month variety they wanted earlier.

I wondered if this was in retaliation for Bill fighting the eviction because it had drawn the whole process out longer than they had planned. Earlier they had talked about getting him out into assisted living in March.

Meanwhile, Bill said, "It's like somebody has thrown away the key to my life!" He then had to rush off the phone because they were making him drink extra water because his kidney function was impaired and that was about the best they could do to treat it. He probably wouldn't have had this problem either if they had gotten him into hydrotherapy.

Jake's lawyer friend, George, had actually met Bill once about five or six years earlier when he and Jake were in Northfield for Jesse James Days. "George has a brother who has almost exactly the same leg problem as Bill," said Jake. "His legs swell up and his feet get very large. He goes to the Mayo Clinic about once every six months or so where they put him into some kind of a pressure suit and squeeze all the fluid out of both legs and feet. With a diuretic it all ends up as urine and takes about eight hours or a little more. This is probably what Bill could use now but he can't get it in Anoka."

On another phone call, Bill said, "I'm so angry I can hardly contain it. I can't stand being here. I don't know what is going on and the staff doesn't tell me anything. I don't know if I have a guardian or not or whether I have an apartment or not. My shoulders hurt like hell almost all the time and now I'm getting neck pain along with it. My ankle is fucked up too. No one has taken x-rays or even palpated my shoulders in an effort to find out what the problem is. I can't sit in my wheelchair because the padding is inadequate and they can't find my $550 orthobaric cushion. Now, with my shoulder pain and ankle pain, I don't transfer well. So, it is either laying flat on my back in bed or sitting for a short period in my wheelchair. My pulse rate is down to 48. No TV in my room, no radio, no clock. The food tastes like shit and if I can't get up in time, I go without. I need someone to get me out of this hell-hole snake-pit."

Everything he said was consumed with rage and with a desperate cry for help. I didn't blame him a bit. Bill was given pain pills at times, but not enough to stop the pain. Experts in treating pain all indicate that enough medication should be given early enough so that they get ahead of the pain intensity, not end up chasing it after it gets so intense that nothing will help.

I finally received a response from the Office of Health Facility Complaints regarding the complaint I had filed with respect to Bill experiencing adverse side-effects from the Abilify he was forced to take. I didn't know it when I submitted the complaint, but they were really the Center for Medicare and Medicaid Services . They said they could only investigate a complaint if it establishes the potential for a significant health or safety deficiency under federal requirements.

"We do not mean to imply that your complaint is not important, or that the incidents you describe did not occur. Under the Medicare law we can authorize complaint investigations against accredited hospitals only in the circumstances described above. The complaint must be so serious that, if substantiated, we would take action to remove the hospital from the Medicare program and stop all Medicare payments. We do not have the authority to impose lesser penalties on hospitals."

They went on to say "We are making the TJC [The Joint Commission on Accreditation of Hospitals] aware of your complaint. However, we will not reveal your identity to the TJC. Should you wish to write to the TJC directly, the address is: TJC, One Renaissance Boulevard, Oakbrook Terrace, Illinois 60181."

When I worked for the VA, I went through a Joint Commission inspection and I remembered it was a big deal for administrators. They, of course, expressed their anxiety by having all of us underlings practice for weeks for possible questions that might be proposed by the examiners. It was known that the commission kept records of complaints from patients and followed up on previous areas of inadequacy to see if they had been corrected. So I suspected and hoped that this might actually have some effect.

I went through the *Minnesota Patient Bill of Rights* and used that as a guide for writing my letter, after soliciting any comments from others that were trying to help Bill. I sent a copy to the Minnesota Ombudsman for Mental Health and they, of course, made no response whatsoever.

In my letter, I cited the forced drugging and the adverse side-effects it had on Bill and the deprivation of hydrotherapy which had played such a major role in maintaining his physical and metabolic functioning in the past. I pointed out that the institution had also prohibited Mr. Tollefson from getting chiropractic treatment for his back pain, even though he was able to arrange an appointment locally in Anoka, arrange for transportation and get coverage approved by UCare, his Medicaid provider. I reminded them that the *Patient Bill of Rights* required that *"Patients shall have the right to appropriate medical and personal care based on individual needs."*

Referring to the rule that *"Patients shall have the right to a prompt and reasonable response to their questions and requests,"* I pointed out that Bill had been having constant shoulder pain for at least three weeks and his requests for evaluation were ignored by his medical physician.

I mentioned that Bill's arms had been bruised by use of an improperly sized blood pressure cuff or keeping it on too long, that he was supplied with a too-narrow wheelchair with an inadequate seat, so that he was in such discomfort that he could not sit for long and had to return to bed for relief, foregoing any opportunities for entertainment or distraction.

I asserted that Bill had been subjected to emotional abuse. He had been roused in the morning and assailed by a nurse sounding like a mad fishwife for not making it to breakfast in time. He had been told when he was in bed with pain from his shoulders so severe that he could not get up, "Well, you'll just have to go hungry then!" He had been disrespected and treated callously by his doctors and treatment staff. They had been indifferent to his pain and desire to be listened to rather than just being told he was "delusional" or "paranoid" (both of which were blatantly false). According to the *Minnesota Patient's Bill of Rights*, *"Patients have the right to be treated with courtesy and respect for their individuality by employees of or persons providing service in a health care facility."*

I mentioned that Bill felt totally in the dark about what was being planned for him regarding his health care and that I, his power of attorney and health care representative, was not involved in the planning of Bill's health care. According to the *Patient Bill of Rights*, *"Patients shall have the right to participate in the planning of their health care. This right includes the opportunity to discuss treatment and alternatives with individual caregivers, the opportunity to request and participate in formal care conferences, and the right to include a family member or other chosen representative, or both."*

In conclusion, I wrote, "I consider this inadequate care, both medically and psychologically, and a violation of the state's own *Patient Bill of Rights*. I ask that you investigate these complaints, include them in your next review of the facility, and ensure that appropriate action is taken by the facility to correct them."

I received an email from Jake. "Just got done watching the first half of a long video called: *The Marketing of Madness: The Truth About Psychotropic Drugs*. You've probably seen it. Scary. And Bill fits right into that picture with an imaginary disease classification (NOS) being treated by a drug with not much science behind it. Bill's case reminds me of the old Soviet Union where dissidents were declared mentally ill and shipped off to the Gulags to rot in silence out of the way. And all it took for Bill were a couple of imbecilic judges, incompetent lawyers, and a vindictive land lady in combination with a clown for a social worker all conspiring against him. Thinking about this is starting to piss me off."

I hadn't seen the video but after I did, I sent the web address to everyone I knew that might be interested in it. Seems like every week there is some new expose about evil doings in the drug industry, especially with regard to psychiatric and cancer drugs. Those two areas are where the money is. Abilify costs about $16.44 per pill and has a $4 billion per year market. The manufacturer appeared to be trying to grow the market by advocating its uses as an adjunct to other medications, such as anti-depressants, claiming it had some sort of synergistic or potentiating effect.

Jake saw an ad for Abilify on TV with a bunch of children running around in the background and he wondered if they were trying to push the drug for use in children. Cynically, I replied, "Well they just have to grow that market. The psychiatry industry has been expanding the market for all sorts of things, not just the drugs. Once they have a diagnostic category, they can then hold seminars and consult with all those folks who aren't in the know, even if it is a totally made-up disorder. The people can become experts in that area and form dues paying associations, get some political clout, then require that anyone practicing in that area be specially certified or licensed. Then the practitioners have to pay fees for training, certification testing, and just to help out the state budget! I even know a child psychiatrist who admits to being 'a pimp for the drug companies' since they pay him to go around lecturing general practitioners about uses for their drugs. It's a great racket if you can live with yourself afterward."

Coincidentally, I received my newsletter from the Health Sciences Institute in Baltimore asking the reader, "If a powerful drug has the potential to kill the people taking it, wouldn't it make much more sense for the warning box to be a thick red line and the font five times the size of the minuscule font used in the rest of the insert? THAT would be a serious, eye-catching warning for a drug such as Abilify (for bipolar disorder) that may actually cause dangerous increases in blood sugar levels that have been associated with coma and death in some patients."

The article went on to report that a Stanford University study found that black box warnings did not appear in all the drug labels in the same drug class. Most drugs which were eventually withdrawn did not carry required black box warnings prior to their withdrawal and those withdrawals usually didn't occasion black box warning for other drugs in the same class. The time lag from when a drug class received at least one warning to when the warning was extended to other members of the class ranged from a few months to 14 years. Thus, corporate profits appear to have higher priority than patient safety.

Jake reported the Anoka Treatment Center to the Medicare fraud e-mail site.

On April 19, just a month after he had been started on Abilify, the drug was stopped, not by Dr. Quack but by his supervisor. Apparently, Dr. Quack had left the hospital for parts unknown. I didn't know if they had received a "back channel communication" from the Medicare Complaints Office (whom both Jake and I had contacted) or from someone at the Joint Commission (who had been sent my complaint about the forced drugging from the Complaints Office) or if they just finally realized they were killing Bill with an inappropriate medication.

I received a request from the Joint Commission for my permission to use my name in confronting the institution with my complaint on May 5, which I granted. It was not until June 7 that I received word from the Joint Commission that they had received the hospital's response and that they had accepted it. They do not tell complainers what the response was, so it is difficult to know what transpired. Well, at least Bill was off the damn drug even if they still weren't doing anything for his bunged-up shoulders and ankle and his sore butt!

About that time, Lucy attended a hearing on a somewhat similar case in Minneapolis and talked with a couple of lawyers who were present. She told them about Bill's situation and they agreed with her assessment that Bill had been screwed over by the mental health-legal cabal. I talked on the phone for about 45 minutes with one of these lawyers who did not sound like he was a bottom-feeder.

After I briefly described Bill's situation and the failure of the court to ensure that his legal rights were maintained, he said, "Public defenders in Minnesota cannot be sued in criminal trials and I suppose the same thing is true in civil cases. Judges and county prosecutors are also immune from prosecution for their errors or violations of the law.

"With regard to the medication problem," he said, "it is hard to challenge a judge on any matter. The whole thing might be challenged if the public defender was incompetent but the time for appeal of the original hearing is past.

"About the only thing that can be done at this point is to work with the six month review of the commitment. Since they are already trying to find some way to get him out of the hospital, the best thing is probably to wait and let them move him out."

He said that just for him to look into it would cost about $2500. We could probably have scraped up that amount but it would all be wasted if he couldn't go further than just "looking into it."

I asked about suing the hospital for Medicaid or Medicare fraud under the False Claims Act. This is a law passed after the Civil War intended to stop the flood of false claims that were being made against the government for war-related expenses. Recently, cases had been won where hospitals were found to be treating patients who did not have the disorders claimed or used drugs known to be ineffective. The government fined those found guilty in the amount of three times the amount for each charge made on government accounts. The person making the allegation of fraud, the "whistle-blower," would also collect a fee for each charge. The lawyer didn't seem to know anything about that kind of legal action.

"And what is this about Rice County charging exorbitant fees for court records? That has to be obstruction of justice and discrimination against poor people doesn't it?"

"Maybe, but they seem to get away with it," he said.

Jake talked with his lawyer friend, George, again. George had talked to another lawyer, Dan, in Minneapolis who had been doing commitment defense for about 20 years. He said Hennepin county didn't use public defenders for commitment hearings because they were all too busy in crime cases. On the other hand, in the county seat where George practiced, they didn't have any public defenders since there was just not enough work to keep them busy. The county had a list of lawyers on call when needed and they rotated the names. Furthermore, in most of the counties in northern Minnesota that were all on the verge of bankruptcy, they could barely afford to provide any defense at all.

That last point made me wonder if Bill's rights to a second opinion and to appeal were denied because of Rice County budget problems. It wouldn't surprise me at all but I thought the public defender, the prosecutor, and the judge would have to at least implicitly conspire to do it, i. e., they would all have to agree not to bring these matters up. In theory, all officers of the court are responsible for ensuring that the law is followed, which includes seeing to it that the defendant's rights are protected.

Jake said, "Dan told George that since Rice County had a report from a licensed psychologist recommending commitment, Bill was pretty much out of luck and any pursuit of negligence claims aimed at the county would be quite expensive and unfruitful. Ninety-nine percent or so of people committed can't afford to fight it due to the high costs (expert testimony, legal fees, etc.). And when Bill told someone that he stopped taking all his drugs because God told him to do so, (what I think he meant with that answer was, 'screw you--none of your business') his goose was cooked since that remark ended up on his chart at the hospital or the police report. Any law suit would require a ton of money and a big up front fee to pursue the thing."

In 2013 Emory University School of Law conducted a study (reported in an article by Marshall Allen and Olga Pierce in *Pro Publica*, Jan. 6, 2014) called "Uncovering the Silent Victims of the American Medical Liability System" in which 450 attorneys were surveyed . The study found that about 95 percent of patients harmed by medical malpractice would find it impossible to obtain legal representation. Monetary damages were the most important factor in a lawyer refusing cases. Assuming that the chances of winning a case were 95 percent, virtually no attorney would take a case if the damages were expected to be less than $50,000; more than 50 percent of lawyers would refuse a case if the expected damages were less than one quarter of a million dollars, no matter what the probability of winning. For people without assets or much income (children, unemployed mothers, the elderly, the disabled and the poor) who are unable to cough up the money for basic expenses to bring a suit to court (which might be from $20,000 to $50,000), the attorney would have to do so. And because disbursement on a successful lawsuit is based largely on "real" damages (economic losses like foregone wages, medical bills and future costs), the return on this investment of time and money might be slight (unless punitive damages were also likely). Thus, members of these disadvantaged economic groups are least likely to find an attorney to offer them their services. Stephen Daniels, a research professor at the American Bar Foundation summed up the attorney's perspective by saying, "the juice isn't worth the squeeze."

In order to fix the economic discrimination, the study authors suggested providing a financial incentive for lawyers by increasing public funding for these kinds of legal services, having defendants who lose a case pay the plaintiff's attorney fees, or setting up an administrative system composed of neutral adjudicators and medical experts so attorneys would not be needed.

I updated Bill's friends by email with the subject line: "How much does it cost to get justice in Rice County?" Inside, the answer was, "If you have to ask, you can't afford it."

Jake saw a video on hoarders and wondered if Bill might not have that problem, even though, he admitted, Bill would have to be considered a mere amateur compared to the folks shown on that program. I watched the program and wrote back.

"A couple of my wife's friends, who are both bright but unconventional people, shudder to think that what has happened to Bill could happen to them. One is a "collector" that has her attic above her garage & house filled with stuff, but she successfully plays the stock market. She has a couple of siblings who would both like to get their hands on her money and would love to declare her incompetent to do so.

"The other is a woman with a chronic physical disease who isn't exactly a hoarder but has a hard time throwing stuff out. She lives in what she considers 'a lot of clutter' and is afraid to have any inspectors see her apartment for fear they will try to take control of her life.

"My dad had a friend in Northfield - a bachelor farmer - who used to collect Cadillacs and cloisonné that would probably now be worth millions. He had lots of money and built garages to store his collection of Cadillacs but his house was so filled with cloisonné pottery it was hard to navigate in some rooms. He was never locked up and reportedly willed all his stuff to a waitress who was nice to him at the Big Steer out where Highway 19 intersects with the freeway.

"Unfortunately, the mental health education system is producing technocrats who know nothing and appreciate little about the range of different types of people there are in the world. Psychiatrists are probably the worst of the lot since they have retreated back into biological medicine, which in the mental health realm is nothing but pseudo-science. They don't even bother to talk with their patients anymore, let alone try to understand them."

Jake visited his semi-retired lawyer friend in Albert Lea again and had this to report:

"I showed him one of your write-ups about how Bill got the shaft from the Rice County Courts and the Anoka place. He could hardly believe his eyes and told me that he had some experience in Hennepin County with commitment hearings. In Hennepin County public defenders are only used for criminal cases. For commitment hearings, a three lawyer panel is used for the defense. And these guys aren't just some clowns just out of law school. They are practicing attorneys who have been specially schooled in mental illness. They are required to take a bunch of psych courses at the University all dealing with mental illness issues. They are then certified by the county to act in such cases. They get paid by the hour so they like to drag things out a long time. NO ONE ever goes to the Anoka joint unless they are beyond any doubt crazy as a hen and a danger to themselves or the community. In Bill's case, the judge probably would have made him join an AA group. Nothing else."

Wow! This was very interesting because, since civil commitment is a state law, should there not be uniformity across counties in the manner in which the law is implemented? According to the Equal Protection Clause of the 14th Amendment, the laws of a state must not discriminate in the way they are applied: an individual in given conditions and circumstances must be treated in the same manner as other people who are in similar conditions and circumstances. A violation occurs when a state grants a particular *class* of individuals the right to engage in an activity but denies other individuals the same right. The Supreme Court tends to find a classification defined by the state as constitutional if the state can prove that the classification has a "rational basis" and is necessary to further a "legitimate state purpose." If the classification obstructs fundamental rights, such as First Amendment rights (freedom of religion, speech, the press, assembly, petitioning the government for redress of grievances), it is likely to be found unconstitutional.

I reasoned that the same principle should apply at the county-state level: the law, and in particular the laws regarding civil commitment, should be applied or implemented equally in different counties. If so, what branch of government would take up that matter? Would it have to go to the state supreme court? Is it a federal matter? Rice County and Hennepin County appear to be so different from each other that they could be on different planets.

I called Bill's non-profit lawyer about another matter but prevailed upon his willingness to answer legal questions.

"Shouldn't state laws be applied the same across the state?"

"The law is the law," he said. "The procedures should be more or less the same in all counties."

"Is there a government agency that can make courts behave or can they do whatever they damn well please?"

"You might try Watch Minnesota. Here, let me give you their address. Here it is: http://www.watchmn.org/court-monitoring."

After I got off the phone, I put the address in my web browser and clicked "Go." The web site stated that their mission was "to make the justice system more effective and responsive in handling cases of violence against women and children, and to create a more informed and involved public." I sent them an email to find out if their domain of operation included cases of civil commitment. I never received a response.

I found a blog on the Internet by someone calling himself Mr. Magoo who answered a question by an individual about equal application of the law. His response, while not what I wanted to hear or believe, was informative:

"I guess you haven't figured it out yet. The Constitution and the Bill of Rights are little more than a Madison Ave. snow job. It's money that gives you rights in the US. Those who pay more, have more rights. Take the case of Hal Turner. Accused of threatening the lives of 2 judges because he expressed that they deserved to be killed on his blog, Turner was twice tried and both times the trial ended in hung juries. On the third try, Turner, by now broke and forced to rely on public defenders, was convicted in less than 2 hours. Now if Turner had said that Joe Blow down the street deserved to be killed, nothing would have happened. But because he said it about judges, all of sudden it's a crime, First Amendment notwithstanding. So where's your equal application of the law? And furthermore, Turner was an FBI informant who had been encouraged by his handlers to make inflammatory comments on his blog and radio program. The bottom line is that if the government wants to destroy you, they will simply hound you into bankruptcy. Only those with very deep pockets can fight back. Do you really think that when our founding fathers legislated against double jeopardy that they intended for people to be tried over and over again because of a hung jury and run into the poor house? I don't think so."

I wrote Jim Gottstein, the lawyer in Alaska, and asked what he thought of the 14th Amendment argument as well as some other rights violations according to state law and he replied as if he were Mr. Magoo's twin: "People's rights are violated as a matter of course in these types of proceedings. See *Involuntary Commitment and Forced Psychiatric Drugging in the Trial Courts: Rights Violations as a Matter of Course*, 25 Alaska L. Rev.51 (2008). I don't know how strong the equal protection argument is, but I like the other ones. The problem is in getting lawyers to aggressively pursue people's rights."

At this point I was thinking that we would never get any justice out of the legal system and began searching for different avenues to have an impact on Bill's situation. Maybe we could marshal public sentiment to express outrage at what had happened to Bill. Most publications accept only very short "reaction" type letters to the editor for items that are already news, not fresh material. I couldn't imagine how I could adequately explain Bill's situation in 450 words. I looked at the submission requirements listed for the *Minneapolis Star Tribune* and *St. Paul Dispatch* and even the *New York Times*. The Star Tribune allowed for slightly longer submissions, so I wrote up a 700 word essay. But when I was finished, I couldn't see how it would be especially persuasive or of any direct help to Bill.

I considered developing a Facebook page for Bill under their "causes" section since that would allow a longer exposition of what happened and why it was important. Not being up to speed on all the new social media technology, I began to write up some copy for a page while studying how you go about creating one.

I also thought that maybe if an investigative reporter got involved, he or she might do a story on Bill and others who were in a similar predicament. I identified a couple of prospects at the two major papers and my friend at the Twin Cities branch of Mindfreedom suggested a reporter who had done an article about mental health matters at the *City Pages*, a popular Twin Cities newspaper. She also suggested going to the local TV stations. I looked on the web sites for National Public Radio and Michael Moore and both had avenues to submit ideas for possible stories.

The problem was that all of these places had thousands of people clamoring to get their pet project publicized so why should they pay attention to a fat, wheelchair-bound 70 year old fisherman who got locked up in a state hospital? They wouldn't believe he had his rights violated and the hospital hadn't killed him yet, so what's the big deal?

I sent an email to Gloria, one of Bill's high school classmates. Gloria had always been a dynamic woman, starting out in show business after high school and later returning to get her college degree and work herself up the ladder of school administration. We used to go to dances together back in the 1950s when they were held in the old National Guard Auditorium. She was a great dancer. I had two left feet. We had reconnected a few years back on a web site devoted to finding old classmates.

I told Gloria what had happened to Bill and asked if she had any ideas on how we might help him or if she knew of any of his old classmates that would care to get involved. Gloria said the hospital where Bill was being housed sounded like something from an old movie – *The Snake Pit*- and she found the uncaring attitude expressed by staff disheartening.

"It boggles my mind,"she said. "I have a theory that bullies and people with abusive and sadistic personalities gravitate to jobs in prisons, reform schools, and mental hospitals because they then have access to people who are captive and at their mercy, people who have lost their rights, freedom, voice for help, and access to safety and recourse to justice just by being where they are. The same theory takes in pedophiles who become priests because that is where the young, innocent, and unprotected are. Because of the priest's position, he gets away with it or, at least, used to get away with it."

Gloria acknowledged that none of Bill's friends had the kind of money required to fight the matter in court. She suggested starting a letter writing campaign to improve Bill's treatment at the hospital. She had a lot of pride in her high school class.

"We were a class with which to reckon. We were a class that was cohesive and that accomplished things. I am going to ask the class to come together again to help one of our own. Each one of us at this point is a snowflake. Together we become a snowball. Once we start contacting and enlisting others, we start rolling down hill gathering momentum and size as we roll. Finally when we all start sending our letters, we become an avalanche of opinion and demand. Hear us roar! A single snowflake has no power. An avalanche can take out everything in its way. Hopefully, when being bombarded with letters, the state hospital administrator will figure they have to take some positive actions with Bill. Let's get this avalanche started!"

Gloria sent out emails to her classmates trying to enlist their help while I called a man who had known Bill since the two of them were in college together. A retired social worker, he proved to be a delightful man.

"I have a brother who is a lot like Bill in temperament," he said. "My brother started out his career with a 2500 mile canoe trip! I know Bill is a non-conformist, but that doesn't make him crazy. In fact, I am proud to call Bill a friend." He wanted to help even though he was contending with a serious life-threatening illness himself.

A high school classmate of mine who knew Bill when we were all growing up in Northfield volunteered to help in any way he could. He had completed a year of law school before deciding it wasn't for him but had worked in an administrative position in a law school for a number of years. I figured he had more knowledge than the rest of us about legal matters.

I made out a list of all the issues involved in Bill's case to be sent around to those who decided to join the effort. Then I organized a list of links to websites we might want to contact: media (television, radio, newspapers); state laws regarding civil commitment, guardianship, civil rights, Medicare fraud; agencies such as The Joint Commission and state department of human services; advocacy groups and information sources (e.g., Psychrights, Mindfreedom).

The response to Gloria's passionate plea to recruit classmates to help Bill was overwhelmingly positive. Only two out of thirty-three people preferred to be de-listed from the group. Most were puzzled that such a thing could happen in Minnesota and especially to one of their own that most remembered quite well. One person who had moved away years ago wrote, "That's pretty disgusting. I remember Minnesota as a civilized place, growing up in Northfield."

Some voiced the assumption that there must be something wrong with Bill or he wouldn't have been committed. Several wanted to know more details about just how debilitated he was, what were his physical and mental limitations and what would be his requirements for independent living. Most knew about his long history of being overweight and several had suggestions about what to do about that. Several who had known him since grade school wondered why his siblings weren't doing something to help.

I told them about the ill-fated trip to Florida, the problems with the drug amioderone, the fact that he was largely confined to a wheelchair, the problems with the apartment manager and her legal shenanigans, the inadequacy of his court-appointed lawyers, the failure of the court to ensure his legal rights, the consequences of the forced drugging and other inadequacies of care at the state hospital, the frustrations in getting any help from state agencies and the financial infeasibility of hiring a lawyer to defend him or even getting transcripts of the court proceedings so we could document the ways in which the court failed in its duty to uphold the law.

I informed the members of the "Free The Fisherman Network," as I called our group, that one of Bill's lawyers said Bill was in a kind of Catch-22 situation since arriving at Anoka. If he contested their claim and asserted that he had no significant mental problems, that would be interpreted as him being "in denial" and therefore he must be mentally ill. If he didn't contest the accusation, then that would be taken as an admission that he was mentally ill and needed to be penned up with the other wild animals. There was no way for him to win. It had been the same way with the medication that was making him ill: if he stopped taking it without his doctor's permission, he must be crazy and a danger to himself; if he continued to take it, he could be dead.

One person responded, "Just amazing! This information sounds like it is taken from some conspiracy novel, not real life and actually happening. I am shocked. This type of legal abuse and misuse of power isn't supposed to happen in the USA. Where is 'Equal justice for all'? It is just one more area in which poor people are screwed. They have no voice so they are easily dismissed and pushed around."

Most of the suggestions for action were ones we had already tried or considered. Several people suggested contacting various agencies that are supposed to help people with legal troubles but do not have funds to hire an attorney. One person who had a son with one year of law school under his belt said that Bill's lawyer could be disbarred for failure to represent his client competently due to the things he did not do, like file an appeal when asked to do so, not challenging items presented, not advising his client that he had the right to a second opinion, and possibly other things. He suggested we take our facts and file a complaint with the

Minnesota Law Bar Association against him for inadequate and incompetent defense with the hope that another hearing could be requested.

My old high school buddy with one year of law school, but also considerable experience working in or with government agencies, thought it might be possible to put pressure on certain points in the system (e. g., facility administrator, politicians, ombudsman for mental health) to get them to see that it was in their best interests to get Bill out of the hospital. Now that we had a respectable size group, I thought, we might be able to do that. If there was another court hearing, we could all show up and demand to be heard.

One especially kind person volunteered to be Bill's guardian and provide him a home in the northern part of the state where he used to work as a fishing guide, but it was unlikely that it would be approved by the court. A few people wrote about their own fights with imperious agencies and corporations.

"A personal care provider company lost it's license last week. Many people including my mom and uncle need help with daily living and are now without help. They transferred to a new provider so people would still get help, but the insurance company won't accept that because they save much money by making us shop for a new provider, and going through two months of background checks and much paperwork. Meanwhile, innocent elders and disabled have no one to help with very important daily stuff. The Prime West Insurance lady said if I need help placing them in a nursing home, to let her know. Sure. Medicare probably pays for that, eh?.... So yes, it is crazy what's happening to those who can't help themselves. Selfishness and greed govern those who have power."

Another woman lamented the loss of her long battle with a county planning and zoning commission which decided in favor of a private corporation whose activities would jeopardize the environment, town buildings and the mental health and serene nature of their small community.

Shortly after she began, Gloria had to cut back much of her involvement in order to care for a loved one who was in dire straights. I then became the one to respond to most of the inquiries from members of the group. These were reasonable enough requests for information to help them think about the problem, decide where they stood on an issue, and try to come up with suggestions. I had been spending about one third of my waking hours trying to do something about Bill's predicament: trying to track down potential sources of help on the Internet, doing research on laws, responding to emails from members of the group and talking with Bill on the phone. I was getting tired and neglecting other things I should have been doing or wanted to do.

The expressions of concern and sympathy for Bill from the group were appreciated but I had hoped that having many minds working on the task might help divide up the work and give me a break. That was not to be. Since I didn't know exactly where we were headed, the task was not one that could easily be broken down into "assignments" for different members. With a few notable exceptions, no one volunteered to do anything on their own and, I suspect, didn't know what they could do.

We couldn't find the name of the director of the hospital (it wasn't listed anywhere) and I was doubtful that sending a bunch of letters to him or her would be fruitful anyway. I remembered in the VA when an activist patient sent complaints to the regional office and they were just bounced back to the facility chief of staff, who blew them off for a second time. Even when this particular patient compiled a number of complaints from different patients and documentation of them into a packet and sent it to the "secret" address for the Secretary of Veterans Affairs, at the suggestion of someone in his office, the information just "disappeared." No, I think any kind of letter writing campaign would have to be directed at someone at a higher level than a hospital director.

From my point of view, the shinning star of the group was Jake, who lived in a town about half way between Anoka and Northfield. He traveled hundreds of miles to visit Bill in the hospital, encouraged him, brought him things he needed, and checked on the status of his apartment and possessions. He studied on the Internet to better understand Bill. He did some detective work to get information that helped us make sense out of what was happening. Several times he traversed the southern part of the state to get legal advise from a lawyer friend and he made the effort to attend some of Bill's hearings at the Rice County Court House. Jake was a bright self-starter and the kind of guy you could always count on.

In early May, Bill was slated for another hearing in which the prosecutors were going to ask that he have a permanent guardianship. This would leave him totally under the control of a couple of women in Owatonna who had formed themselves into a company to handle all of a ward's money, determine where he lived, decide whether medical treatment was needed and who was to provide it, and, basically, make the ward do whatever they wanted. Bill was so debilitated by pain in his butt that he could not make the trip to court and his lawyer made no effort to obtain a continuance. Thus, the judge decided in the prosecutor's favor.

GERALD D. OTIS

6 A DYSFUNCTIONAL SYSTEM

Bill is not the only person who has ever been ensnared by the dysfunctional mental health – legal system. Just how large is the problem? It is hard to come by accurate statistics since many hospitals and states do not keep records of civil commitments. One frequently cited estimate is that 1.5 to 2.0 million U. S. citizens are subjected to involuntary incarceration in mental hospitals each year. This figure is extrapolated from the figure for the state of California, which does keep statistics, and has 10% of the U. S. population. However, there may be considerable variation between states. Oregon, for example, has seen a 50% decline in commitment rates over the last 20 years even though its population has increased substantially over the same period of time. The decrease is thought to be somewhat dependent on a change in the operational definition of "dangerousness" but primarily due to the decreased number of acute psychiatric beds available in the last two decades. If the state legislature does not fund state hospital beds, there are, as if by magic, fewer psychiatric commitments.

How much does all of this cost? Colorado's Representative Patricia Schroeder, Chair of the House Select Committee on Children, Youth and Families presided over hearings in Washington, D.C. on various psychiatric industry abuses in 1992. Using an estimate of $940 per day for hospitalization and treatment (Bill's was $910 per day), each commitment cost $16,700 although some costs were as high as $35,000. This is the average cost for the typical patient who is discharged before 28 days when the usual insurance plan stops paying benefits. For Bill, who spent eight months in confinement, the cost of his erroneous commitment was estimated at over one quarter of a million dollars! For the 1.5 million people committed yearly, the annual cost to the nation is estimated to be about $25 billion. And who do you suppose pays the bulk of this cost? Why, of course, it is you and I, in the form of higher insurance premiums, higher prices passed on by employers who pay for insurance, and higher taxes to pay for all the machinery that keeps it going.

Representative Schroeder summarized her committee's findings as follows: "Our investigation has found that thousands of adolescents, children, and adults have been hospitalized for psychiatric treatment they didn't need; that hospitals hire bounty hunters to kidnap patients with mental health insurance; that patients are kept against their will until their insurance benefits run out; that psychiatrists are being pressured by the hospitals to increase profit; that hospitals 'infiltrate' schools by paying kickbacks to school counselors who deliver students; that bonuses are paid to hospital employees, including psychiatrists, for keeping the hospital beds filled; and that military dependents are being targeted for their generous mental health benefits. I could go on, but you get the picture."

Back in the 1970's, during the depths of the Cold War, the Committee for State Security, or KGB, had co-opted Soviet psychiatry and created a group of special mental hospitals to treat a condition known as "sluggish schizophrenia" which afflicted about twice as many individuals in the Soviet Union as it did in Great Britain. The symptoms were so subtle as to be detectable only by the trained eyes of KGB-tutored psychiatrists. The classic symptoms of sluggish schizophrenia were found in political dissidents, who believed they could reform the governmental system. They were rounded up and consigned to these special hospitals for psychiatric treatment.

The international community condemned this political abuse of psychiatry. In order to keep from being expelled from the World Psychiatric Association (WPA), the Soviet organization of psychiatrists quickly resigned from the WPA. The WPA, knowing the western idea of "mental illness" was not much different from that of the Soviets, took a conciliatory approach asking only that the Russians "ameliorate" the abuse in order to again be in good standing. The UN Commission on Human Rights dithered about their recommendations until the Soviet Union disintegrated, so that the final version of their "Principles for the Protection of Persons with Mental Illness and for the Improvement of Mental Health Care" adopted by the United Nations General Assembly in 1991 is primarily designed to protect the rights of voluntary patients, not involuntary patients.

On March 23, 1976 a multilateral treaty created by The International Covenant on Civil and Political Rights (ICCPR) and adopted by the United Nations went into effect. It committed its 72 signatories and 167 parties to respect the civil and political rights of all individuals, "without distinction of any kind." Included in its Article 18 are the right to life; to non-coerced freedom of thought, conscience and religion; to freedom of speech; to freedom of assembly and electoral rights; and to rights to due process and a fair trial. The Covenant states that beliefs may be manifested in worship, observance, practice and teaching with the only limitation being with regard to manifestations that endanger public safety, health, or the rights of others. But, according to a conference of international jurists, other people's rights only have precedence if they are "more fundamental" than the right to manifest a belief. In other words, the sole justification for constraining any person's liberty is a "pressing public need" to prevent harm to others. The individual's "own good" is not a sufficient condition to do so. The pledge is meant to protect the rights of all individuals including those labeled mentally ill.

An Australian writer deduced from the wording of Article 18 that involuntarily treating a person claimed to be schizophrenic would probably be a violation of the pledge because it constitutes coercion that would interfere with the patient's freedom to adopt a belief of his own choice. Drug treatment, in particular, could be seen as impairing freedom of thought by obstructing the higher thinking functions of the brain.

On March 3, 2013 Juan E. Mendez, the Special Rapporteur on Torture of the UN Commission for Human Rights gave a speech to the 22nd session of the Human Rights Council. He specifically considered forced treatment in psychiatry as torture and/or cruel, inhuman or degrading treatment. He recommended that "States should impose an absolute ban on all forced and non-consensual medical interventions against persons with disabilities, including the non-consensual administration of psychosurgery, electro-shock and mind-altering drugs, for both long- and short-term application. The obligation to end forced psychiatric interventions based on grounds of disability is of immediate application and scarce financial resources cannot justify postponement of its implementation....The prohibition of torture is one of the few absolute and non-derogable human rights, a matter of jus cogens, a preemptory norm of customary international law." A group called Alliance Against Torture in Psychiatry called on all state and federal legislators to immediately declare void all special laws that legalize forced psychiatric treatment.

In the United States, the Supreme Court considers involuntary commitment a "massive curtailment of liberty" that requires the protection of due process. Involuntary commitment is not constitutional unless proper procedures and standards of evidence are followed. The standards of evidence are not at the level of "beyond a reasonable doubt," but must be *more* than a preponderance of the evidence. The accused must be found to be dangerous either to himself or to others. According to the Supreme Court, simply being unable to adequately take care of oneself, unless it is a matter of life or death, is not adequate grounds for a finding of dangerousness. If the otherwise non-dangerous person, with the help of family or friends, is capable of surviving safely in freedom, he cannot be confined against his will. In addition to dangerousness, there has to be an additional matter of concern, such as "mental illness." It seems to be generally accepted that, if there is a "less restrictive alternative," it should be chosen over commitment, although the Supreme Court hasn't specifically made that statement.

Minnesota statutes regarding civil commitment, if they were actually to be followed (and they were *not* followed, in the case of Bill), provide a number of safeguards for the person claimed to be in need of psychiatric incarceration. In a typical commitment procedure, a screening team from the county, excluding the petitioner, is supposed to conduct an investigation to include personal interviews with the proposed patient and others who have knowledge of the condition of the proposed patient. The specific alleged conduct must be identified and investigated. Specific reasons for rejecting or recommending alternatives to involuntary placement must be identified and explored. The capacity of the proposed patient to make decisions regarding administration of neuroleptic medication is supposed to be determined as is his likelihood of consenting to administration of the medication.

The court may order the patient taken to a treatment facility for evaluation, treatment, and, if necessary, confinement, when there has been "a particularized showing by the petitioner that serious physical harm to the proposed patient or others is likely unless the proposed patient is immediately apprehended."

If a petition is filed, the patient has the right to a court-appointed attorney and the right to request a second examiner to be paid for by the county at a rate of compensation fixed by the court. The patient has the right to attend hearings, and the right to oppose the proceeding and to present and contest evidence.

A patient has the right to be represented by counsel at any proceeding governed by the law. This would include any examination by any psychiatrist, psychologist or mental health official. The attorney is expected to prepare for all hearings and be given adequate time to do so. He is required to consult with the person prior to any hearing and be a "vigorous advocate" on the patient's behalf. He is to continue to represent the person throughout any proceedings governed by this statute unless released as counsel by the court.

The petition for commitment is supposed to provide the name and address of the patient's nearest relatives and give the reasons for the petition. It must contain factual descriptions in behavioral terms, excluding judgmental or conclusory statements, of the proposed patient's recent behavior, including a description of where it occurred, and the time period over which it occurred. Each factual allegation is supposed to be supported by observations of witnesses who are to be named in the petition.

All of these safeguards are expensive and time consuming, however, so a cheap short-cut second route by which a patient may be committed was created via the emergency hold or so-called "72 hour hold." (In California, about 60% of involuntary commitments occur by means of these emergency detentions). According to statute, any person may be admitted or held for emergency care and treatment in a treatment facility with the consent of the head of the treatment facility upon a written statement by an examiner who is knowledgeable, trained, and practicing in the diagnosis and treatment of mental illness. He must be of the opinion that the person is mentally ill, developmentally disabled, or chemically dependent, and is in danger of causing injury to self or others if not immediately detained. The patient has to have been examined not more than 15 days prior to admission and *it must not be possible to obtain a court order in time to prevent the anticipated injury*, i. e., the anticipated injury is "imminent." The statement is supposed to be made in behavioral terms and not in conclusory language, and it must be sufficiently specific to provide an adequate record for review. It should include direct observations of patient behaviors, reliable information about recent and past behavior, psychiatric history, past treatment and any current mental health providers. If danger is alleged to be toward specific individuals, the statement must identify those individuals.

Often the emergency hold is used when there is no actual emergency, thereby sidestepping the judicial process and depriving the person of rights that would otherwise be due him. This was true in Bill's case – there was no "imminent danger" either to himself or to others. The Northfield doctor simply did not like the fact that Mr. Tollefson did not take his medication as a doctor had ordered and took his statement about consultation with God (praying) as a presumptive indicator of psychosis. If he was concerned about Bill harming someone, he was required to specify who those persons were and he did not. If he was concerned about Bill's physical health, he should have examined and treated his legs, which was the presumptive reason for him being brought to the hospital in the first place. He did not do that either.

While being held, the person may be pacified using anti-psychotic medication and his behavior when so affected can be used in subsequent court procedures against him. Likewise, if he was brought in by police, their reports can become part of the patient's medical record. Also during these 72 hours, the person may be coerced into signing himself in voluntarily in order to avoid the threat and stigma of involuntary commitment, thereby giving him the illusion that he is in the hospital by his own volition and able to walk away whenever he chooses. If he tries to do so, however, he is likely to be involuntarily committed by his doctor and relatives. So the "voluntary admission" is really just a sham.

Individuals have been confined in hospitals for years as a result of the commitment process. If they do get out, it may be a conditional release where their guardians determine where they live, how much of their own money they are allowed to have, and what treatments they must accept. If the person objects, they can send him back to the hospital. (In California there were over 22,000 guardianships from 1990 to 1991).

At the time of admission, the patient must be informed in writing of the right to leave after 72 hours, the right to a medical examination within 48 hours, and the right to request a change to voluntary status (providing the head of the treatment facility agrees). If the person requests it, the treatment facility shall assist him in exercising these rights. Bill was not informed of any of these rights.

Minnesota statutes also specify certain rights that patients are, in theory, supposed to enjoy. Restraints are not to be used unless the head of a treatment facility, staff or a licensed police officer determine they are necessary for the safety of the patient or others. If they are used, the reason for so doing must be made part of the clinical record and signed by the head of the facility. "Administrative restriction," which includes separate and secure housing ("solitary confinement") can't legitimately be used for staff convenience, retaliation or as a substitute for actual treatment and must not include any further deprivation of privileges than is necessary. If the patient is placed on administrative restriction, his attorney must be notified within 24 hours.

A patient has the right to receive visitors, correspond freely without censorship and make phone calls. Any limitation on phone calls or visitation must be justified and made a part of the clinical record. The patient has the right to practice his religion and to meet with or call a personal physician, spiritual advisor or legal counselor at all reasonable times. All of these rights were interfered with at one time or another in Bill's confinement.

The patient has the right to periodic medical assessment and continuing care and the right to prior consent to any medical or surgical treatment, but not for non-intrusive mental illness treatment. For intrusive treatment for mental illness (electroshock and neuroleptic medications), a competent voluntary patient must give his written informed consent. Otherwise, neuroleptic medication may only be given if there is an emergency ("... necessary to prevent serious, immediate physical harm to the patient or to others.") lasting up to 14 days; if there is a court order in which it is determined that the patient is not aware of his situation (including reasons for hospitalization), understands the possible benefits and risks of taking and possible consequences of refusing neuroleptic medications, and understands the alternatives to such medications; or if the patient can communicate a clear, reasoned choice that is not based on delusion. *"Disagreement with a physician's recommendation is not evidence of an unreasonable decision."*

Coercive drugging requires a specific court order in Minnesota but the degree to which the judge evaluates the evidence (or is capable of doing so) is questionable. He is likely to just defer to the doctor who recommends it and, as in Bill's case, the patient is allowed to suffer the consequences. In Alaska the State Supreme Court considers forced medication to be just as intrusive as lobotomy and electroshock treatment. Human rights activists around the globe regard forced drugging as a violation of the prohibition against torture and some think it should be prosecuted as a hate crime. In any event, the coercive environment in which the drug is administered can traumatize the patient and, paradoxically, have the opposite of the desired effect.

A patient has the right to receive proper care and treatment aimed at making further supervision unnecessary, i. e., the objective of treatment is supposed to be improvement in functioning such that the person can reenter society. The facility must devise a written "program plan" which describes in behavioral terms the case problems, specific goals, expected duration of treatment and actions to be taken to effect the goals. The program is supposed to be reviewed and modified with the patient, if necessary, at least quarterly and recorded in the clinical record. If neither the agency nor the patient participate in the review, the reasons must be stated in the clinical record. The patient's rights may be exercised on his behalf by a legally authorized health care proxy, agent, or guardian.

These international, national and state bodies all talk a great game on paper. But in Bill's case, nearly all of the high-minded proclamations at all levels were ignored. In fact, it seems to be happening all over the country. Lawrence Stevens, JD commented: "There are a few groups in particular who tend to be the target of America's involuntary psychiatric commitment laws. Included in these are the young, the old, and the homeless. Sometimes old people are placed in mental hospitals just to get them out of the way. In most cases, nursing homes would be more appropriate, but often nursing homes are not preferred by the family because they are more costly and must be paid for by the family. Involuntary psychiatric commitment laws are used to get homeless people off the streets and sidewalks. Adolescents are committed by parents as a way of shifting the balance of power towards parents in intra-family conflicts, parents usually being the ones who have the money to hire psychiatrists to incarcerate their family member adversaries and define their opposing views and disliked behaviors as illnesses."

How is this possible in a democracy presumably governed by laws? Jim Gottstein at Psychrights.org says the judicial process is circumvented in a number of ways. Judges often execute ex parte (one-sided) orders to have people picked up and taken to a hospital without any inquiry as to the validity of allegations or whether it is really an emergency that justifies incarceration. Due process, on the other hand, requires that the accused be given adequate notice of the factual basis of claims made against him and opportunity to tell his or her side of the story before an impartial decision maker. If he is not, it becomes a case of "ambush litigation" that was, in theory at least, eliminated in 1938 by the Federal Rules of Civil Procedure.

As Gottstein says, "Instead of automatically taking a person into custody through the use or display of force when there are concerns about their behavior, someone should go and talk to the person, explain the concerns, and work on de-escalating the situation. Inquiry should be made into what difficulties the person might be experiencing, and, if possible, assistance should be offered." Gottstein cited a doctor he knew who, over the course of 40 years of practice with psychotic patients, attributed his never having had to commit anyone to the fact that he established rapport in his relationships based on trust and respect rather than the use of brute force.

Of course that is not the way it goes down in many, if not most, situations. Instead, the person is handcuffed and/or drugged and carted off to some building occupied by people he does not know that presume he is crazy. He is frightened and thinks people are out to get him but his accusations are interpreted as paranoia, taken as proof of his craziness, and dismissed. Whether he fights to maintain his freedom or just puts up token resistance, he is labeled violent and dangerous, thus justifying his incarceration in a manner reminiscent of a self-fulfilling prophesy.

Although state laws, such as in Minnesota, often require that courts use proper evidentiary standards in presenting information to be used against the defendant, they may also allow for the acceptance of hearsay (something heard from another, which in nearly all other legal proceedings is not accepted as testimony) into the proceedings, thereby abrogating the very safeguard against erroneous deprivations of liberty the law was meant to uphold. This appears to be the case with Bill Tollefson. In fact, there was virtually no attempt to obtain valid information from friends and acquaintances and there was an actual attempt to exclude those sources of information. Proper distinctions between true evidence and hearsay may not be maintained once the accusations are accepted as part of the court record, so that hearsay then ends up carrying as much weight as observed behavior.

Another type of evidence allowed into the proceedings is expert testimony. Professionals recognized as "experts" in some field can present either scientific findings (e. g., the results of empirical studies assessing the effectiveness of different drugs or modes of treatment) or findings based on the personal experience of the professional (e. g., clinical experience of a psychiatrist). Scientific evidence, the ideal of objective knowledge, is regarded as yielding unbiased and impersonal results (although even that has been questioned more and more in recent years). Expert testimony based on personal experience is considered "opinion" or "clinical judgment" and can vary widely from one professional to another, depending upon their training, intelligence, years of experience, range of patients of different types and any number of other factors. Unfortunately, a psychiatrist may be considered an expert in both types of evidence even though he may not be qualified to be so regarded. In fact, he may provide a "top of the head" opinion about an individual without being able to distinguish extreme values on normal personality dimensions from actual behavioral disorders. His experience may have all been with people in psychiatric institutions or settings and he may never have studied the wide range of behaviors that fall under the "normal" heading. He may confuse a super-enthusiastic extraverted intuitive type with a person with bipolar disorder simply because both can generate a host of ideas in a short period of time.

Clinical judgment has been the subject of scientific inquiry for many years. With respect to judgments about "dangerousness," which is usually required in a commitment hearing, the majority of studies indicate that psychiatrists and other mental health professionals are no better than the average man or woman in the street. In fact, their predictions are no better than chance and they are biased to predict violence when such behavior does not appear. The American Psychiatric Association has itself claimed that "the professional literature uniformly establishes that such predictions are fundamentally of very low reliability." They made this argument to the Supreme Court in self-defense because their members were under threat of being sued in cases where patients committed suicide or violent acts.

In 1973 psychologist David Rosenhan performed an experiment that eerily anticipated the fate of Bill Tollefson some 37 years later. Rosenhan had eight normal persons - a psychology graduate student in his twenties, three psychologists, a pediatrician, a psychiatrist, a painter and a housewife - each present themselves for admission at a psychiatric hospital. The twelve hospitals were in five different states and included public hospitals in rural areas, well-regarded university-run hospitals and one expensive private hospital. The pseudo-patients disguised their occupations and used false names but reported other aspects of their histories accurately. Each reported just one symptom: hearing an unclear voice of someone of their same sex saying the words "empty," "hollow," or "thud" and nothing else. They claimed to have no other psychiatric symptoms and acted friendly and cooperative if admitted.

All of the pseudo-patients were admitted to the twelve hospitals. At eleven hospitals the patient was diagnosed as schizophrenic and the remaining patient was diagnosed as suffering from manic-depression. They were kept in the hospitals from seven to 52 days and were discharged with their original diagnosis and the tag line "in remission." Rosenhan regarded that as evidence that hospital staff thought of mental illness as an irreversible lifelong condition and stigma. Although none of the hospital staff recognized any of the pseudo-patients as impostors, 30 percent of the true psychiatric patients expressed an opinion that the pseudo-patients were sane and possibly journalists or researchers, apparently due to their frequent note taking (which staff regarded as "pathological writing behavior").

The pseudo-patients were not given a "get out of jail free card" although an attorney was retained in case it looked like the person would never be released. The phony patients were supposed to get out of the hospital by convincing the hospital to release them. But the only way that

94

happened was if they agreed with the psychiatrist's diagnosis that they were mentally ill and if they agreed to take neuroleptic medications. They actually flushed the medications down the toilet without being detected by staff.

All of the pseudo-patients felt dehumanized when even apparently well-meaning staff engaged in extended discussions of them in their presence as if they were not there and avoided any but the most trivial direct interaction. Their possessions were searched without their permission and their privacy was invaded by observing them using the toilet. There were some incidents of verbal and physical abuse by some staff when they could not be observed by their colleagues. The average time that pseudo-patients had contact with their doctors was 6.8 minutes per day.

I remember when news of this study first began to circulate. Hospital administrators all over the country were afraid of getting embarrassed by falsely admitting fake patients. Those who were on the front line of the patient stream were warned to be watchful for any "ringers." One famous research and teaching hospital, full of academic hubris, challenged Rosenhan to see if he could get any of his pseudo-patients past their gatekeepers. Rosenhan agreed to send at least one pseudo-patient to the facility during a three month period providing the staff would rate every incoming patient as to whether they were an impostor, a suspected impostor, or a genuine patient. Actually, Rosenhan sent no false patients, yet 44% of 193 patients were considered to be either impostors or suspected imposters. Obviously, the validity of the diagnostic process was severely limited.

Reliability of psychiatric diagnosis is a limiting condition for the validity of any kind of diagnostic system and assessment procedure and has been widely recognized to be a problem ever since World War II. Most studies from then until the publication of the Third Edition of the *Diagnostic and Statistical Manual of Mental Disorders* (DSM III) in 1980 found agreement rates between different psychiatrists judging the same patients to be in the 50% range. A study of the stability of diagnoses over a four year period with the same cohort of patients in the 1990s in the United Arab Emirates found that concordance rates varied from one diagnosis to another. With schizophrenia it was 74% while with the neuroses it was only 38%.

The DSM-III departed from earlier diagnostic systems in that it included relatively detailed, explicit criteria for many psychiatric disorders derived from structured interviews and operational criteria that had been previously used in research projects. Nevertheless, one group of researchers claimed that data from the field trials used in developing DSM-III, if analyzed carefully, did not show what the authors of the manual said it showed. According to their analysis, the reliability of psychiatric diagnosis was no better than with the earlier version and possibly worse.

In the diagnosis of psychosis, one of the "gold standard" criteria used to be the presence of hallucinations, the auditory type being the most frequent, e. g., "hearing voices". (Note that in the Rosehan study, above, all of the pseudo patients reported just this one symptom and were diagnosed with schizophrenia). However, a 1983 study of 375 college students revealed that 70% of them admitted to hearing voices at least once in their lives. Forty percent reported hallucinations when waking or just before falling asleep. And a 1991 study by the National Institute of Mental Health found that five percent of 15,000 Americans who had experienced auditory hallucinations, heard them for a complete year, but only one-third of these respondents met the criteria for a psychiatric diagnosis.

Hallucinations are now frequently studied in the context of the broader phenomena of "source monitoring." The idea is that we ordinarily attach a "tag" to incoming information indicating where it came from but, at times, either storing or retrieving this tag somehow goes awry and we mistake, for example, something we just thought from something we actually said or heard. Experimental psychologists are beginning to tease out some of the variables that control when the mis-attribution occurs. The point is, however, that even dramatic "symptoms" can occur frequently in the population of normal people.

In empirical studies, the reliability of psychiatric diagnoses using DSM-III and its successors DSM-IV and DSM-5 seem to have improved because of better research design, less ambiguous criteria, and the use of structured interviews in assessment. However, the same cannot be said for its use by everyday practicing clinicians. Diagnoses for clinicians who are not engaged in a research project can vary for a lot of different reasons, some due to patient characteristics, some due to clinician characteristics and some due to indeterminate aspects of the diagnostic system itself.

Some patients may not be able to report information about themselves accurately due to cognitive impairments like poor concentration or memory defects while others may have disorganized thoughts, be fearful or wish to deny certain unpleasant facts. Still others may withhold certain information because of shame, concern about possible legal consequences, or the desire to avoid particular treatments. It has been said that most patients do not fit the classic psychiatric diagnoses for one reason or another and thus requiring the clinician to select only one category may contribute to diagnostic unreliability. (This may be more a limitation of the diagnostic system, however, than a problem with the patient's "atypical presentation"). If the clinician has to rely on someone else, such as a family member, to provide information, that person may have a personal interest in minimizing or exaggerating what he reports. The quality of the information he or she reports is also dependent upon the degree and nature of contact with the identified or proposed patient.

Clinicians differ in training, experience and theoretical orientation so that some of them overuse a particular diagnosis, e. g., a biological psychiatrist explains a symptom as due to a "chemical imbalance" while a dynamic psychiatrist explains the same symptom as due to a childhood trauma. It is a case of "When you have a hammer in your hand, everything looks like a nail." Most clinicians do not use a structured interview and focus, in their low-reliability routine interview, on the most pressing problem behavior that brought the patient to their attention, to the neglect of other symptoms that might implicate a different kind of disorder. The use of the routine interview in assessing such areas as dementia or intellectual impairment is particularly prone to error, as was the case with Bill. If clinicians have a heavy workload and are pushed for time, they are disinclined to do a very comprehensive assessment or give diagnoses for all of the conditions a patient might have.

Some clinicians choose a diagnosis because it is reimbursable by insurance or Medicare, Medicaid or CHIPS. Institutions may provide incentives or put pressure on clinicians to diagnose so that reimbursement rates are maximized. To say that a patient is feeling blue or is disposed to being moody or high strung will not earn the clinician or the institution a plugged nickel. The magic words to unlocking the coffers of insurance companies or of government benefits are in the DSM: change those words to *Adjustment Disorder with Depressed Mood*, *Bipolar Disorder* and *Anxiety Disorder*. All mental health professionals have to list the diagnostic code number in the DSM along with the diagnostic category on claim forms in order to get paid.

The clinician may just want to be helpful to the patient by providing a diagnosis that will provide needed benefits. This was the case back in the 1960s when I was in my internship. Staff members often told us that they gave a diagnosis such as schizophrenia in order to allow a patient to obtain VA benefits and enable their transition to non-hospital life. (Of course, some patients either feigned symptoms or denied symptoms in order to either get out of or stay in the hospital, depending upon their particular motives. It was a two-way street).

The inadequacy of the psychiatric nomenclature itself was the reason for diagnostic unreliability in 62.5% of cases in one study conducted in 1962. Diagnostic criteria are still stated in a quite vague verbal manner that is difficult to translate into specifics in particular cases. However, a survey of 28 clinicians in 2007 found that 63% of the causes for diagnostic errors were attributed to clinician factors and only 15% of the reasons cited were for problems with the diagnostic nosology, while 22% were attributed to patient factors. In any event, there are plenty of reasons to doubt the reliability of psychiatric diagnoses, even in the day of the DSM-IV or DSM-5.

The authors of the DSM themselves say that the manual should not be used for forensic purposes. Nevertheless, judges, attorneys and social workers, often out of ignorance of the subject matter and methods, are intimidated by psychiatric nomenclature and treat the abstract concepts of the DSM as if they were real things – an error of *reification*.

The mental health care system provides many opportunities for unscrupulous providers. In 2004, the U.S. Defense Criminal Investigative Service (DCIS) issued a report stating:

"The DCIS has found an increase in fraud in the delivery of mental health services, including those provided by hospitals, clinics and private practitioners. A review of recently completed and ongoing investigations suggests that psychiatric and psychological services are vulnerable to abuse, particularly in the following areas: billing for 'phantom' psychotherapy sessions; billing for excessively long hospital stays for inpatient psychiatric care; providing kickbacks to physicians; and grossly inflating the number of psychotherapy hours provided to obtain thousands of dollars in over-payments from government and private insurance programs."

Texas State Senator Mike Moncrief testified: "…We have uncovered some of the most elaborate, creative, deceptive, immoral, and illegal schemes being used to fill empty hospital beds. ... This is not just unreasonable. It is outrageous. And it is fraudulent."

Criminal charges against psychiatrists and hospital directors ensued, continuing up to the present time. One conviction resulted in psychiatrist Robert Hadley Gross beginning a one-year jail sentence in April 2004 for billing patient services he never delivered, and for accepting $860,000 in patient referral "kickbacks" in the early 1990s.

The scandal caused a domino effect in the United States with numerous other private for-profit psychiatric hospitals paying tens of millions in refunds, penalties and settlements. In 2000, the U.S. Justice

Department investigated the private psychiatric hospital chain Charter Behavioral Systems, Inc. for fraud and abuse. That year, the company agreed to pay the government $7 million to settle allegations regarding overcharging Medicare insurance and other federal programs. One of my psychologist friends who practiced in Albuquerque during the 1980s and 1990s told me that the Charter Hospital there was paying a finder's "head fee" for patient referrals. A school social worker in that city told me that the hospital recruited kids for their adolescent unit and then bled the family's insurance companies until the limits of coverage ran out, after which they would discharge the kids to the streets.

In May 2004, New York psychiatrist David Roemer was sentenced after pleading guilty to a charge of felony conspiracy in a prescription drug scam that defrauded the government's insurance scheme and flooded the streets with millions of dollars in highly addictive narcotics and other drugs, including the tranquilizer Xanax. Roemer worked with four accomplices who recruited Medicaid insurance recipients from the streets and drug treatment centers. On the ride to Roemer's office, the recruits were given money and told what drugs to ask for. Roemer then "sold" them the prescriptions, which they took to pharmacies and filled using their Medicaid benefits. The pills were handed back over to the recruiters who sold them on the black market. Roemer was sentenced to 10 1/2 years in prison and ordered to pay more than $340,000 in restitution to the Medicaid program.

In 2003, financial audits discovered that Kedren Community Mental Health Center in California had misspent $1.4 million in funds, including paying for its president's Land Rover vehicle and Cadillac, and for some employees' theater tickets and trips to Las Vegas, New Orleans, Georgia, Washington, D.C. and London.

In 1990, a U.S. Congressional committee issued a report estimating that Community Mental Health Centers (CMHCs) had diverted between $40 million to $100 million to improper uses. Various CMHCs had built tennis courts and swimming pools with their federal construction grants and, in one instance, used a federal staff grant to hire a lifeguard and swimming instructor.

The misuse of funds continued despite the congressional report. In September 1998, Medicare barred 80 CMHCs in nine states from serving the elderly and disabled after investigators found patients had been charged $600 to $700 a day for watching television and playing bingo, rather than receiving any care. In New Mexico in 2013 the governor halted payment of federal funds to many mental health providers in the state claiming they had filed millions of dollars in fraudulent claims. The attorney general would not release the details of the investigation, however, so it is impossible at this time to ascertain whether the charges are true or if it was just a ruse to make a political payback to corporate supporters in Arizona (who subsequently took over the facilities).

Public Citizen reported that in the last two decades drug companies have paid out nearly $20 billion in False Claims Act penalties and most of those occurred from 2006 to 2011. *BMJ*, in an article published on 18 December, 2013, reported that civil and criminal penalties paid to federal and state governments by pharmaceutical companies from January 1999 to July 2012 amounted to $30.2 billion. More than half of that amount was for either illegal promotion of drugs or illegal overcharging of government programs for drugs. The author said that having companies sign corporate integrity agreements (CIAs) for five years would be a deterrent only if the size of the penalties was greater than the companies gains while violating the law and only if the CIAs were enforced, neither of which conditions currently obtain.

Pfizer paid $2 billion for illegal marketing of their painkiller Bextra and now has RICO (Racketeering Influenced Criminal Organization) status. Eli Lilly, Glaxo-Smith-Kline and Schering-Plough forked over $10.5 billion in fines over the last 20 years. Medicaid was overcharged by as much as 12 times the cost of a drug in some state programs. The drug companies appear to just regard the fines as a "cost of doing business."

Psychiatry was not always the way it is today. When I was in graduate school back in the 1960s, one of my clinical mentors was a past president of the American Psychiatric Association. Looking a lot like Charlton Heston with a mustache, he was a fantastic instructor and compassionate human being with the rough hewn demeanor of a WWII army neuropsychiatrist. I remember one time, after returning from our "traveling clinic" to Bisbee, Arizona, when we were drinking Scotch and reviewing cases at his house. He said that he had been approached by a drug company a short time before to give his advice about them developing a drug that would reduce anxiety. He told them that he thought it would never sell because it would do away with a patient's motivation to improve. He laughed at his naiveté when he confessed that a competing drug company had subsequently made a bundle on their anti-anxiety medication while his name had become Mudd with the company that sought his advice.

Psychiatrists in those days were dynamicists. They knew the disorders that were then considered to be due to some kind of organic pathology, but they also knew something about human nature and psychodynamics.

Many of them were trained in psychoanalysis or in the social psychiatry of Adolf Meyer and other neo-Freudians. For them, the life history of the individual, environment and social factors were the most significant elements in the etiology of mental illness and drugs were merely an adjunct to psychotherapy. This was before psychiatry "returned to its roots" in biology.

I was working in the psychiatry department of a medical school when this transformation began to take place. The first chairman of the department was a classically trained psychoanalyst, although he did not practice or teach in the classical manner. He was more eclectic and social-psychologically oriented and placed psychologists and social workers, along with psychiatrists, in major positions in the department. One of his popular courses among psychiatric residents was based on the study of classic works of fiction.

After his departure from the department, there was an 18 month delay before the acting director was finally confirmed as chairman. The new chairman believed he saw the writing on the wall: psychiatry had to change if it was to bring anything unique to the treatment of mental disorders. With power in his hands, he reclaimed for psychiatrists as many of the critical departmental positions as he could. Education became more medically and pharmaceutically oriented and psychotherapy was de-emphasized. Several years later, I learned from one of my former psychologist colleagues that psychiatric residents were actually surreptitiously seeking him out in private practice in order to learn how to do psychotherapy.

Dr. Nathaniel S. Lehrman, a psychiatrist who started his work in the post-WWII years, has criticized current-day psychiatry in an interview titled *Psychiatry: 60 years in an increasingly corrupt specialty*. This followed a paper he read in Israel in 1984 because he could not find anywhere in the United States to present it. It was titled *The Prostitution of Psychiatry: 1930's Germany, 1980's America*. It is Lehrman's view that:

"Over the past fifty years, this primary treatment role in psychiatry [the patient-doctor relationship] has gradually been taken over by medication – first for psychotics and now for everyone else with psychological symptoms, both grave and trivial. The result has been horrendous... The specialty can indeed help many troubled people – both the disabled and the merely distressed – by examining and helping to correct their attitudes, relationships and behavior, as I've done for years. But when pill-pushing eclipses examining a patient's life problems, the situations often worsen."

101

Dr. Joanna Moncrieff, a London psychiatrist and author of *The Myth of the Chemical Cure: A Critique of Psychiatric Drug Treatment* (2009) expresses similar sentiments and exposes the vested interests of psychiatry, pharmaceutical companies and politics in maintaining a dangerous fraud.

The pharmaceutical industry is the most profitable industry in the world and psychiatric drugs generate some gigantic revenue. The active ingredient in the popular antidepressant Prozac, for example, costs 11 cents for 100 tablets while it is sold to customers for $247.47 (a 2250% profit). The corresponding cost for Xanax, an anti-anxiety potion, is 2.4 cents for 100 tablets while the cost to consumers is $136.79 (for a whopping 5700% profit). And this for drugs that are likely to be of modest benefit at best. Irving Kirsh obtained 42 clinical drug trials submitted to the FDA from 1987 to 1999 using a freedom of information request. He found that the majority of trials for drugs like Prozac, Paxil, Zoloft, and other selective serotonin reuptake inhibitors - SSRIs) showed no improvement in the patients' conditions compared to placebos.

The drug industry pays for 40% of TV advertising in the U.S. and it is the largest contributor to political campaigns. According to Dr. Marcia Angell, psychiatrists receive more money from the drug companies than any other medical specialty. They also keep lengthening the list of diagnoses for which drug companies can create new drugs. And these definers of the new categories themselves have financial interests in the industry: 56% of the members of the working groups doing research for the new DSM-5 had such interests. Lab fellows from Harvard's Edmond J. Safra Center for Ethics have compiled 16 articles dealing with Big Pharma corruption in five areas: systemic problems, medical research, medical knowledge and practice, marketing, and patient advocacy organizations (such as NAMI). The articles are now online and will appear in *The Journal of Law, Medicine & Ethics*.

Dr. Lehrman believes psychiatric drugs are dangerous, increasing suicidal risk and injuring brain and endocrine systems. He uses them only for short periods, when a patient is acutely upset, and gradually weans him or her from the medication while using psychotherapy to work on the individual's goals. He sums up by saying:

"Psychiatry, a formerly-honest medical specialty, which tried to help patients with the problems causing their symptoms, is now dedicated almost entirely to drugging them for their symptoms and ignoring their problems. One result has been a five-fold increase, since the introduction of these drugs fifty years ago, in psychiatric disability, as measured by Social Security disability statistics. In the mid-1800's,

Dr. Ignaz Semmelweis recognized how physicians produced childbirth fever in the women they delivered – for failing to wash their hands. Psychiatry's current focus on symptoms and drugs, while ignoring problems and 'side-effects,' is causing similar harm to those it treats."

Sometimes the court subverts the cause of justice by failing to truly embrace the adversary system. This system includes a "vigorous defense" that contains thorough cross-examination, presentation of contradictory evidence, and careful instruction on the duty of proving a particular position, a failure in the performance of which duty calls for judgment against the party on whom the duty is imposed. The court-appointed defense attorney or public defender, who has little financial incentive for mounting a strenuous defense, may assume his client is guilty of the behavior claimed by the prosecutor and present a perfunctory defense, calling few if any witnesses and asking few probing or challenging questions of the witnesses, social service personnel or expert witnesses standing for the prosecution. This is exactly what happened with Bill Tollefson.

Gottstein believes the defense counsel should understand the legal processes of involuntary commitment but also the alternative options for care that are less restrictive than incarceration. He should conduct an initial investigation in which he acquires the accused's medical history, relationship to his family and friends and to current and past medical professionals. He should interview his client early enough to permit adequate preparation, not show up just as he is going into the court room. He should have available an independent expert witness, a second professional opinion chosen by the defendant or his representative, for the initial commitment hearing. The defense attorney should have family, friends and employers available to testify as to specific facts in the case. He should remind his client that he does not need to waive his right to remain silent in any hospital interview by a psychiatrist. He should inform his client that he is there to be an advocate for the client's interests, perspective and wishes. And he should remind himself that he is not empowered to decide what he thinks is best for the person he represents but to "vigorously argue to the best of his or her ability for the ends desired by the client." Bill's two lawyers failed in all of these ways.

Although all members of the court are charged with the responsibility of seeking justice, they may engage in a "silent conspiracy," where none of them raise questions about the patient's rights even though they know they are being ignored or disregarded. Thus, in the case of Bill Tollefson, he was never asked if he wanted a second opinion by a physician of his

103

own choosing and the question of an appeal was ignored, including by his own attorney when he was specifically asked about it. The court may accept dishonest or distorted testimony, condescendingly thinking that "it is for the person's own good." The standards of evidence may be ignored even if they are specified in state law. In Bill's case, rumor, innuendo and hearsay unattached to any specified observer were contained in the prepetition report and not even questioned by his attorney.

According to Jim Gottstein, "This combination . . . helps define a system in which (1) dishonest testimony is often regularly (and unthinkingly) accepted; (2) statutory and case law standards are frequently subverted; and (3) insurmountable barriers are raised to insure that the allegedly 'therapeutically correct' social end is met . . . . In short, the mental disability law system often deprives individuals of liberty disingenuously and upon bases that have no relationship to case law or to statutes." He believes that the judicial system is most dysfunctional in the adequacy of legal representation for defendants in psychiatric proceedings. It is the ethical responsibility of the person's lawyer to vigorously represent his or her civil and human rights.

Unfortunately, people such as Margaret Koch-Nabialczynk ("Justice: An impossible Dream" at www.tulanelink.com/tulanelink/impossibledream-04a.htm) who have looked into what others have had to say about unethical lawyers have found "no good news there." As the author says, many books have been written about the inadequacies of the law and lawyers: *Jurismania: the Madness of American Law* (Paul F. Campos); *Law Against the People: Essays to Demystify Law, Order, and the Courts* (Robert Lefcourt); *Verdicts on Lawyers* (Ralph Nader and Mark Green); *Injustice for All: How Our Adversary System of Law Victimizes Us and Subverts True Justice* (Anne Strick); *Crisis at the Bar: Lawyers Unethical Ethics and What to Do about It* (J. K. Lieberman); *Lawyers on Trial* (Philip Stern); *With Justice for None: Destroying an American Myth* (Gerry L. Spence).

In his *The Lost Lawyer: Failing Ideals of the Legal Profession* Anthony K. Kronman said, "Every year produces a fresh crop of scoundrels and renewed doubts about the ability of the profession to police itself, along with familiar complaints about the undue power of lawyers (which any democratic society is bound to regard with suspicion)."

Mary Ann Glendon, a Harvard professor of Law stated that "a significant advance of arrogance, unruliness, greed and cynicism in the legal profession is of more concern than similar developments [in other professions]." And Robert Bork remarked, "Men and women given unaccountable power will often use it to further their own ends, not ends of the polity which they exist to serve....Our courts are behaving badly and the public, to the degree it can be brought to understand that, will exact force for reform that must be structural as well as intellectual and moral....[lawyers] become cynically accepting of a system they do not admire but have learned how to work, or at least live, with."

Forty some years of academic tomes decrying the sad state of the legal profession has resulted in substantially no change. According to Richard Zitrin and Carol M. Langford in *The Moral Compass of the American Lawyer: Truth, Justice, Power and Greed*, "These are perilous times for Americans who need access to the legal system. Too many lawyers blatantly abuse power and trust, and engage in reckless ethical misconduct, grossly unjust billing practices and dishonesty disguised as client protection."

Gottstein and many mental health professionals think that most people who are claimed to have a psychiatric disorder are not being confined in institutions because they are in fact dangerous or grossly disabled. Rather, it is because people dislike their behavior or lifestyles, because they are bothering their relatives or others, or because it is an expedient way to get them off the streets "for their own good." Alternatives to drug treatment are ignored because it is cheaper (depending upon your method of accounting and the time period over which it is applied) for a hospital to hire a psychiatrist with a prescription pad than to employ all the psychologists, social workers, nurses, occupational therapists and vocational counselors it might really take to treat a cohort of patients adequately. Except for his one month of forced drugging (which can be considered torture by UN standards), Bill Tollefson received virtually no treatment while he was in the hospital.

7 <u>FREEDOM ON A LEASH</u>

So there sat Bill Tollefson - once the apple of his mother's eye; once a "wild and crazy guy," a frat rat and party animal; once a mortician, businessman and a member of the chamber of commerce; once a skilled fisherman and candidate for the National Freshwater Fishing Hall of Fame; once a proud husband and father; once a benefactor of the poor and homeless who, as a mayoral candidate, wanted to rejuvenate old city buildings for the benefit of the poor and downtrodden – not at all the kind of history one expects in someone claimed to be schizophrenic.

I remembered him as a childhood friend, always jovial, good-natured and ready to try something new. We used to hike out to the woods about a mile behind my house to go squirrel hunting, go out to the old archery field range to hone our skills with bow and arrow, gawk and jawbone with our WWII hero mentor at his gun-smithing shop, ride our bikes down to the lakes on the Carleton College campus to fish where Bill invariably would make a haul of sunfish, crappies or bluegills, or hang out at Tiny's Pool Hall. One time, while swimming in one of those lakes I managed to wear myself out, got leg cramps and was about to sink to the bottom when up comes Bill like a huge barge, asking, "You need some help there Bud?" He provided a supportive hand and quickly got me back to the shallow water where I could stand on the muddy bottom. Always at home in the water, Bill displaced enough fluid by his size so that he could float without moving a muscle and would even fall asleep while floating on his back in the summer sun.

We lost contact for a few years as we went our separate ways after high school. He visited me once when I was in graduate school in Tucson and he was passing through on a trip to California. I saw him sporadically when I would visit our old home town. Bill always had a story to tell about some interesting person or event that occurred in his life. One time he told me stories about his trip to Norway on a tramp freighter, the unusual people he met along the way, and his love affair with a girl he met there. Another time it would be about some gigantic party he and his friends had thrown or about how he crashed his Sun Beam sports car while street racing in Minneapolis.

For the last ten years or so, I would visit him every year when I came to town to visit or bury relatives or attend reunions and for the last couple of years I had maintained regular telephone contact. I knew that he had gone through a couple of marriages, the breakups causing him a lot of anguish and I knew that his career as a fishing guide had been brought to a halt by orthopedic and foot surgeries that had not gone well. But he continued to socialize with friends, rolled himself downtown in his wheelchair to fish off the river bank, would try to help out those he met who were suffering bad economic or emotional times, and continued to try to come up with ideas that he thought might allow him to make money and reduce his dependence on disability payments. In 2004 he decided to make a run for mayor of Northfield, not so much because he thought he could win but to have a forum from which to promote his ideas about what could be done with the old city hospital and the old high school building (use them as centers for youth activities or respites for the homeless) and to resist town governance being totally dominated by the two colleges.

So Bill still had a life – not exactly the one he wanted but still an active engagement with the world of ideas, the community and the future. Yet here he sat in a state hospital over 50 miles from his friends, his butt sore from an inadequate cushion in his wheelchair, his shoulders paining him from an injury caused by an improper method used to transfer him, his legs swollen and hurting from cellulitis and fluid retention due to unavailability of his aquatic therapy, harangued by a nurse for failing to get up on time even though his clock had been stolen, made fun of by his doctor and treatment team as being delusional, paranoid or in denial, his home of ten years lost due to a scheming landlord, his possessions stored in some unknown location, his income confiscated by court-appointed guardians. What a fix!

Bill felt he was going into a physical tailspin and his friends seemed to sense the danger. Louise said, "I'm afraid that it may be a matter of time now for the end for Bill."

Big Jim expressed his dismay that, "Our friend is literally falling apart and we can't seem to countermand the kangaroo court's decision or hire a mouthpiece who has the balls to fight these bastards. Bill has been a friend to so many, I can't even estimate the totals, but none of us has the wherewithal to enter into the battle."

Bill's youngest sister, who lives on the west coast, told me that the two of them have similar kinds of bodies and both have chronic bone spurring in the back. She also said they have similar kinds of temperament - both being socially outgoing and needing people around them to maintain their normally upbeat attitudes.

Jake suggested that a hyperbaric chamber might be helpful to Bill. He said his friend's brother, who has a fluid retention problem similar to Bill's, had stopped going to Mayo Clinic because they didn't have pressure cuffs large enough for his feet and legs. Instead, he found a place in his home town that had a hyperbaric chamber that could hold up to eight people at a time and could raise the ambient pressure while also raising the oxygen level to 25 percent. "The higher pressure sort of squishes the fluid out of the legs and feet. One and a half atmospheres is like being at about 10 feet under water. In fact, I bet one of the reasons Bill got much relief in the pool may have been the increased pressure on his feet. Too bad he's not 10 feet tall and could stand in the deep end."

Bill and I had talked about the possibility of his getting treatment for his chronic infections in a hyperbaric chamber prior to his ill-fated trip to Florida. The theory was that treatment with antibiotics at an elevated pressure would force the drug into bodily spaces with restricted blood flow, where the bacteria could hide, that did not occur at ordinary atmospheric pressures. At that time, his physicians were talking about surgeries to replace his artificial hip and knee joints. The very expensive surgeries would require that Bill be laid up for a year, mostly in bed and, of course, subject him to the risks associated with any surgery and long-term care. He had checked with Mayo Clinic but the gatekeepers to the hyperbaric chamber there vetoed his request. He checked with Hennepin County Medical Center, which also operates a hyperbaric chamber, and the chances for admission appeared greater. But then the opportunity to return to his beloved fishing grounds in Florida beckoned, and he took the chance.

Brian Landers notified Bill that, after his landlord managed to manipulate the court into effectively evicting Bill, he could no longer represent him because his was a non-profit legal clinic that received federal funds and he was not allowed to sue anyone for money. He did, however, send information to the lawyer who represented Bill in the guardianship action, telling him how Bill could file for civil damages since HUD regulations had been violated. One of Bill's friends, Sandy, suggested contacting the American Center for Law and Justice. I checked them out on the Internet and discovered they do not represent individuals and only deal with matters of constitutional law.

Patients on the ward where Bill was housed had two telephones but one of them was never answered. I called the only number where I had ever received an answer. It rang about 100 times before I gave up. Eventually Bill called me and asked for me to call him back at the number I had just called. I did so and it again rang many times. Finally, Bill picked up the phone after hearing no rings and knowing I was going to call him right back. He checked around the phone wires and found that someone had turned off the ringer. Since there was no incentive for patients to turn off the phone, I suspected some staff member had done so in order to keep from having what they considered an unnecessary added duty, answering the patient phone.

Bill told me he was scheduled to take a look at a place in St. Paul on Monday for a possible placement. The social worker told him that she knew of someone who lived there who had been taken to the Courage Center for treatment. Bill thought that getting out of Anoka was the only way he was going to save his life and he was really desperate to do so.

Unless it is a real dump, I thought, he'll probably take it. If he does get out and is able to get to the Courage Center, it is probably the only way he is ever going to get back into condition to direct his own life. And if he is able to get stronger, both physically and emotionally, he might be better able to fight this corrupt system that ran him into the ground. If he stays there in Anoka, it will kill him.

Of course, Bill would still be under the control of his court-appointed guardian and the only way he could rid himself of that burden would be to file a petition for a Restoration of Capacity. Chances of succeeding at that looked fairly dim. It would be up to him to prove that he was sane and able to take care of himself. Jake's lawyer friend in Albert Lea said such a petition is often successful if the claimant says that the hospital cured them of their mental illness. However, if they admit to having mental problems, it can limit any future legal action they might be able to take. And, of course, if they deny they ever had any significant mental problems they must be "in denial."

I wrote to Jake, "I think it is more likely that Bill would say that Anoka gave him Post Traumatic Stress Disorder rather than that they cured him of anything! At least they didn't waterboard him. I expect to hear from him tomorrow after he gets back from his "tour." He was hoping that he could stay at the new residence and never have to go back to Anoka. That probably won't happen. He will have to go through "discharge" procedures, just a little more torture, before they let him go. If he files for Resoration, he should hire his own lawyer and not any of these rummies that the court hires!"

Bill got up early, all psyched up about his trip to a possible residence in St. Paul. When I talked with him afterwards that night he said, "It turned out to be a bummer, Bud, with old folks smoking their brains out and trash laying all over." So it was a "no-go" and he was back in Anoka. The social worker that was working on it was leaving the facility for good in a couple of days so Bill would be starting anew with someone who probably didn't know anything.

In the meantime, he wanted to get back into the water and the closest place to do so was the Courage Center. They have pools in Golden Valley, Burnsville, Coon Rapids, Eden Prairie, Hudson and Stillwater, the last two probably being the closest. I gave them a call the following day to see if they would accept him for treatment. They said he needed a doctor's orders and the facility would have to submit an application. Bill thought he would see if he could get that at Anoka but I doubted that they would be very cooperative.

The next contact I had with Bill was a message he left on my answering machine. "Hey Bud, I'm going outside to have a cigar and a shot of whiskey." He left his new phone number and said he would call again if I didn't catch him.

He sounded upbeat and the remark about "a cigar and a shot of whiskey" was his kind of joke. I thought maybe he had talked himself into the Courage Center as an inpatient. I called his new number. "Bill's phone" his roommate answered. He said Bill was outside but he would give him a message. About 11:30 pm Minnesota time Bill called back. He said he had had a great shower that helped his shoulders and he was feeling good. He did not sound as though he had been drinking. He reported that he was in the Golden Living Center in St. Paul, the place he had inspected on Monday and had found to be wanting. Now he seemed overjoyed to be there.

Bill said that earlier in the day he was surprised when his captors at Anoka told him that he was moving in 1 hour. He asked for some time to pack his things but soon about 15 people came in, pinned him to his chair and dragged him 40 feet down the hallway. He claimed to have witnesses who observed him being abused. I wasn't sure what really had happened and suspected he was leaving something out of his story. I speculated that they had decided to get rid of him, perhaps for financial reasons, perhaps because he was trying to organize the patients and had called the office of the governor with some complaints. Some smart-alec staff member had taunted him as he was being ushered out, "So you think you're some kind of politician, huh?" The inspection of the place on Monday had just been a sham to give him the impression that he had some choice in the matter when, in fact, he had none. They were not straightforward with him, didn't give him time to get used to the idea and ended up using unnecessary force, which he probably resisted.

If there had really been abuse, I could amend my letter to the Joint Commission to include a description of the event and the names of any witnesses since I had an open complaint with them. Both Jake and Big Jim thought the hospital should be held accountable for the manner in which they discharged Bill. I did too. At the least, they could be accused of psychological abuse since they led him to believe that he had some choice in the matter and then told him he had no choice, but there could be even more to it. It might involve actual physical abuse. Of course the fact that they pushed him out with little warning made a farce of their argument that they were "keeping him safe" or that he needed to be there in the first place.

But Bill sounded evasive when I asked for details and said he just wanted to enjoy his first day of freedom. I could understand how he felt after nearly six months of captivity, forced drugging, and humiliation. I decided to bide my time and get a better account of what had happened after the dust had settled. He was happy to be out of Anoka and thought he might be able to get hooked up with the Courage Center as an outpatient. If so, I thought, he might be able to get a free psych evaluation from them, which could help in filing for Restoration of Capacity.

Jake visited Bill in his new digs. "It seemed clean and with no unusual odors. Bill met me in front of the place where they have a good size patio with chairs. It faces mostly east and gets great morning sun. Nice little park just across the street with a small lake and fountain shooting water about 15 feet high. A sidewalk circles the lake. The north side of the building is a grassy area with a picnic table and an open sided cabana. The neighborhood has seen better days but it's not too bad. Tons of big leaf maple trees all around the place. Probably looks really great in the fall. Bill sounded and looked about 1000% better than he has in a long time."

Within days of getting out of Anoka, Bill was, as Jake said, "back to his old self, dreaming and planning for future events." He wanted to go to LaCrosse to visit Big Jim and celebrate his birthday. He had already checked on three possible ways to get there with AMTRACK being the most likely since there was a station only about a mile away.

Bill was always on the lookout for business opportunities, a habit he developed early in life. He liked thinking about the possibilities in a situation - developing a vision of *what could be* and calculating what it would take to bring it about. Thus, he complained about how his new residence was being run and, simultaneously, how he would like to buy it and turn it into a first rate facility. The chances of him actually doing so were next to nil and he knew it, but he enjoyed the mental exercise of figuring out the changes that would be needed and how and from whom he would get financing. I had seen or heard him engage in this kind of activity numerous times over the years. Jake considered it one of Bill's most endearing and fascinating qualities. Of course, mental health professionals unacquainted with the context, history and function of Bill's creative ideation might consider it rather peculiar if they didn't go overboard and jump to the conclusion that it was a sign of madness.

Bill wanted to throw a party for some of his new house mates and planned to buy fifty pounds of shrimp and cocktail sauce for the occasion until Jake advised him that the price of shrimp had gone up considerably since he last had purchased any. He was unable to cash a check because someone had stolen all his IDs in his hospitalizations, so he established a charge account at a nearby fast-food restaurant and treated one of his new friends. Then he fretted about his "name being shit" because he was unable to get rapid access to cash to pay his tab. A loan from Jake took care of the problem.

The biggest plan Bill was working on was marriage to Jackie, a woman he had known for at least 30 years. She was the type of woman who liked the outdoors, camping and fishing. Bill knew her brother, a retired fishing guide, and her son and grandson. Bill and Jackie had shared a number of activities over the years but had never gotten romantically involved. Recently, Bill had proposed marriage to her and she had accepted. I asked when this marriage was supposed to occur and he indicated some time in the indefinite future. I asked him if there was any possibility that Jackie would back out and he said, "Of course, it's always up to the bride - when, where or if."

It didn't sound like he was really counting on a marriage taking place but considered it another "possibility" that he enjoyed fantasizing about. I considered that he might just be trying to figure out some way of getting around the guardianship situation. The prospect, if realized, would make life easier for him in that he would have a residence and a function in life, namely to make her happy. Consistent with other audacious shindigs Bill had organized in the past, he imagined Big Jim and I arriving as dual best men riding a motorcycle with a sidecar. Bill had always liked being a prankster and an entertainer.

While I thought it was fine that Bill was amusing himself with harmless diversions after a long period of stress, I was getting a little perturbed that he wouldn't devote some time to matters that were important in his legal situation. When I tried to get a straight story about what exactly had happened when he was discharged from Anoka, he wouldn't cooperate, even claimed he couldn't hear on his phone when the reception was crystal clear. I explained that we had an open complaint with the Joint Commission that could be added to if he provided the details. He wanted to put it off and enjoy his "freedom" (although he wasn't really free and had only 60 days to appeal the Court ordered "Guardian of the Person and Temporary Conservator of the Estate"). I reminded him of that and also suggested that he might want to ask for a change of venue since, if he presented evidence of dereliction of duty by the Rice County Court, they would not be able to render an objective judgment. He didn't want to hear about it. Previously, when I asked him to go over the allegations in the prepetition report so that charges of making false statements on an official document could be filed with the Attorney General's Office, he also was elusive. And when I asked him to go over his notes about the trial so we could add some more examples of his lawyer's inept representation of him to present to the Minnesota Bar Association, he never got around to it.

It crossed my mind that he might be "playing me" for some reason of which I wasn't aware. That had occurred a couple of times in my career as a psychologist but it was so rare that I thought it unlikely. (Some of my colleagues were so frightened of being taken advantage of that they were hyper-skeptical of anything said by their patients. I figured that such a strategy would interfere with establishing a working relationship and, in any event, I thought that I would be able to survive any chagrin I might experience if a patient ever put one over on me.) More likely, I thought, Bill wanted to maintain some control over the time and way that events unfolded in his life after having been under someone's thumb most of the time during the last six months. Even before he was committed he had never liked to be pushed into anything. During his incarceration I had gained a great deal of respect for his ability to modulate his feeling state and husband his emotional reserves under very trying circumstances, rolling with the punches so as to be able to fight again another day.

During my next phone call with Bill he was spitting bullets. He had been going through his old medications to see what he could use for a "take-along emergency pack" when he would travel and a nurse saw him, grabbed them away from him and ran off down the hall. Then some of the nurses came in and went through the stuff that was brought up from storage the day before by his guardian, scattered it all over his bed and left it there when the clock struck 5:00 and their shift ended. He tried to explain what he was doing and got into a battle with them. They threatened to send him back to Anoka if he didn't go along with what they were telling him. He called the police but they refused to come to his aid.

I told him to make a formal complaint to the manager about the manner in which the nurses conducted the investigation. I told him that it is not unusual for places like that to restrict medications brought in from the outside. In fact, most care facilities are like that. They didn't know if he had drugs with a street value that he was trying to sell or if he was trying to commit suicide with them. They were probably searching the stuff the guardian brought for contraband. He just didn't know the rules and was learning the hard way. However, threatening to send him back to Anoka might be construed as assault if it was an act that would cause him harm. Unfortunately, he had no witnesses to support his version of events and he would be assumed to be the guilty party.

Shortly thereafter Bill had a flare-up of his cellulitis. The nurses had taken all of the medications in his possession and wouldn't give him any that they had available. They called in a contract psychiatrist who presumed his agitation was a sign of his mental illness and told him he had to start taking Abilify again. He refused to take it. Jake reported, "Bill was not a happy camper and while I was on the phone he was shouting and cussing at some nurse in his room. He told me he can't get from his bed to the bathroom without the cellulitis meds."

I looked "cellulitis" up on the Internet and got a good education about it from the "medicinenet" web site. Armed with a little knowledge and uncertain that what Bill was experiencing was really cellulitis, I asked him about his symptoms, but he was not in a mood to listen to anyone. He was trying to throw his weight around (figuratively speaking) and doing his Bombastic Bushkin impersonation, which only made him sound more whacko than actually was the case.

I told Jake, "Well, Bill managed to get himself hauled off to St. Joseph hospital on a 72-hour hold after making a big fuss about the lack of treatment for his cellulitis at the nursing home and refusing to take Abilify prescribed by the shrink. They just thought he was being crazy and non-compliant and decided they didn't want to put up with that shit! When he goes off like this, he just digs himself in deeper!"

I got a phone call from the nurse that was called in to do the admission for Bill at St. Joseph's hospital. She was the first person who sounded at all reasonable in five months of dealing with Bill's caregivers. I gave her information on Bill's chronic problem with cellulitis and his adverse reaction to Abilify. She actually seemed to listen. I told her I had made a complaint to the Joint Commission about the adverse reactions he had to the drug Abilify and that the hospital finally stopped administering it to Bill. I told her I had also made a complaint to the ACLU because there were all sorts of illegalities involved in his incarceration. She was trying to figure out who had the legal rights to make decisions for Bill's health care and was trying to find an email address where I could send my certificates appointing me Bill's Power Of Attorney and listing me as the responsible party for his Advanced Directives. I told her I thought what Bill really needed was for someone to actually listen to him and not blow him off as being some sort of nut. She said they would listen and try to make the best judgment they could. In the meantime she would do some blood tests and figure out how to treat his cellulitis and/or swelling in the legs.

Damn, I thought. Maybe he'll get a legitimate evaluation this time. I was disavowed of that notion by my next call from Bill. They were shooting him full of Abilify again and his speech was slurred after just two shots, one at 1:00 pm and the other at 9:15 pm. Muttering to myself, I said "This is nutso time again!"

I found out the name of the psychiatrist who prescribed Abilify for Bill and wrote her an email explaining that Mr. Tollefson had developed adverse reactions to the drug when it was forcibly administered to him at Anoka. I included a copy of the letter I had sent to the Office of Health Facility Complaints prior to discontinuation of the medication. The email came back as undeliverable from an outside source. I did manage to get it through to a so-called "Patient and Family Advocate" who said she would make it available to the treatment team.

In a few days Bill called and I updated Jake on the current status of our friend. "The latest (as of Wednesday) is that Bill was going to be sent back to the Psych Ward at St. Joseph's. A social worker came in yesterday and gave him a paper saying that his discharge to Golden Living Center was rescinded and that his needs could only be met in a state facility, i. e., he is going to be sent to a state hospital someplace (but maybe not Anoka). He can appeal but he needs a lawyer to do so. I haven't heard anything from him today and don't have a number for him. They did treat his leg and apparently it was cellulitis. They gave him an antibiotic and elevated the leg for a few days and he said he was able to walk down the hall using a walker further than he has been able to in

several years. He said that they had not given him Abilify the last couple
of days. Hospital staff were supposed to get back to me but they haven't
yet and I don't expect they will. Bill said three people told him they were
going to call me but none of them ever did. I think they are all a bunch of
bull-shitters and incompetents!"

The next day Jake sent an email filled with a sense of foreboding, He
had called St. Joseph's Hospital, the nursing home and Anoka and got no
answer at any of them. "I hope ECT isn't in the works here. God only
knows what these clowns might try." He had just read a letter from Anais
Nin to Henry Miller in which Nin said she had gone to Switzerland
"where I am not trying to find sanity but the power to conceal my
madness." Jake thought that was what Bill needed to do when he ran into
medical people but he added, "I've always found his madness to be his
most endearing characteristic – his constant planning for the future with
all sorts of great ideas. If that's madness, then it would be ideal if a lot
more people had it."

I told Jake the new phone numbers where Bill could be reached.
"They are on him like a hawk when he is on the phone - only give him
about 10 minutes. I don't know what they have planned for him but I sent
an email saying I expected to be informed. They'll probably ignore it but
then that is just another complaint to go to TJC." I said I thought of Bill's
madness as "ideational fluency" and gave him the link to The Icarus
Project, "a network of people living with and/or affected by experiences
that are often diagnosed and labeled as psychiatric conditions. We
believe these experiences are mad gifts needing cultivation and care,
rather than diseases or disorders." I added a joke: "By the way, if you
think you are not depressed, it is a sign of a thought disorder."

I decided to call St. Joe's and learned that Bill had been moved back
to Anoka. I let Jake know right away. "This will give them a second
chance to kill him! Of all the dumb things to do, I guess they chose the
dumbest. Haven't heard from him yet but probably will unless they have
him so doped up he can't talk." I couldn't believe the arrogance of these
doctors!

Bill was placed on a different unit from the one he was on when
originally admitted to Anoka. The first time I called they had the ringer
turned off and so I got no response. Same for second, third, & fourth
times. Finally, I called the main number and got a message sent to Bill to
call. I called him back when he was sitting right there at the phone and it
didn't ring. He finally noticed the ringer switch and turned it on.

He said he was feeling "like a whipped puppy." They came to him at
breakfast at St. Joe's and told him he was going to leave in one hour to go

117

back to Anoka. He said he thought Golden Living Center was behind the move to send him back to Anoka. I thought they just didn't want him around because he was too much trouble to deal with - too big, too hard to move, complained too much, threatened legal action, and so on. Running a nursing home would be easier without him around. And St. Joe's didn't want him around because they weren't going to make any money on him.

So, we were back to square one. There was a court date on the 21st and it was conceivable that they could give him an add-on to his "sentence." He might be stuck with the same old lawyer again. I suggested he request a change of venue (to Hennepin County or even to Dakota County where it all started) and refuse to have Mr. Pecor represent him because he was going to bring charges against him to the Minnesota Bar. Bill said he didn't want Pecor, then he said he might consider him if he signed a contract, then he said he didn't want him under any circumstances. His roommate received the same kind of treatment from Rice County Court and was also represented by Pecor. He was assigned the same guardian too, whom he hated. Bill said his roommate would be interested in filing a joint complaint to the Minnesota Bar Association about Pecor.

"The more the merrier," I said.

Hospital staff found the money Bill had hidden in his wheelchair and confiscated it. He was told he would get it back a little at a time.

"What with the way your belongings seem to disappear in hospitals, I wouldn't count on it," I said.

As it turned out, both Bill and his roommate decided to give Pecor another chance. I asked Bill why he was doing that and he just beat about the bush. I gave him the names of a couple of lawyers able to practice in both Minnesota and Wisconsin that I found on the Internet, but I doubted that anyone was going to rush to take his case.

For some reason – perhaps to confront him with his distortions of information - Bill wanted to be able to call Dr. Quack as a witness. I thought it would be dangerous to have him around, spewing out more bull shit. After all, the judge took the MD's word as gospel and would probably rule against any attempt to show him up as a fraud. I mentioned that he should try to get a change of venue but he was just as evasive as he was about what sort of a plan he had if the marriage thing didn't work out. I asked what Pecor's strategy was and he didn't know except that the lawyer wanted to call Bill's prospective bride as a witness.

Bill's case sounded all very nebulous and weak. What I thought he should be doing was to present some plan to live in an assisted living place for a while and get the physical and perhaps psychological therapy he needed. If he told the court that he was going to live on his prospective bride's property or live in some old motor home or camp out, they would just think he was being unrealistic. He hadn't talked with Jackie directly, only with her granddaughter. I told him that if Jackie was going to testify on his behalf, he had better talk with her beforehand and if not, then she was irrelevant to his defense.

I had a sense of dread regarding Bill's future and was completely taken aback when I got the following email from his new psychiatrist:
June 17, 2011

Dear Dr. Otis,

At Mr. Tollefson's request, I am sending this note to inform you of our Treatment Team's recommendations as of today. Our treatment team is of the opinion that Mr. Tollefson is currently on no psychotropic medications and that his difficulties at present cannot be attributed to an active Axis I psychiatric diagnosis. We therefore at present do not believe that commitment or continuation of commitment be pursued on a psychiatric basis.

Sincerely,

William B. Smart, MD
Psychiatrist
Anoka Metro Regional Treatment Center

"Holy shit," I said out loud. I couldn't believe it. Somebody had finally listened.

That night I talked with Bill and he told me about how Dr. Smart had interviewed him and discussed with him the material I had presented in my letter to the Minnesota Attorney General. He said that Dr. Smart and other people on the treatment team made the effort to go through the records and listen to what Bill was telling them. One member of the team counted that the previous psychiatrist had referred to Bill as "Mr. Johnson" on five different occasions in court. When Bill tried to object, his "public pretender" told him to be quiet. Dr. Smart asked Bill a lot of questions and let him know that he thought he did not belong in a mental hospital. He shared with him his own enjoyment of fishing and his predilection for Walleyes. Bill said he offered to give the good doctor some advice on how he might increase his catch. Needless to say, Bill was overjoyed at his vindication and the prospect of getting out of the hospital.

I responded to Dr. Smart's email, expressing my relief that someone had finally recognized what many of his friends had been saying since this ordeal began – that Bill may be unusual but he is not psychotic or dangerous and in need of hospitalization. I informed him of the Free the Fisherman Network and conveyed the appreciation of all of us to him for his diligence in his work. I ended the note with, "May you have good fishing!"

Jake said, "Glad to see Anoka has finally seen the light. I have reconsidered my position. If Bill gets married I will not eat my hat-- stranger things have happened. And if the Courage Center can do anything to help him regain the use of his legs then that's where he should go. Hope everything comes out OK with the Rice County Court next week. "

"I hope it goes well too," I told Jake, "but I just don't trust those assholes and I pray Bill will keep his mouth shut or at least not stick his foot in his mouth. With his new psychiatrist's statement, the court should just drop the matter. But, you never know with these bastards. He should also be in a good position to get a lawyer to sue the snot out of a bunch of these jerks plus file criminal actions against the original accusers. We will see. I will be sending another update to the network about the last abomination of the system that got Bill sent back to Anoka. Thank God he's got a psychiatrist with a brain!

"The Courage Center did a lot for him back in the mid to late 1990s and going to the pool in the Northfield Senior Center kept his joints from freezing up. My wife and I go to a pool at a physical rehab place twice a week and the instructor is an overweight guy with back problems and deep-vein thrombosis who says that being in the water has kept him from being immobilized. The trick was for Bill to talk his way in there. Now that his shrink said he wasn't currently nuts, they shouldn't have any objection, if they have the space."

As it turned out, Bill didn't need to even go to court. Dr. Smart sent a letter to Mr. Pecor who presented it to the court and the judge immediately rescinded the commitment, effective the 27th of June. After seven months of incarceration, Bill was free - sort of.

I sent an email to all the members of the Free the Fisherman Network, informing them of what had happened. Big Jim was the first to respond. "Yee-haw! We finally got a shrink that agrees with us. Its about time. You made my day,Bud."

Dawn sent a one word reply, "Fabulicious!"

Louise responded, "My goodness! I can't believe that someone finally woke up and discovered a mistake had been made."

"Great news," said Will. "Is anybody putting together a small fund to help him get back into his normal life? You can count on me for $100 if a fund gets organized. I haven't laid eyes on Northfield since 1960, but I still have great affection for the town and its people."

Jeannette commented, "It is great to finally hear some good news about Bill.

I liked what Gloria said, even though it was overly generous: "Thanks to you, Bud. A good end after all and due 99% to your dogged, never-give-up, hard work fighting the system. You are a great friend indeed."

"Yay," said Sonia. "Finally! I am so happy for Bill. He deserves this...poor guy. I hope everyone that screwed him over pays for it! Then justice will be served. Bill is lucky to have a friend like you, Bud."

Everyone was joyful that a little bit of justice surfaced amidst all of the madness of the last few months and they were happy for Bill. But he still didn't have a place to go since his home had been dismantled and his belongings stored somewhere out of his reach. The hospital no longer had a right to hold him there against his will and they probably couldn't keep him there for long since he wasn't "qualified" to be there, but they might be able to buy him some time for "discharge planning." In spite of his new status, the ward staff were still treating him like a committed patient and chasing him off the phone after a short period, so I still hadn't gotten the full story. But at least the psychiatrist and treatment team appeared to be willing to work with him.

Jake called the Courage Center to see what Bill needed to do in order to get admitted and whether or not they had a hyperbaric chamber, since it worked so well with his friend's brother. He learned that they had no hyperbaric chamber but was told that getting admitted as an inpatient was not a big problem as there seemed to be plenty of room. But he needed a doctor to write the order and make all the arrangements. Bill said that the doc and the treatment team at Anoka were all supportive of him going to the Courage Center.

The status of Bill's admission to the Courage Center was up in the air for many days. Bill thought it was his court-appointed guardian that was standing in the way of his admission there. I wasn't sure but thought it a definite possibility. I wrote an email to Bill's court-appointed lawyer:

"Dear Mr. Zimbledon,

I am contacting you on behalf of Bill Tollefson regarding the guardianship that he was placed under in recent months. The guardian apparently is standing in the way of Mr. Tollefson's admission into the

Courage Center in Golden Valley for unknown reasons. I have talked on the phone with Mr. Tollefson's new doctor, Dr. William Smart, who is trying to help Mr. Tollefson in this regard as he did with regard to rescinding the original commitment. We agree that it is imperative that Mr. Tollefson regain his physical health after the ordeal of being unjustly incarcerated for seven months and we see the Courage Center hydrotherapy program as instrumental in bringing that about. However, the problem appears to be a legal one requiring a legal solution. Is there an action you can file to rescind the guardianship? Since it was all based on the now discredited commitment procedure, there is no basis for a guardianship existing at this time.

"Mr. Tollefson is now at Anoka on a voluntary basis because there is nowhere for him to go and neither social workers nor guardians have been working with him on placement. Dr. Smart tells me that since he is a voluntary patient, placement is more difficult because the patient would be free to leave a residence whenever he wanted - a strange Catch 22 situation to being a "free" agent. In order for him to be totally free, as he should be, this guardianship arrangement should be terminated immediately."

Mr. Zimbledon responded that, in order to get rid of the guardian, a petition for Restoration to Capacity had to be filed with the court. In the meantime, I learned that Bill's sister had contacted the Courage Center and they were just waiting for the social services people at Anoka to submit an admissions package for Bill. The social worker had not done it, he told Bill, because his guardian didn't want him to go to the Courage Center. I told Dr. Smart that if the guardian was the one standing in the way that she was practicing medicine without a license.

Finally, after enough people complained, an application for admission to the Courage Center was submitted for Bill. It was turned down and it was their policy to give no explanation for their decision (which could probably be contested under the *Americans with Disabilities Act*). Jake was the one who found the newspaper article that explained what we were up against. The article included an interview with someone from the Courage Center who said that they did not want to receive any more "state patients" because they ended up losing money on them and, in the current economic situation, they could no longer afford to do that.

8 PRETTY PLEASE, GOVERNOR DAYTON

Jake checked with Valley View Assisted Care in Northfield and found that there were a few rooms open right away. It all depended on the financial arrangements. Cash payers could get in within one day. All others, like Bill, needed to go through all the proper channels, which usually took a couple of weeks. Openings would pop up quite often because residents died or moved to a higher level of care. At Valley View, Bill would be about a mile from downtown and would need to take the bus to do any shopping rather than just rolling his wheelchair down the street as in his previous residence. However, he would be able to get transportation to the Senior Center to do his own aquatic therapy.

Jake worried that Bill's Owatonna handler – the guardian – might not want Bill to return to his home town if she believed all the trash from the first hearing. "The way they railroaded him in that hearing still boggles my common sense," he said.

Jake didn't know if Bill's former landlord had blackballed him from getting into Valley View, as Bill thought. "Think I'll head down there Friday late morning and talk to the administration. I'll mention the name Bill Tollefson a few times and see if I get a response. Then I'll ask if he's banned from the place because of the lies told by Laura Biggs. I would think they would give me a straight yes or no."

When he executed his plan, he learned that the administrator had never heard of Bill Tollefson or of anyone ever being blackballed from admission. "Bill has to stop talking about his law suits. These outfits are deathly afraid of a suit and even if it's groundless, the insurance companies go nuts. I'm going to deliver this admissions request form to Bill next week with a stamped envelope so he'll have no reason not to send it to Valley View."

While there, he talked with one of the residents, an old friend who had been there about three years and someone who knew Bill. "He likes it although he finds it hard living on $85 a month. They give you a bed if you need one or you can bring your own. Also, clean sheets once a week, weekly room cleaning, do the laundry, TV and computer cable in each room. They give free rides to any doctor's appointments or physical therapy. The shuttle bus to town stops three or four times a day and costs $1.00 each way."

The resident Jake talked with had an interesting tale to tell about his experience with Rice County Social Services. "He liked where he was living before he came to Valley View, but a social worker from Rice County kept showing up to inspect his apartment and telling him that he had too many books. She'd been trying for almost three years to get him booted and into a place like Anoka. She even complained about how he dressed and combed his hair. Then one day the Northfield cops showed up and hauled his ass to the local hospital for no good reason. He would have been headed to a mental hospital except for the fact that the doctor who examined him had taken piano lessons from his mother when he was a kid living in Northfield. She found nothing wrong with the guy except 'depression'. He thinks there's a collection of social workers in Rice county who like to show how important their jobs are by railroading people any way they can get away with."

Bill called me and was "livid." He said he received a notice that the guardian was getting rid of all his property except for personal effects within 10 days. This had to be a purely vindictive move on her part since he had just been officially declared not crazy enough to be committed to a state hospital. Bill was wondering if it might not be brother Gary that was behind it. I thought that it might be that or it could be that the guardian was seeing the Bill portion of their gravy-train slipping away and wanted to sell his stuff and take the money for themselves. They had already tapped his bank account for $2000 or more. I didn't see any honorable faces on that side of the fence.

I contacted the attorney of record for this aspect of the case and requested on Bill's behalf that he file a protest, since there was now no basis for him having any "guardian," or having his property and residence confiscated. I sent copies to Jake and Big Jim to act as witnesses that the attorney had been notified of his client's request. Zimbledon finally talked with Bill (after avoiding his phone calls from the previous week) and he agreed to file the protest.

The attorney who had represented Bill in the eviction matter, Brian

Landers, had sent some information to Zimbledon about how Bill could go about suing if the guardian or Laura Biggs did anything with his property, so Bill called Brian right away to find out what it was. Bill didn't know what all he had in his apartment but thought much of it was of significant value, at least to him. If his possessions really weren't worth anything, I thought, then Bill could value it at whatever he wanted and sue them for that amount plus punitive damages. I had read that, when an eviction occurs in Minnesota, there has to be an inventory made of all property. I was pretty sure that had not been done when Bill's property was moved from his residence.

I was thinking there were a lot of people who should be sued and maybe it could be done all at once in a kind of reverse class action, the class being all the people who contributed to Bill's pain and suffering. Bill was damaged in a lot of ways: loss of liberty, loss of residence, loss of possessions, loss of income, loss of health, psychological and physical pain and suffering. Add them all up to get a total amount and let a jury decide on how much each party should pay. I figured Rice County had overall responsibility for the damages that Bill suffered but the psychologist and Vulnerable Adult Social Worker could also be sued for malpractice.

Bill needed a lawyer who knew the ins and outs of mental health law and how to work for his client while not being baffled by the disinformation of workers in the mental illness industry. While browsing the web, I ran across a reference to an attorney who had won $3.4 million for unjustified commitment of a man in Georgia. I found his web site and learned that, in 1999, he had cases in process for unjustified commitment in Boston, New York, Chicago and Atlanta. This sounded like just the guy Bill needed to represent him. I sent him an email inquiry but he never responded. I was about to call him when a friend suggested I contact someone closer to the scene of the crime, another professor at Hamlin University, who might be able to help.

I sent an email to the professor, briefly outlining what had happened to Bill and asking if she or someone she knew might be able to represent Bill. I was about to give up on her when I received an email reply. She said she had been tied up in hearings and other matters that delayed her answering my inquiry. She explained that she did not accept clients from the general public and did not practice in the relevant area of law. She suggested that I contact one of her colleagues who had some expertise in that area and might take Bill's kind of case, or would be likely to know some attorneys to whom she could refer me.

I immediately sent an email inquiry to this new lawyer, mentioning who had referred me to her, and at the same time sent a thank-you email to the professor. This "hot prospect" never did reply to my inquiry, even with just an acknowledgment. I then generated a list of potential lawyers in the Minneapolis area with specialties in civil law, elder law, elder abuse, mental health law, legal and medical malpractice from whom Bill might be able to recruit an attorney. I told Jake what had happened with the ones I had contacted so far. He contacted his lawyer friend to get a professional opinion about the chances of Bill getting an experienced lawyer to handle his case.

"My friend said it would be tough to find one that would do it on a contingency basis," Jake reported, "since there would be a lot of research and time required. Plus the expense of depositions from the many people involved in the suit. And since Bill doesn't have a lot of lost wages, or any, the case would be only on negligence and pain and suffering etc. I asked him to mention Bill's case to the guy in Hennepin county who has done a ton of defense work in commitment hearings to see if he had any ideas. I will let you know what he has to say."

Bill was still having a lot of trouble with his shoulder that was screwed up from trying to transfer him with a rolled-up blanket and he was having a lot of butt pain because he didn't have that $550 pad for his wheelchair. The shoulder pain had lasted for two or three months and I suspected there was something major wrong.

Big Jim sent an email. "Hey Bud. I just spoke with Bill and he really sounds bummed about still being stuck in that shit hole. He said that the fiduciary ripoff artists are still controlling his funds and want to stick him into a nursing home and he needs to go to the Courage Center, and see a chiropractor and they won't let him out to do any of that, not to mention, the fiduciaries are recommending that he stay put 'til he finds a permanent residence, and with a 10 minute phone limit and only $85 in hand, it makes it damned near impossible to do anything over the phone. After he gets out, and that's assuming that he gets into the Courage Center, he will need a place to live. I suggested he move to LaCrosse. He said he'd give it some thought."

It was a Friday that I had last talked with Bill. He was very discouraged. He had had a pain in his butt for some weeks now and his medical doctor wouldn't do anything about it. His bed went to hell and they gave him a new one that he didn't think was any better. He said it was like a concrete slab. He knew he had to tell Zimbledon on Monday to file the Restoration of Capacity motion but he was hesitating because he had nowhere to go. He had not yet heard the outcome of his protest of the planned disposal of his property. He did not call me and, when I called him, he would not take the call. This lack of communication went on for about a week and finally Dr. Smart called me. When I called back, there was no answer because the state government had been shut down.

Eventually I got through to the doctor and he told me Bill had been denied for inpatient treatment at the Courage Center although there was a possibility that he might be seen as an outpatient. Since then, Bill had become very morose and uncooperative. Dr. Smart said he had gotten him four different beds because of Bill's complaints but his patient was not satisfied with any of them. He had offered to take Bill to a pool where he could exercise but, surprisingly, he even refused that. Bill would just get up, eat and go back to bed. I mentioned Bill's reputation in his family for being bullheaded and Dr. Smart said that it was as if he was dealing with a child who was going to hold his breath until he turned blue unless he got his way.

Because Bill did not meet the criteria for incarceration at the state hospital, Dr. Smart's team had been trying to get him placed in one of several nursing homes, including one that had a pool. However they had been turned down by seven different places. The problem, it seemed, was that the nursing homes liked to have a legal hold on their patients so they could not just choose to live somewhere else if they didn't like the facility. Since Bill was not legally committed, he was no longer a desirable patient because he could, in theory, just walk away.

It appeared to me that Dr. Smart was really trying to help Bill regain his normal life but he feared what would happen when he left the facility and more imperious staff members - people like Dr. Quack - took control. Dr. Smart was a locum tenens doctor, which meant he was working at the hospital on a temporary basis and would be leaving in three weeks. When he left, if Bill kept on with his bullheadedness, he would eventually wear out his welcome and might be seen as unmotivated or not really being able to take care of himself. He could get recommitted or shipped off to some nursing home to die. Dr. Smart did not want that to happen and wondered if I might say something to him that would shake him out of his obstinacy. He said that, if Bill continued to refuse my calls, I could send him an email letter that he would print and convey to his patient.

When I didn't hear from Bill, I composed a letter and sent it to Jake to see if he thought it might press the right buttons and avoid pressing the wrong ones, then I sent it to Dr. Smart. I started off with a some mild guilt induction, saying that, after having written a ton of letters on his behalf in the last seven months, I never expected to have to write to him in order to communicate.

127

"It has been a long battle for you these last seven months and you have been disappointed many times along the way. Maybe you don't want to get your hopes up again, expecting that they will be dashed like all the other times. I can understand that you are tired of fighting and I can understand that you are angry with everyone and would like to punish them. I don't blame you for feeling that way, but continuing in that mood is not going to get you back to any semblance of a normal life. It will only dig you deeper into the pit you are in right now. That kind of "story ending" will inspire no one who finds themselves in a similar situation; it will just be another horror story."

I reminded him that Dr. Smart would be leaving the hospital shortly and that he had been the only mental health professional that Bill had run into in Minnesota that had recognized and been willing to stand up and say that he should not have been committed in the first place and did not belong in a state hospital. I let him know that I knew he was thwarting Dr. Smart's efforts to help him and encouraged him to use his talent as a problem solver to achieve what was possible in the current context. I threw in a little fear threat: the next doctor may not be so competent and might decide you really do need to be there.

"There are a lot of your old friends that are rooting for you. Don't let them down by sinking the boat just before it gets to the dock!"

My appeals, threats and guilt induction didn't seem to work. I heard nothing back from Bill. Jake, in the meantime, had heard from the administrator at Valley View. She said that she had a Physical Assessment Coordinator going to Anoka to do assessments of three persons and would have her do one on Bill Tollusfon while she was there. Afterward, the Valley View administrator called Jake and told him that Bill had too many medical problems for them to be able to adequately care for him. I informed Dr. Smart and he responded:

"Thanks for continuing to follow-up on things. Our hope is to find an appropriate nursing home that can attend to Bill's needs medically and with PT and, in addition, one where outpatient pool therapy would be possible, either at a Courage Center or similar pool. I will share your e-mail with our social worker as well. Bill's next challenge will be to go to court on August 5th to try to save his belongings. I have encouraged him to do so. Our Social Worker is arranging transportation and looking into the possibility of having either the case manager or guardian meet him at the storage locker to look for his seat cushion and leg lifts.

"To answer your second concern, Bill has refused any interventions that are not Pool Therapy, including working with our on-site physical therapist as well as outpatient consultation with Orthopedics/ pain medicine even though we are willing to arrange these appointments and provide transportation. We will continue our efforts. Unfortunately tomorrow is my final day here, but I do believe that all the team members have Bill's best interests at heart.

With sincere regards,

Dr. Smart"

Damn, I thought. It's anyone's guess what kind of shrink will replace Dr. Smart. It's too bad Bill is doing this crap right now. I suppose he will get some kind of crack-pot psychiatrist that will give him a diagnosis of Major Depression so they'll be justified in keeping him there forever.

Both Jake and I were worried that Bill would undercut his legal position by continuing his obstinate stance and refusing treatment that was offered. I wrote Jake, "The judge is the same guy that ordered the Abilify. I hope Bill shows up but if he weren't such a bull-headed SOB, he'd be able to get some coaching on what to say. I'm betting he won't show but if he does, he'll probably just wing it or try some cockamamie thing that will backfire on him. What he needs to do is work out a plan about how he would manage his property and/or pay for the storage. If by some strange stroke of luck Bill got a decent lawyer, he probably could force the county to pay for it since it was their error that resulted in his false incarceration. And he probably could collect damages for the illegal eviction. But with Bill undercutting his legal position by taking dumb stances and refusing treatment, it probably won't happen. And if he gets accusatory towards the judge, he is sunk (even if he is right!)."

Jake wrote back, "It could be interesting. Laura Biggs has had to pay the storage charges up until now - I think that's the law. The judge will probably decide that if Bill will pay the storage charges from now on himself--then he can keep his stuff. BUT, what kind of person is Bill's brother Gary? He could let Bill keep his stuff there for no charge if he wanted to do so. However, a few weeks ago Gary told me that all of Bill's stuff is junk and should go to the dump, the same claim he made when he threw him out of the house he shared with his mother. It could be a long time for Bill to get out of a nursing home and rehabbed to the point where he could move to assisted care, and in assisted care you usually don't have much room to bring your stuff--other than a bed, desk, and a few clothes or maybe a chair or TV. Jane once said she'd pay for the storage but I doubt if she will now. Also, I think Biggs has a legal right to sell the stuff to re-coup the storage and other fees which they have spent so far with the eviction....which may or may not have been legal. I'm looking forward to the fireworks."

I thought neither Gary nor Jane could be trusted any further than I could throw Ames Mill. Jake was unable to get to the hearing because of car trouble but called the court clerk to get the results. "Bill got a 60 day continuance from the judge. Hopefully, he will soon be in a nearby nursing home so he can go look at his stuff and find what he needs. I've got my fingers crossed just in case. He might end up in Bum Fuck, Egypt if his bad luck continues."

Bill's youngest sister, Irene, called and asked what had happened to her brother. She had called the hospital and was told that he wasn't there and they could not tell her where he was because of the new privacy laws. I said I didn't know as I hadn't talked with him for about a month. She said that her niece had been taken off life support and either was expected to die or already had died and she wanted to inform Bill. Earlier, she had called the hospital and Bill had given her the same routine as he had given me, "Leave a message." Somehow Irene was under the assumption that Bill had been thrown out of the Golden Living place in St. Paul because he went drinking. I corrected her on that, informing her that he was taken to St. Joseph's because he complained about his cellulitis and then complained when they tried to give him Abilify again. I supposed that Jane had tried to recruit Irene to her side in the continuing dysfunctional family saga by telling her that Bill had been thrown out for going to bars.

It was several days before the social worker at Anoka got back to Irene to tell her where her brother was. Irene called me and reported that Bill was at another Golden Living Center in a suburb of Minneapolis. "Bill is more depressed than I have ever heard him," she said, "with sparks of rage every now and then. He complains about the food and how they aren't doing a damn thing to help his physical problems. The social worker from Anoka is trying to get him into the Courage Center as an outpatient."

I called the number Irene had given me and was able to talk with Bill briefly. He was very depressed but at least he was responding. He complained about the food and not being able to relate to anyone at the place. I looked up the place on the Internet and the pictures they showed weren't too bad (but, of course, they wouldn't show the bad ones in a promo for the place). I suspected that he found it difficult to relate to the other patients because many of them had Alzheimer's disease.

I talked with Bill again the following night and he was still down and couldn't focus enough to do much problem solving. I asked him what he needed first, second and third and he couldn't answer. I asked if getting to aquatic therapy was most important and he couldn't say. I told him to give some thought to it and we'd talk again. I asked who was in charge of him and he said, as a joke, "Some mouse in the dinning room." I later learned that the facility had been cited for a "rodent problem" by state inspectors.

I told Jake, "I don't know if he is still under the control of the witches from Owatonna or not. He said his roommate urinated all over the place! He did not know that Zimbledon got the continuance on the hearing regarding his stuff. I think he just shut off about a month ago - he says he is just in survival mode, which I think means not getting his hopes up and not expecting anything good to happen. It may take some doing to get him back out of that state of mind."

One day I spent about 6 hours calling Bill's phone number, accumulating hundreds of rings, in total, and got no response. Maybe the place burned down, or they had a tornado, or terrorists took it over, I thought. More likely, was that they had no one answering the phone on Sundays and maybe all weekend. I thought there should be some regulation that covers this circumstance and started browsing the Internet for nursing home regulations. In the process, I found the Medicare assessment for the nursing home where Bill had been placed. Their rating was "Much Below Average" and it was enclosed in a bright red box.

Under the section labeled "Repeat Violations" was the following: "1) Make sure that residents who take drugs are not given too many doses or for too long; 2) make sure that the use of drugs is carefully watched; or 3) stop or change drugs that cause unwanted effects. Develop a complete care plan that meets all of a resident's needs, with timetables and actions that can be measured. Develop/implement required procedures for the administration of immunizations. Do a new assessment after any major change in a resident's physical or mental health. Give professional services that follow each resident's written care plan. Make a complete assessment that covers all questions for areas that are listed in official regulations. Make sure that each resident who enters the nursing home without a catheter is not given a catheter, unless it is necessary. Make sure that the nursing home area is free of dangers that cause accidents. Make sure that the nursing home area is safe, easy to use, clean and comfortable. Properly mark drugs and other similar products. Store, cook, and give out food in a safe and clean way."

Oh-oh, I thought This is *not* good news. Bill has an amazing ability to survive in difficult circumstances, but with all his physical problems and lacking his usual will power and inventiveness, this incompetent place could kill him. How the hell are we going to get him out of there?

Somehow, I received an email asking me to sign a petition for some

GERALD D. OTIS

poor woman in Georgia who was being prosecuted for not using a crosswalk after her child was killed by a drunk driver after getting off a bus. The nearest crosswalk was a mile away. I was about the 140,000th person to sign the petition and before long the prosecutor relented. Then there was a petition to force the state to put in a crosswalk where the tragedy had occurred.

Hot damn! Maybe I can do something like that for Bill, I thought. It doesn't cost anything, which is in my price range, and it might put some pressure on those idiots in Minnesota that started the whole damn thing and are keeping it going.

I went to the web site that sponsored the petition, Change.org, and checked out the kinds of petitions that were there and how one went about implementing one. Figuring that Bill's situation fit best in the "Human Rights" category, I began to formulate my petition to Mark Dayton, Governor of the State of Minnesota.

The web site suggested that the petitioner focus the "ask" question on a rather specific thing, e. g., "Tell Mark Dayton to Get The Fisherman into a therapeutic pool!" or some such thing that it is possible to accomplish. The web site could send an email to the "target" (e. g., Dayton) each time someone signed the petition. If you got a large number of respondents, that could crash an email program. I thought, at the time, that that might happen if some of my Facebook friends who had thousands of friends of their own all asked their friends to sign up. So I didn't think that alienating the guy I was asking something from was the way to do it. Instead, the signatures could be collected online and presented in person or by regular mail. I believed I could write the "description" section ("Why should I sign this?") by summarizing some of the other things I had written. I considered the possibility that the governor might not be the best "target" but figured it would be handled by an aide anyway, and he or she could decide how best to rout it within the administration. After I had a draft petition, I sent it out to a number of Bill's friends who were acquainted with his plight for comments and suggestions. The final document was called "Tell Governor Mark Dayton: We Want Justice for Bill The Fisherman!" The image on the first page was a picture of the then 71 year old Bill superimposed on a picture of a young Bill standing on a dock in front of a boat on a lake. The text of the petition read:

"The Minnesota court dismantled his home, consigned his property, income and bank account to a company acting as a 'guardian,' forced him into locked confinement in a state hospital where he experienced psychological abuse, assaulted him with a drug that caused him severe adverse side effects, deprived him of the kind of therapy that had been effective in maintaining his physical functioning, and squandered an estimated quarter of a million dollars in Medicare/Medicaid funds on ineffective custodial care that wasn't even needed. As a result of his confinement, his condition has deteriorated and he is not, at the present time, able to return to totally independent living. There was nary so much as a "Sorry about that" when the commitment was rescinded after a new psychiatrist declared that he did not have an Axis I disorder and therefore did not meet the requirements for compulsory incarceration. Give Bill Tollefson, "The Fisherman," the justice he deserves.

"Bill Tollefson is a 71 year old former fishing guide who became physically disabled from his occupation after hip and knee surgeries and has been dependent on a wheelchair for several years. A jovial and entertaining extravert, Mr. Tollefson had relied on Social Security income and lived in HUD subsidized housing until December of 2010. Shortly before Christmas, he slid down on the seat of his wheelchair and was unable to reposition himself due to pain from cellulitis in his leg. Because he weighed 350 pounds, police were called to assist. Against his wishes, the officers forcibly subdued him with sedatives and took him to the local hospital. Bill had earlier discontinued some medication because he believed it was adversely affecting him and reasoned that God would not want that for him. The examining physician, angered by Bill's rationale, decided to "trump" his patient's religious views by placing him on a 72 hour hold. Mr. Tollefson was spirited away to another hospital 50 miles away from his home where commitment procedures were initiated. Thus began one of the most shameful and disgusting episodes in the history of Minnesota mental health jurisprudence.

"There were many violations of state law in the handling of Mr. Tollefson's case including denial of his right to have a second opinion by a doctor of his own choice, denial of his right to appeal, and failure to abide by the rules of evidence specified by state law in the charges made against him. His legal representation was incompetent and unethical. There was gross incompetence by the psychologist who evaluated him: she made several major errors of fact, numerous unfounded inferences and she lacked adequate data to support the assertions and conclusions in the report. The psychologist did not do any psychological testing of any sort and no MRI, EEG or physical tests were conducted, yet she diagnosed him with "Cognitive Disorder, NOS" and an unspecified organic brain disorder. She did not moderate her conclusions because of the lack of empirical evidence. In doing so, she violated tenants of the Code of Ethics of the American Psychological Association and ignored professional guidelines for psychological assessment of elderly persons.

"The first psychiatrist who supervised the "treatment" of Mr. Tollefson claimed that Bill was paranoid schizophrenic, not on the basis of any behavior demonstrated by Bill on the ward but on the basis of the defective initial court records. A short while later he changed his diagnosis to "Psychotic Disorder, Not Otherwise Specified," a garbage can category for psychoses that don't fit into typical symptom patterns. He obtained a court order to prescribe the drug Abilify despite affidavits from expert witnesses, citing 50 years of research, that such drugs are ineffective and often times harmful, especially for patients with Bill's kind of medical problems. In his court testimony, the doctor referred to Mr. Tollefson as "Mr. Johnson" on five different occasions and Bill's attorney 'shushed' Bill from making any objections to this colossal attributional error.

"The drug was forcibly injected into Mr. Tollefson while more than a dozen staff members held him down in a hallway of the state hospital. Bill subsequently developed several adverse reactions to the drug and one of his supporters sent a letter of complaint to the Joint Commission on Accreditation of Hospitals which included several other aspects of neglect of Bill's physical problems and psychologically degrading treatment. The hospital finally discontinued administering the drug. However they simultaneously denied him medication that he needed and kept him from continuing the aquatic therapy which had kept him mobile for the last 15 years. Through use of an improper method of transfer, they injured his shoulders and he continues to experience pain several months later.

"Appeals to several state agencies that are supposed to help in such situations were met with indifference and lack of action.

"After five months imprisoned in a locked ward, Bill was discharged to a nursing facility in St. Paul. He complained of leg pain due to his cellulitis but his requests to see a physician were ignored and he became more vocal. Instead of calling a physician, they called a contract psychiatrist who apparently decided Bill was going crazy (because he was complaining loudly) and wanted to drug him again. He protested even more and they summoned the police to take him to St. Joseph's Hospital in St. Paul. There they treated his leg and it improved. But they continued to believe the untruths in his record and sent him back to the state hospital.

"Fortunately, this time he was admitted to a different ward and assigned to a new psychiatrist, Dr. William Smart. The doctor read a document that had been written about Bill by a friend of 60 years duration, who also happened to be a retired clinical psychologist, that had been submitted to the state attorney general. Dr. Smart evaluated the patient himself. He and his treatment team decided Bill did not have an active Axis I diagnosis and the commitment was therefore not justified. When confronted with this new information, the court immediately rescinded the commitment.

"The immediate problem then became one of placement. Bill was convinced that what he needed was to go to the Courage Center in Golden Valley where he had been after his surgeries. They specialize in aquatic therapy and Bill credited them with having saved his life when he was a patient there before. However, they did not admit him this time and they do not divulge reasons for denial. An evaluation for admission to an assisted living facility in his home town indicated that his physical problems were too great for that facility to be an appropriate placement.

"After several placement efforts failed, Bill finally gave up the fight, becoming depressed, morose and pessimistic about ever returning to his previous level of functioning, or to his home town. Then the psychiatrist who had been his champion left the hospital. Shortly thereafter, Bill was discharged to another nursing home in St. Louis Park, MN, one with the lowest possible Medicare rating: *Much Below Average*. Because they have many Alzheimer patients there, Bill can find no one to relate to – a fate worse than hell for a person of his personality type. His roommate is given to "urinating all over" and acting threatening. Bill is forced to either sit in his wheelchair or lie in his bed because no other appropriate alternative seating arrangement is available and there is no room for the electric lift chair he has in storage.

"The justice that is being requested for Mr. Tollefson, The Fisherman, is the following:
1. Relocation to an appropriate nursing facility rated by Medicare as at least Average until such time as he may resume independent or assisted living.
2. Assistance in locating and moving to a permanent address when that is possible.
3. Involvement in a program of aquatic therapy to restore his level of physical functioning to the point where he can take advantage of other types of physical therapy and regain mobility.

4. Storage of his possessions until such time as he is able to take possession of them and decide about their disposition.

5. Financial compensation, upon which no claims by any agencies can be made, for having been unjustly imprisoned in a state hospital and the attendant complications of his physical and mental conditions and disruption of his living arrangements.

6. Required remedial education for all members of the Rice County Court and any public defenders or contract attorneys used by the court in civil commitment cases, the content of which shall include all International Conventions regarding human rights and all Federal and Minnesota statutes involving civil commitment and civil rights of person's living in the United States of America.

7. Prosecution of all individuals who entered false statements in documents used in the court actions taken against Mr. Tollefson."

After the first day we had 46 signatures for the petition including some from Ireland, Portugal, and British Columbia as well as the USA. One of Bill's old classmates suggested that, in dealing with the court system, I should not have asked for justice but rather for mercy. "If you ask for justice you will get the short end of the deal." I pondered why that might be true. I had done some research back in the 1980's on "Justice & Care Considerations in Making Moral Judgments" in men and women of different psychological types. The two Jungian psychological types studied were those preferring "Thinking" and those preferring "Feeling" in making decisions. Thinking decisions are ones made by using more or less rational, objective standards, where the decision-maker's own interests and sentiments are left out of the picture. Feeling type decisions put those personal considerations right into the center of the picture and the decisions are made are the basis of personal appraisals of like/dislike or compassion.

About 60% of men have a Thinking preference while 60% of women prefer Feeling but when the data is adjusted for psychological type, the sex difference in decision-making style disappears. There was also an effect according to the context in which the decision had to be made: business situations pulled more Thinking decisions while the context of relationships between intimates pulled the most Feeling decisions.

So, I would have to think that the friend's observation would be true if judges prided themselves on being objective decision-makers and didn't think they could be flat-out wrong, i. e., if they were blinded by their own arrogance. If you ask for mercy, on the other hand, you are appealing to their "other side" and they might grant your request because they feel less confident in that arena. While it may have thus been more diplomatic to phrase the petition in terms of mercy, it was already "out there" in the justice format and it would have been difficult to retract it and start all over again. Besides, I am a Thinking Type and I think Bill's situation is basically a matter of injustice, although no one has shown much mercy along the way either.

I remembered being at a conference on Psychological Type many years ago where a few judges from California were in attendance. They were instructors from the state "Judges College," and were actually trying to teach new judges how to make good decisions. They wanted to learn about the different perspectives of different personality types and how the different types go about making decisions. They thought they could apply it to both the judges (i. e., getting them to recognize their own particular biases) and to the clients those judges served (understanding the different perspectives taken by the parties to a dispute). The military was trying to do the same kind of thing at the Army War College, focusing primarily on how to form effective work groups, which meant having knowledgeable and "fair" leaders of those groups. I think the military correctly implemented the ideas but don't know how it turned out for the California judges.

When I talked with Bill on the phone, our conversations covered a lot of ground besides the latest abhorrence wrought by the "system" which still held him captive. I tried to keep him connected and up to date with what was happening in our home town by relating topics covered in the online version of the local newspaper. One of the long-time columnists for the paper, still writing at age 90, wrote retrospectives starting at 100 years ago and proceeding by 25 year increments. If there was something that occurred during our lifetimes, I would mention it to Bill and we would reminisce about it and the people involved. We also discussed articles about city government, since he had a long-time interest in the direction the city was taking, and I would report the latest obituaries. Bill knew many people in town and there were frequent deaths of his old apartment mates, including his former mother-in-law with whom he maintained a friendship during the time he was incarcerated.

One of my former classmates, Hank, a man that both Bill and I had known nearly all of our lives, had eventually become a very skilled substance abuse counselor. Hank and I, after graduating high school, had roared off to Colorado on my old 1940 Harley Davidson EL61 to seek our fortunes, it turned out, as migrant farm workers. It was a trip filled with adventure and a lot of fun, but we both knew there was not much of a future in it. We returned home to attend St. Olaf College and later we transferred to the University of Minnesota with two other classmates, together renting a dilapidated old McKinley-era house on the west side of the Minnesota River.

Hank got a part-time job as a psychiatric hospital orderly and there met his future wife, Eva. We lost track of each other for a few years after graduation but met up again at a class reunion. Hank was working in a substance abuse clinic and he and Eva lived with their two children on a hobby dairy farm they owned on the western edge of Wisconsin. A few years later they moved to southern California for a job and they both became volunteers for AIDS patients in hospice care. Eventually they returned to live on the farm in Wisconsin and Hank started a private practice in a nearby town. The couple had been married for nearly half a century when Eva was diagnosed with a rare medical disorder and died after a long illness.

About a year later, Hank made a trip to the west coast and stopped by to see me on his way. He was planning on seeing some old friends and then looking up his high school sweetheart, who was widowed. It wasn't but a few months before I received a phone call from Hank. He was going to get married, not to his old girlfriend but to his deceased wife's best friend and he wanted me to be best man. I agreed because he asked me but, privately, I wondered about the wisdom of his choice. The woman had become a paraplegic at a young age after falling off a cliff on a camping trip party. Marriage to her would mean that Hank would be looking forward to a lot of medical care-giving without an end in sight, this after he had spent many years in that role with his first wife. It didn't make sense to me that he would want to face that grueling kind of duty again unless, perhaps, it was the case that he and his new wife were still in mourning for Eva.

In any event, they married and lived in southern California during the winter months and on the Wisconsin farm during the summers. But three years after their marriage, Hank began to have problems with dizziness and falling. After a brain scan and biopsy, he was diagnosed with brain cancer of the type that felled Ted Kennedy. Hank called me with the news and we talked on the phone for several weeks as he underwent surgery, chemotherapy and radiation. My wife and I contacted two physicians we trusted and scoured the worldwide web looking for information. We learned that the standard medical treatment had a success rate of 1-2% while a new treatment, not yet approved by the FDA, was having a 50-60% success rate. If Hank could get into one of the FDA clinical trials, he might make it and I suggested it to him. But he trusted the party line his doctors gave him and decided he would try the alternative method if the standard treatment didn't work.

No surprise, then, that Hank got progressively worse. He was still quite lucid and knew that his condition would be fatal. He wanted to go home after he had completed his series of treatments, but his new wife wouldn't allow him to return. She was afraid that she wouldn't know what to do if he had another seizure and her sister had convinced her that she had to think of "protecting her assets." Hank said to me, "You just don't know who you've married until something like this happens. I promised I would be with her to the very end but I guess she is worried that she won't know how to dial 911 if I have a seizure."

Hank couldn't stop crying when he thought about "The Losses" - all the family events he would miss by being dead. He was critical of the nursing care he was receiving, knowing from first hand experience what should be done, and couldn't hold his tongue about these inadequacies in the interest of not alienating his care-givers. His care-givers chalked his "rages" up to his brain lesion, of course, and didn't give a thought to the possibility that Hank might be right about his criticisms. He thought about suicide and when he voiced his despair, they had him carted off to a psychiatric facility for the elderly.

I told Hank about Bill's plight and I told Bill about Hank's situation. Both of them had more than the usual acquaintance with the complexities of death and dying – Bill as a mortician and Hank in his work with AIDS patients. Each of them could understand the situation of the other and sent their wishes, prayers and encouragement to their counterpart. Neither of them had committed a crime, yet both were incarcerated by the powers that be "for their own good." I couldn't figure out what that "good" was and neither could they. Hank knew he was going to die shortly and just wanted to go back to the farm and die lying on the floor of the barn with his beloved old dog. But no, he had to remain institutionalized and the last dollar of his benefits had to be extracted from him. Bill did not face an imminent demise but could feel his life ebbing away, prevented from getting appropriate medical treatment and enjoying, as best he could, his last days, weeks, months or years by fishing, enjoying the outdoors, and entertaining his many friends. I began to appreciate that the self-interest, lack of compassion, illogic and bizarreness of the cancer industry was equally as bad as that of the psychiatry industry.

GERALD D. OTIS

9 THE GOLDEN YEARS

In the early days of Bill's incarceration, I had run across, on the Internet, a reference to Mindfreedom International, an advocacy group for those individuals labeled with a psychiatric condition. I had given Bill the phone number for the branch in Minnesota and he had called them and talked with one of its members. While nothing ever came of it, since Bill was not a dues-paying member, he was encouraged by the discussion and vowed to pursue it further when he was able to do so.

Mindfreedom International (MFI) is a coalition of numerous grassroots organizations that grew out of the civil rights and psychiatric survivors movements in the late '60s and early '70s and includes as members thousands of patients, family members of patients, ex-patients and sympathetic mental health professionals from fourteen nations. The late Judi Chamberlin was an eloquent spokesperson for the movement in her 1978 monograph *On Our Own: Patient Controlled Alternatives to the Mental Health System.* Mindfreedom International was chartered as a non-profit organization in 1990 to fight compulsory medication, use of physical restraints and involuntary electro-shock treatment. Directed by David W. Oaks until he was disabled by a tragic accident, the organization endeavors to protect the civil and human rights of people who have been given a psychiatric label. It receives no funding from governments, drug companies, religions, corporations or the mental illness industry. The United Nations recognizes it as a non-governmental human rights organization with Consultative Roster Status.

MFI has challenged psychiatry to produce unambiguous evidence that mental illness is a brain disorder, as they claim. Of course, the psychiatrists have been unable to do so. Mindfreedom has criticized the financial and political influence of Big Pharma on mental health care, including that industry's direct lobbying for laws allowing forced administration of psychiatric medication in the community without involuntary hospitalization, their payment of psychiatrists to hawk their products, and their corruption of research on the effectiveness and safety of their products. They have publicized instances of forced electro-shock treatment and lobbied for cessation of such practices. They have compiled survivor stories from people who have been abused by the psychiatric system and achieved stability by other means. The Gesundheit! Institute and its famous founder, "Patch" Adams, upon whose life the movie starring Robin Williams was based, is a sponsoring member of Mindfreedom. Patch is honorary head of the International Association for the Advancement of Creative Maladjustment.

The Solidarity Network of MFI has a Shield Program which provides organized, constructive nonviolent action (publicity, media alerts, passive resistance) to help members who are being harassed by courts or treatment officials with use of involuntary drug treatment or the use of electro-shock. It was in connection with one of these actions that I became involved with Mindfreedom.

A former school teacher had been forcibly subjected to electro-shock treatments on an outpatient basis by yet another Minnesota court. After about 15 sessions without evidence of any improvement and with increasing memory impairment, the woman and her husband decided to no longer submit to the procedure. The court was notified by the doctor and they had the sheriff haul the woman off to Anoka Metro-regional Treatment Center, the same place where Bill had been warehoused back in December of the previous year. Mindfreedom called for an alert and a letter writing campaign to the two Minnesota senators, Amy Klobuchar and Al Franken, and the representative from her district.

In my letter, I asked the State of Minnesota to halt this torture conducted under the guise of "psychiatric treatment." I asked them to investigate the well-being of the woman and referred them to the Mindfreedom web site for further information. I also suggested they read their local newspapers and included a recent article by David Brown in the Washington Post entitled "FDA panel advises more testing of 'shock-therapy' devices." A majority of an 18-member panel advising the FDA said that electroshock machines should undergo the same rigorous testing for safety and effectiveness as any new medical device coming on to the market. This had never been adequately done since the advent of the device back in 1938.

Jim Gottstein, head of Psychrights in Alaska, had written a letter to the FDA in January 2011 summarizing the evidence that use of the device can cause permanent memory loss, cognitive deficits, and brain damage and that it tends to increase mortality while lacking convincing evidence that it is effective. In searching the Worldwide Web, I found that some 45 residents of Hennepin County alone were being subjected to involuntary electroshock. I wondered how many poor souls were having their brains zapped "for their own good" in the whole state. I concluded my letter with the statement, "For the State of Minnesota to allow this barbaric practice to continue is tantamount to being complicit in the commission of a crime."

The campaign appeared to work, since the state gave up their persecution of the woman and let her return home. She wrote a letter to Mindfreedom thanking them for their efforts on her behalf.

During this period, I became acquainted with Bonnie Nelson, director of the Mindfreedom branch in Alaska. A delightful woman with wide-ranging interests and friends all over the planet, she became interested in the saga of Bill and thought she might be able to put me in contact with someone who could help. I had sent her the first few chapters of this book and she mentioned briefly the idea of doing a movie or documentary based on Bill's story and she knew someone who had the skills to do so. Bill himself, when he was in the hospital, had talked about making a movie using patients to play themselves. He even had thought of an old building in Minnesota where it might be filmed. Bonnie liked the idea and thought Bill might be fun to work with because of his creative thinking.

Of course, Bonnie was well acquainted with Jim Gottstein, head of Psychrights which is based in Anchorage. Gottstein had placed stopping the forced use of antipsychotic drugs on children as his top priority. He had won a number of cases in Alaska and one case was coming to the Court of Appeals in Seattle on the 8th of September. Not surprisingly, the drug companies were all aligned against him. He was arguing a qui tam case based on the False Claims Act which was passed after the Civil War. Basically what he was claiming was that those who prescribed such drugs were engaging in fraud against Medicaid and CHIPS (children's health services) because the drugs are not approved for off-diagnosis use in children. The other side was arguing that "everyone is doing it" and therefore it has been heard before. On appeal, Gottstein asserted that it was not just like other cases for a number of reasons. If he were to win, it would mean billions of dollars for the US government and a bad market for all the drug companies.

143

Bonnie connected me with another dynamic woman living in Vancouver, Washington who had started a support and training program for people who wanted to act as advocates for individuals with mental problems. Also a member of Mindfreedom, she called her new organization Movement of Mothers and Others Standing Up Together or MOMS, for short. I shared chapters of this book with her and she began using some of the material in her training program. One of her students applied for a start-up grant to create a film focusing on the corruption and harm that pharmaceutical companies and guardianship laws cause for foster kids, young adults and the elderly. I will have more to say about that later.

On a conference call, Bonnie introduced me to James Audlin, a prolific writer living in Panama who is interested in human rights. He thought what had happened to Bill sounded "Kofkaesque." Frank Blankenship, head of Mindfreedom in Florida, thought Bill's story was one of gross injustice but not unusual in his experience with the mental health jurisprudence system.

It turned out that another person to whom I was introduced, Al Galves, president of the International Society for Ethical Psychology & Psychiatry, lives in the same town where I live, Las Cruces, NM. After hearing the story about Bill, he said he would gladly sign the petition. Al said that Minnesota was notorious for mental health abuses and reported that he and some other people had put on demonstrations in the state a while back. His organization was about to have a convention in Los Angles where the keynote speaker was to be Thomas Szasz, the psychiatrist and author of the iconic book debunking psychiatric diagnosis, *The Myth of Mental Illness.* In that volume he argued that mental illness was a metaphorical construct defined by culture and society, not a biological illness.

Joe Carr, an Alabama attorney, thought Bill needed a good lawyer. He referred me to Abigail Turner, a woman he had worked with in Alabama who had moved to Minnesota and was second in command of Mid-Minnesota Legal Assistance. The organization was supposed to serve clients who could not afford a regular lawyer but they did not take any public funds, so they could "sue the bastards," at least in principle. He spoke very highly of her and said to mention his name when I talked with her.

I called Mid-Minnesota Legal Assistance and talked with their answering service. They had no listing for her and had no institutional memory of her. I looked on the Internet and found that she had won an award for her pro bono work in Hennepin County and the article I found referred to her connection with the Legal Service Advocacy Project. Their answering service didn't work right so I called a couple other places in the Twin Cities area. One of them was a woman at a Civil Rights Organization who had recently called Ms. Turner about a political campaign. She said she had moved to Virginia and she gave me a number where I might reach her. I thought, "What's the point. She won't be able to help Bill from there." Then I thought, "Why not give it a try. She probably knows the legal community in Minneapolis and might know someone who would be willing to help Bill."

When I finally reached the attorney, she listened carefully and politely to my brief account of the situation with Bill and then thought a minute about her Minnesota contacts. "It might be a long-shot," she said.

"That's the only kind of shot we have," I responded.

She referred me to an attorney in Minneapolis who practices "elder law." "If that doesn't pan out, you can always try Mid-Minnesota Legal Assistance where I used to work." I was totally surprised when she closed the conversation by saying, "Thank you for trying to help your friend." I don't think I had ever heard an expression of appreciation for someone doing the right thing from a lawyer before. I hoped this lawyer she referred me to was going to be like her. Maybe we did have a shot!

Of course, I checked out the woman she referred me to on the Internet before I called her. She was a share-holder in a three-person legal office with a good resume and lived in a three story house with her father and disabled son. That sounded like a good sign. Maybe she had some personal experience dealing with social agencies and would have some empathy for Bill's situation

My call to the Minneapolis attorney was answered by an aide. I explained Bill's situation to her in some detail and she said she would call back after she presented it to the attorney. When she did so, she said that the attorney would only take the case if she were presented with $5000 up front to begin with and that there would likely be additional expenses after that. This was about twice the amount an earlier lawyer had asked for just to "look into" the matter. It was clearly outside the scope of Bill's resources and it was evident that she did not want to take any risk at all in the interest of "justice" or "compassion." Maybe this kind of case would just be too hard to win in Minnesota. After all, even in a clear case of medical malpractice resulting in death, the chances of getting to court were less than one in a hundred.

I was beginning to think that our only hope was if the governor intervened in some way as a result of the petition. We now had about 60 signatures, one of the most recent from Switzerland. The people in the governor's office probably wouldn't care what people from out of state or out of country thought, but I was hoping that some local reporter might pick it up and make a story out of it.

I received an email from Jake who had just sent out requests for signatures to 61 people who gave email addresses in his high school reunion book and only three did not go through. He also found a list of the class of 1961 and planned to send requests to those with email addresses the following day. "I hope they sign, but many people will never sign a petition for fear it's some kind of scam just to get valid email addresses." I found a list of my classmates with their email addresses and sent the request email out to them. I had received some messages back from the first group I had sent requests to that the link I had provided didn't connect them with anything, so I added an email address as an alternative way to get to the petition. I also added on to the request letter the statement, "Since neither Bill nor his friends have the kind of money required to retain a decent attorney, we have resorted to trying to shame the governor into doing the right thing for Bill."

It wasn't long before Jake and I received an email from Bill's sister, Jane, in which she reiterated her old song about wishing that Bill would "take responsibility for something." She refused to sign and claimed that the petition "makes Bill a victim and doesn't lead to any realistic action now." She then proceeded to ask for help to dispose of Bill's belongings. Taking the stance of a commanding general, she said Jake was to go through Bill's stuff and decide what could be thrown away and, as for me, "your part would be to gain Bill's cooperation in the form of permission." In other words, Jake and I were to victimize Bill even further by revoking his choice about his property and conning him into giving his consent. I didn't respond to the email.

Soon I received another email from Jane saying that Jake had agreed to sort through Bill's stuff and again asking for me to convince Bill to allow Jake to do so. She ended the letter with "I am sorry I did not start with saying thank you for all you have done and do to help Bill." Again, I did not respond.

Then I got an email from Jake in which he asked, "Why do I get the feeling Jane doesn't really give a hoot about Bill? Does she not have a dictionary to look up the meaning of 'victim?'" He said he had agreed to sort through Bill's stuff only because he was trying to be helpful but now he was having second thoughts. "I could never presume to know what Bill thinks can be tossed or should be saved. And without a detailed list from him, well, I doubt I'd ever try to make those kinds of decisions."

A few days later, Jake traveled down to a small town south of

Northfield where Gary Tollefson owned a rental storage facility. Gary was even more obese than his older brother and was known as a "big shot developer" in the area. Bill said that, after he ran for mayor, people would come up to him and tell him that he should have run under an assumed name rather than be associated with his distrusted wheeler-dealer brother.

Jane had informed Jake that Bill's belongings were stored there but when Jake asked Gary about the property, he said he didn't know anything about it and wasn't sure where the property was located. Gary told Jake that he was trying to distance himself from the whole thing but then proceeded to tell him how important it would be for Jake to go through Bill's things and decide what was trash and what should be saved. Jake told Gary he didn't have a truck and couldn't take any of the stuff and Gary responded, "Don't worry, I can haul it all to the dump and burn a lot of it."

Jake continued, "Almost everything he said sounded a little fishy. He probably just wants to rent out the storage area for more money to someone else. I told him that you had his power of attorney and were in contact with Bill a lot. He then told me that Bill has this Dr. Otis wrapped around his little finger (better check your little finger). I think I'll forget about Gary and Jane. I won't be going through the stuff just to keep them happy."

I wrote back to Jake, "I think Jane and Gary are two peas in a pod. I guess Gary really likes to haul Bill's stuff to the dump. I don't think Bill will ever forgive him for having thrown him out of the home he shared with his mother.

"I checked my little finger and didn't see Bill there! I'm sure the two of them are rationalizing their immoral treatment of their big brother. They don't seem to want to acknowledge that the major issue is one of civil/human rights and has little to do with whether Bill drank too much or acted like a jerk at times or even a lot of the time. Bill said he told Jane she would think differently if she had her life destroyed by an impersonal, heartless system. I don't think she has a clue what he is talking about! I think your decision to stay out of the sorting business is a good one."

When I next talked with Bill he was still depressed but somewhat objective about it, which gave me some hope. He said he had voiced to Dr. Smart that it felt like his "mainspring" was broken (he was using a pre-digital watch metaphor; he was *not* having an hallucination) and the doctor responded that he probably had a "functional depression," meaning that his disphoric mood was due to all the crap that had happened to him and the lousy circumstances he found himself in. Bill added, "There have just been too many negatives. I try to get my mind in a peaceful spot by meditation or prayer, but then some memory hits me and I lose it. They have destroyed my life." The anger triggered by intrusive memories made me think less of depression than of Post-traumatic Stress Disorder, a condition I had seen a lot of when I worked in a Veterans Administration facility.

Bill continued, "Both the hospital and the nursing home were supposed to be getting aquatic therapy for me but I see no evidence of it." I recalled Dr. Smart, writing before he left, that the social workers at the hospital and the nursing home would be "aggressively pursuing" aquatic therapy for Bill after he left the hospital. It probably would take threat of imminent legal action in order to get that to happen.

Jake visited Bill and reported, "He's depressed and I could barely hear him when he talked. His room is small, like a big walk-in closet. He has to share the bathroom with the room next door. Right now he has to use a portable john because he can't walk or stand as his right ankle is shot and he's afraid to put any weight on it. His roommate still uses the floor as a urinal. His right shoulder looks like it is almost disjointed and he takes Tylenol 3 every six hours. He perked up a little bit after about an hour and even smiled like his old self."

I wrote back to Jake, "That sounds worse than I had imagined! They did the shoulder thing to him in the hospital. The ankle thing is new and even more reason that he should be getting aquatic therapy. I'm bringing my camera over there when I visit and will document everything I can. I talked with him today just after you left. His voice sounded stronger but he admitted to being depressed. Who wouldn't be depressed living in a pigsty, unable to walk and with a fucked-up shoulder!"

My wife and I traveled to Minnesota in mid-September to attend my 55th high school reunion. We stayed with my wife's sister and brother-in-law and borrowed their car to go over to see Bill. We were directed to his room on the second floor and found him close to the nurses station. The room was dark and Bill's portion, maybe a quarter to one third of the floor space, was curtained off from that of his roommate. Behind the curtain pushed up against the wall was Bill's bed, situated over a heat register. A single armless metal chair was restrained by the bed on one side and the curtain on the other. His "closet" was against the wall outside the curtain and was filled with unopened boxes brought from the hospital. I sat on the end of the bed with a view of his roommate urinating in the bathroom. Bill, sitting in his wheelchair, blocked my view so I couldn't tell if his roommate was using the toilet or the floor as the receptacle for his precious bodily fluid.

Bill had cleared it with all the nurses so that we could take him over to the nearest Walmart and get him some new shoes. He was wearing a pair of battered white tennis shoes with a hole in one that he proudly showed us he could put two fingers through. He had been wearing them since he was jerked out of his apartment many months ago and wore them throughout the Minnesota winter. He had mentioned his foot discomfort to his captors at various points along the way, but no one saw fit to get him an unventilated pair of shoes. His guardians and the nursing staff continued the tradition. My wife and I looked at each other, mouths agape in "What the fuck!" disbelief.

We went down to the ground floor and out the front door, Bill greeting people he knew along the way. Once outside, I brought the car up so that we could get Bill and his wheelchair loaded. About that time, a middle aged woman and a tall young man wearing a yarmulke appeared and started yelling at Bill that he could not leave the facility. Bill got agitated and asked for their paperwork that gave them the right to restrict his movements. They ignored his question and kept asserting that he was not allowed to leave. The tall young man, a newly hired social worker, didn't say much and deferred to the older woman to carry on the rant. My wife and I got into the act and asked on what authority they were preventing Bill from going for a ride with his friends. The woman said something about needing a doctor's order for him to leave the premises. I asked who his doctor was and she said she did not know off-hand, that she would have to look it up. They continued their harangue of Bill and Bill kept asking for them to go get the papers that legitimized their demand.

Finally the huge gentleman in the wheelchair made a large sweeping motion with his outstretched arms, starting at the pair from the nursing home and ending behind his wheelchair. At the same time he said in a loud deep voice something like, "Out, damned demons. Get thee behind me. Amen." Everyone was silent for a few moments. I was ready to call it quits and try to find someone above these two clowns in the chain of command. Bill would have none of it and continued to ask them to bring the documentation that they had the right to keep him restricted to the facility grounds. Finally they disappeared into the building. A short time later, they returned and said that whoever they talked to had told them they had no objection to Bill going for a ride in the metropolitan area as long as he returned within a reasonable time.

The matter settled, and the Hounds of the Baskervilles at bay, we loaded Bill and his wheelchair into the Outback and headed for Walmart.

Bill was absolutely gleeful. He was laughing and joking and saying how delightful it was to be with friends and be free of the confines of the hell-hole where he lived. He had not been away from the institution since he arrived and got his bearings by spotting landmarks familiar to him when he lived and worked in Minneapolis. After a while I said to him, "Jeez, Bill, it sounded back there like you were casting out demons."

I glanced over and Bill had that old jokester glint in his eye. "I was. And it worked, didn't it?" All three of us burst into laughter.

"Yeah, I guess it worked alright," I said.

We drove to Walmart and Bill made his way to the shoe department while I went to the bathroom and my wife looked for something she needed. I met Bill as he was picking out the largest pair of shoes they had in stock that met his criteria. He rolled around in the store looking for some other items he needed, like a scissors to cut his beard and a watch to replace the one that had been stolen at the United Hospital in St. Paul, all the time basking in his first opportunity, in the better part of a year, to act like a normal human being. We took the long way back and Bill showed a remarkable memory for places and events from his better times living in the Twin Cities. Bill didn't want to return to "Golden Liver" but he accepted his fate and was still in a good frame of mind when we arrived. We all embraced before we departed and wished each other well.

I told many people at the reunion what had happened to Bill, since nearly everyone knew him, and they were duly horrified by the tale of injustice. Everyone I related the story to would get that look in their eye as they remembered some family member or friend who could have met with a similar fate.

Jane arrived in Minnesota for a visit to a relative who was ill just after my visit. Bill tried to get her to help him get down to Northfield so he could search his stuff for his lost seat cushion and see what items had been stolen but she refused. He then told her not to bother coming seeing him and she didn't. He thought she had just come to Minnesota to see a sick friend and not to see Bill. He told me that he was still having problems with his legs swelling and causing pain.

A short time later I got a call from Bill. He was in Hennepin County Medical Center and said that he was having a recurrence of pain in his legs, like that he had experienced before when he was taken to St. Joseph's Hospital. The people at the nursing home refused to give him the phone number for HCMC until he threatened to call the sheriff, at which point they relented. Then he arranged for transportation and was taken to the hospital. There, like at St. Joseph's, his legs were treated with Lasix, vincomycin and leg elevation, after they ruled out deep vein thrombosis by an ultrasound examination. He did talk with one of the doctors at the hospital about being referred to their hyperbaric chamber for treatment and was told he had to get past a committee but had a good chance of being accepted because they were using the equipment 24/7.

After a few days of treatment, Bill's legs improved and he expected to be returning to what he called "The Mouse House" (because there was a mouse living on his floor at GLC). But, of course, things could not go off without some drama thrown into the mix. Bill had gotten into some kind of tangle with a Dr. High, who he thought was being autocratic and demeaning toward him. He said to her, "Dr. High, you are really low," to which comment she did not take kindly. Dr. High called me and tried to badger me into getting Bill into line. When I didn't simply roll over and yield to her demands but instead asked her what Bill had said to her, she got so angry she had to turn the phone over to a nurse, who tried a more reasoned approach. She claimed Bill had left GLC without a reserved room. This turned out not to be true since Bill had been in contact with the nurses on his floor every day since he went to the hospital. Finally, Bill had a meeting with Dr. High and the patient advocate and things were smoothed over so he could return to the nursing home. But the chances of him ever getting referred to the hyperbaric chamber were reduced to nil. Doctors can be a very vindictive lot, even if a person's life is at stake.

Shortly after Bill was placed at Golden Living Center in St. Louis Park, he asked me to see what I could find out on the Internet about Beverly Corporation, the company that previously owned the nursing home in which he was placed. The Google search turned up some web sites that made what little of my hair that I still retain, stand on end. Much of the history of the Beverly Corporation is taken from an excellent article by Eric Bates titled "The Shame of Our Nursing Homes" that appeared in the March 29, 1999 issue of *The Nation*. Additional information is from a set of web pages called Corporate Health Care (http://www.bmartin.cc/dissent/documents/health/central.html) authored by Michael Wynne. It has several pages dealing with the Beverly Corporation.

Back in the nineteenth century communities regularly auctioned off the poor, infirm, and elderly to families who provided sparse shelter and required their charges to do arduous work. There was profit in it and therefore communities began to operate their own poorhouses or poor farms for those that did not have families to care for them. I remember having my dad point out to me the old "County Poor Farm" as we used to drive to Minneapolis on the old two-lane highway.

In order to keep people of refinement, who had no choice but to be placed in such institutions, from having to associate with the assorted riff-raft that were sent there, reformers began to protest overcrowding and unsanitary conditions in such facilities. The scandals lead to a push to privatize care of the impoverished. The 1935 Social Security Act prohibited payments to anyone in the now disgraced public facilities, thereby providing a huge financial incentive to the new private nursing home industry.

The federal government provided low-interest loans for construction of private nursing homes and made direct payments to them rather than to the individual beneficiaries, making for an immediate and bountiful profit. Medicare and Medicaid, which came along in 1965, supplied a great amount of relatively unrestricted public money for private nursing homes. The nursing homes were reimbursed for mortgages, depreciation, staff and supplies, thus insuring a good return for those who invested in them. Multinational corporations jumped in and by 1969 the number of nursing homes had nearly doubled from the prior two years. Nursing home chains gobbled up competitors and increased profits by cutting staff and wages and increasing the number of patients as well as behind the scenes tactics like swapping properties between subsidiaries to increase costs and therefore reimbursements.

Beverly Corporation was the earliest to arrive on the scene and was the largest, acquiring 1000 homes in less than 10 years. In the early 1980's their average return on investment was 23% but they expanded too quickly and by 1987 had to start selling off properties to prevent a hostile takeover. They moved from California to Arkansas where they were befriended by Governor Bill Clinton and his wife, Hillary, who was working at Rose Law Firm at the time. The company managed to get state approval of $81 million in tax-free revenue bonds which would have allowed them to pay off a lot of debt. However, the governor backed away when his attorney general, Steve Clark, took a courageous stand and refused a bribe from Beverly, publicly calling it "the product of the arrogance of wealth and the arrogance of power." The deal collapsed.

Beverly, like other private nursing homes of the time, relied on Medicare and Medicaid payments for the majority of its income and cut costs by skimping on patient care, number of staff members and staff wages. Some homes had only one registered nurse on duty at any one time and relied on minimally trained and minimally paid nurse's aides or Certified Nurse Assistants to do all the direct patient care. In Arkansas, nursing home lobbyists slipped an amendment into a 1997 funding bill that required taxpayers to reimburse nursing homes for up to as much as

$17 million for any increase in the minimum wage. The state legislature overrode Governor Mike Huckabee's veto.

The nursing home companies made a lot of money on their so-called "ancillary services." These included drugs and medical supplies, which the company bought at a huge discount and billed the government at retail rates. It also included speech therapy, physical therapy/rehabilitation and occupational therapy, also billed at figures substantially above cost. Medicare billings across the industry for such services rose by a factor of six (to $7 billion) in just three years from 1990 to 1993. Beverly Corporation was among those companies that created subsidiary businesses to exploit these sources of revenue from the hapless taxpayers. According to an internal company report, Beverly made a hefty return on their investment in rehabilitative services in the first eleven months of 1994: $671 million on a cost of $360 million.

Another company tactic was to prevent its employees from unionizing to negotiate for better conditions. The General Accounting Office said Beverly was one of the worst violators of labor laws and the National Labor Relations Board cited the company for 240 violations of labor laws in 18 states. The company used threats, coercion and unwarranted surveillance of its employees. It is not surprising, then, that annual staff turnover approached 100%.

As a result of their management practices, official reports soon began coming in about health hazards and squalid living conditions, gaping wounds and infected bedsores and deaths due to negligence or errors in Beverly nursing homes. Grand jury investigations, suspended Medicaid payments, large fines, and prohibitions against opening any new homes were instigated against the company in Texas, California, Washington State, Maine and Missouri. Investigators determined that at least eight patients in Beverly nursing homes died as a result of negligent care in Minnesota between 1986 and 1988 and nine deaths in California lead to a fine and probation for the company.

Some of the stories were pretty gory. One woman was found to have ants swarming over her body and entering her respiratory system through a wound in her throat. An octogenarian with difficulty swallowing choked to death after being fed solid food in spite of a doctor's order to feed her only soft foods. Another older woman died from a heart attack after suffering for three hours before a doctor was called. Ignoring a doctor's orders, a patient was left unattended and suffered a skull fracture after falling off a toilet. A nursing aide dropped a patient, fracturing the person's hip and shoulder, when trying to move her without bothering to ask for assistance. A resident complained of foot pain for 43 days before her foot rotted off her leg. A woman died of an infected bone-deep bedsore the size of a grapefruit. Another woman had to be rushed to the hospital after she was given an overdose of a medication even though the staff had been warned about her inability to tolerate it.

Not content with profits from the industry-wide rip-off of Medicare and Medicaid, Beverly executives got a bright idea: why not charge the government what is good for our bottom line rather than just for the costs we can legitimately claim? After all, they trust us when we send in our counts of the time we devote to Medicare and non-Medicare patients. So, let's just tell the direct-care nurses to pencil in their time sheets with their total time, omitting the distinction between Medicare and non-Medicare patients. Then we will have the Corporate Vice President for that part of the country direct the regional administrator to relay a "targeted number of weighted hours" for Medicare patients to the facility administrator who will, in turn, send those figures to the Director of Nursing who, if she wants to keep her job, will erase the penciled-in numbers and put in the targeted number of hours on the time sheets. What kind of people would come up with this kind of scheme? Mr. Wynne dubs them "successful sociopaths."

Well, luckily there are still a few honest people left in the world and the one who brought down the Beverly empire of fraud was named Domenic Todarello. He worked for Beverly for three years before filing a qui tam action under the False Claims Act in federal court in the state of Arizona. The False Claims Act was passed after the Civil War with the intent of curbing the number of fraudulent claims by individuals who invented government obligations to them. According to its terms, the false claimant is typically required to pay back the sum defrauded plus three times that amount as damages and the "whistleblower" who notifies the government of the crime is entitled to 17% of the recovered funds plus expenses. Because of the False Claims Act and the increase in health care fraud, private citizen whistleblowers had helped the government recover $3.5 billion by the year 2000 according to one article, almost half being in the prior two and one half years. The government collected $1.5 billion in fiscal year 2000 alone!

Together, Todarello and the government claimed that Beverly had provided the Health Care Financing Administration with false claims, records, and statements for the purpose of obtaining payments of $460 million under Medicare and Medicaid programs while using phony time sheets to deceive Medicare auditors. Behind closed doors, the company worked out a deal with the government to settle for $175 million, at that time the largest settlement in any health care suit. But, obviously, this is much smaller than the amount of the claimed fraud, let alone three times that amount which is the traditional penalty under the False Claims Act. Mr. Todarello was to receive $30 million plus $103,000 in expenses.

Not only would Beverly Corporation not have to turn over their last five years of profit, they only had to pay $25 million within a month and pay the balance over eight years by a reduction of $697,000 from each of their 26 annual payments from Medicare. They were also required to hire an independent auditor and submit to extensive monitoring by the Department of Health and Human Services for nine years or the length of time they were obligated to make payments.

Another collusion with the government prosecutors allowed them a clever way of avoiding corporate responsibility for the criminal aspect of the plea bargain. Criminals are by law banned from doing business with Medicare. So what they agreed to was that Beverly would select 10 proxy nursing homes to be the guilty ones - and then sell them!

Adding to their woes, two Beverly shareholders filled a class-action law suit claiming that the company had schemed to inflate billings to Medicare while at the same time telling investors they were within the law and in good financial health. This gross mismanagement of the company was said to be in violation of state and federal securities laws. The suit asserted that shareholders suffered over $1 billion in lost market capitalization while executive officers received millions in wasteful bonuses, stock options and awards based on inflated financial figures between 1990 and 1997.

In 2005 Beverly Corporation put itself up for auction. A group of investors bought it and turned it into a private company, changing their name a few times to try to escape the stink of their bad reputation, finally settling on the name "Golden Living Corporation." However they still maintain a web site whose address retains the original company name at www.beverlycares.com.

If you go to that site you will find that they have six subsidiaries that provide what they like to call "integrated treatment." Their nursing homes are contained in a subsidiary called *Golden Living Centers*. They have 300 locations in 21 states. Twenty-eight of them are in Minnesota, including the one where Bill was placed in St. Louis Park, a suburb of Minneapolis.

Another subsidiary, *Golden Living Communities*, is composed of 16 assisted living residences for individuals who need some minimal help with light housekeeping and preparing meals but are otherwise able to live independently.

AseraCare Home Health is Golden Living's home health care

subsidiary for people who can stay in their own homes but need help that can't be provided by family members. This includes as-needed services from registered nurses or nursing assistants and social workers.

Additional therapy of various types, e. g., physical, occupational, joint replacement, and speech therapy, can be provided on both an inpatient and outpatient basis at the patient's home or in a Golden Living Center or a Golden Living Community facility by another subsidiary, *Aegis Therapies*. They claim to have expertise in balance management, fall prevention, cognitive skills, incontinence management and other medical problems.

If all else fails, *Asera Care Hospice* can ease the transition to a dead state of being. This subsidiary focuses on dampening the patient's physical and the family's emotional pain as the dying one leaves this mortal coil.

To help keep a constant supply of low cost, part-time health care workers while avoiding the pesky matter of unions, Golden Living has its *360 Healthcare Staffing* subsidiary. It claims to be a leader in "per diem, travel, temp-to-hire, and direct placement job placements." If you can't get hired full time at a legitimate health care facility with genuine employee benefits, try this place.

Finally, there is *Ceres Purchasing Solutions*, the Golden Living medical supply and pharmacy subsidiary. Actually, it is an intermediary between the health care provider and the vendors of medical supplies and devices and pharmaceuticals. Being a volume purchaser, they can buy low and sell for whatever the market (or Medicare or Medicaid) will bear and they have a ready market in all the Golden Living nursing homes, assisted living residences and hospice facilities. While they claim it offers providers better control over spending, it actually offers them the opportunity for sharing greater profits with Golden Living Corporation.

Let's imagine this scenario. An elderly or infirm person needs help with some basic activities of living. A family member calls AseraCare Home Health and they send out one or more therapists or aides to help out. If the person's level of functioning deteriorates, he or she might be sent to Golden Living Communities for assisted living. If the patient can't hack it in that environment, he or she might be sent to a Golden Living Center for nursing care. If the patient becomes terminal, he or she can be sent to Asera Care Hospice. All along the way, Aegis Therapies is providing whatever therapies can be justified and drugs are being purchased by the care givers through Ceres Purchasing Solutions while therapy and medications are being administered by part-time employees hired through 360 Healthcare Staffing. If the person somehow manages to improve, the procedure can be reversed. The person can be sent from Golden Living Center back to their Golden Living Community, from Golden Living Community back to their home but, of course, with services from AseraCare Home Health. Integrated care – quite a business model!

Beverly Corporation claimed that Medicaid and Medicare reimbursement rates were so low that adequate care and appropriate staffing could not be provided. This did not prevent them from posting the eighth highest profit margin nationwide. Golden Living Centers has continued the same lament as recently as 2011 when there was a threatened 11% cut in Medicare rates. A director of a Golden Living Center in Pennsylvania asserted that they lost $7000 per year on Medicaid patients. It is probably all rhetoric but, because of their "creative accounting" procedures, it is difficult to determine the actual state of affairs. One commentator said, "They have a set of books that show they're losing money on one side, and yet they're making money hand over fist on the other side."

The rapidly rising costs of nursing home care has spurred Congress to move federal health care programs into managed care, thus putting a cap on program costs. However, this does not improve care and may even make it worse. Elma Holder of the Citizens Coalition said of the nursing home corporations, "The less you spend, the more you make."

A recent (January 11, 2012) article in the Minneapolis Star Tribune by Paul Walsh suggests that the name change has done nothing to bring about any changes in the practices at Golden Living Centers. The Hopkins Golden Living Center is just a few miles from the St. Louis Park Golden Living Center where Bill was a resident and it has a better rating by Medicare: "below average" instead of "very below average." Yet this facility was charged with negligence in the death of a man under their care when the staff failed to monitor his weight and nutritional status for two months. Although the county medical examiner determined the primary cause of death to be pneumonia, inspectors found that dehydration and malnutrition contributed to his 30 pound weight loss. Nursing home staff did not evaluate his fluid levels or weight loss or notify his doctor. They cited a "breakdown in facility systems."

So let's see now. Why is it that Bill doesn't seem to be getting the medical care he needs?

10 <u>THE COMPETENT NEED NOT APPLY</u>

Bill had a burning sore on his backside, apparently caused or aggravated by the absence of adequate cushioning in his wheelchair. His legs were swollen and the muscles were bulging out. I didn't like the sound of that, as it seemed like a worsening of his condition. Penelope, the good nurse on the ward, got some kind of OTC salve with aloe in it along with a Teflon bandage so that it wouldn't tear the skin when he took down his pants to go to the toilet.

Thinking he might be able to make do with his old seat cushion, Bill inquired of the manager of his brother's storage facility whether or not he could look for something medically necessary, like his old wheelchair cushion. She said the rule was he could look but couldn't take anything. So Bill ordered a new seat cushion through a medical supplier, but the order never went through. The medical supplier didn't tell Bill there was a problem so Bill just waited for it to arrive. When it didn't show up, he called the supplier who told him that Rice County said he was no longer a resident of their county and refused to pay for it. The state hospital at Anoka had, apparently, screwed up his residency status when he was placed in the first Golden Living Center and had it listed as Ramsey County. Now, he had to apply to Hennepin County for medical assistance, including medical supplies, and he would have to wait for that to go through before he could get any relief from the pain in his back side.

Trying to get some more immediate help, Bill managed to get an appointment with his old physician in Faribault and arranged for transportation to and fro with a company that he had used successfully for years, one owned by one of my former high school classmates. I was surprised that Golden Liver had allowed him to go, considering the fuss they had made when we wanted to take him to Walmart and their resistance to him going for medical treatment during an emergency. But then I thought maybe they were chastened when he had gotten himself admitted and treated at HCMC. I figured that they didn't want to be embarrassed (or sued) if he croaked or got sick and they were found to have once again obstructed his medical care or didn't do anything to help.

The visit with the doctor went well and she was impressed with the fact that his blood pressure was 110/65. He informed her that it had stabilized in this range after he had stopped taking all of his blood pressure medications, except in the event he should experience atrial fibrillation, which had not happened for a long time. She told him she would refer him to a chiropractor and arrange for him to be seen at the Mayo Clinic in Rochester.

Bill was still in pretty good spirits since our visit and after this appointment. Jake visited and found him in good form. "I got there about 1:20 and they were just getting started with lunch because problems in the kitchen made them late. One of the servers spilled a large metal container full of water on the floor. Bill then shouted out, 'Food fight! Hand me the mustard!' I got a good laugh out of that and so did Bill, but we were the only two people in the room laughing. It's a pretty glum atmosphere around there. I think a lot of medical problems take away the joy. I had an old book of Henny Youngman one-liners, jokes, and bar tricks that I gave to Bill to read. I was going to bring some light bar bells so he could do arm exercises, but I forgot. Bill told me he was going to see if he could get rides to Northfield so that he could use the pool at the senior center for exercise, as he had done for several years.

"While Bill ate, I took a hike around the neighborhood. Nice big park a couple blocks West. Eight tennis courts, two ball parks, and a lot of open space. In the open space I counted 82 Canadian Honkers. Bill showed me a reimbursement check for $296 from the state hospital for property of his that was stolen or lost while he was in the hospital."

Being an extravert, Bill always enjoyed meeting new people and talking with them about their lives. At Golden Liver, most of the tales were horror stories. One of the people he met was a member of the Northfield class that had graduated a couple of years after Bill. She had given her house to her daughter who then proceeded to have her evicted and that resulted in her becoming a resident in the nursing home. Jake knew her from grade school and high school and planned to say hello when he visited next time. Another was a man with a physical disability that made it difficult for him to communicate. The staff would park him in a corner all day and ignore him. Bill managed to establish contact with the man and learned that he had been a swimming champ for my wife's former high school in Hopkins.

On the plus side, Bill's increased activity allowed him to find a small raised garden plot where he could tend and try to resuscitate some tomato and pepper plants remaining from the growing season. He would fill a plastic jug with water and push his wheelchair to the plot where he provided sustenance to the drought-stricken plants. As he was about to harvest the fruits of his endeavors, someone stole the dwarf vegetables he had produced. But he was philosophical about it, considering it to be an experiment, and he was pleased that he had been able to work with the plants and be outside.

Browsing around the facility, Bill discovered a large shower stall and secured the permission of the staff for him to use it. However, for some reason it was required that he be accompanied to and from the shower, and the ward staff to whom that duty fell apparently did not like to do it. So when Bill would ask to take a shower, the guy would disappear or pretend he was occupied with something more important. Bill would have to pester the staff for as long as ten days or more before he could get a shower. When I asked him what they guy's name was, Bill refused to answer because he feared retaliation if the man was called on the carpet. Such are the kinds of games played in "total institutions" that were described so well by Irving Goffman and others back in the 1960's.

Bill believed that the same social worker and nurse who had thrown the fit when my wife and I had visited, were trying to set him up for accusations that he was trying to smuggle a weapon into the place. They had taken him and several other residents out to the Dollar Store to do some shopping and Bill had asked one of the women who were acting as their wardens to hand him a folding knife from the wall display, since he couldn't reach it from his wheelchair. She didn't say anything about this item until he got up to the check-out stand. Then she would not allow the purchase. The next day, the social worker accused him of having tried to steal a cap at the store but Bill explained that he had left the cap at the check-out counter because it was too small.

In spite of his explanations, Bill was excluded from any more group shopping trips. He told me that the people at the nursing home were preventing him from going to Goodwill on a trip open to all nursing home residents. They previously had prevented him from going to Target. When I asked what reason they gave him, he said they told him "because we don't want you to go." Bill said that someone in the nursing home put some kind of alarm device on his wheelchair for when he left the building. He tore two of them off and they installed another one which he also tore off. Who, if anyone, gave them the authority to do that is a good question. I didn't think it could be legal. Later, when Bill brought the matter up in court, they would lie about it, saying they had never heard of that happening.

Bill finally agreed it was time to file for Restoration of Capacity. I sent an email to "Whimp" Zimbledon, his court-appointed attorney, indicating that this was his client's desire and that Bill might also like to talk with him about the disposition of property that had been confiscated from his former HUD financed apartment. I sent copies to Jake and Big Jim just in case he decided to ignore my email. It wasn't long before Zimbledon responded with an email saying that he had sent Bill the forms necessary for filing for a change in legal status. This action, if it were to go through, would free him of the control of his guardians.

State law regarding guardianships is codified in Minnesota Statutes 524.5. Guardians are appointed and removed by the court and have their powers and limitations granted by the court. The court *must* consider whether less restrictive alternatives are available to assist the ward and is allowed to grant to the guardian *only* those powers required by the ward's limitations and needs. The court is supposed to encourage development of self reliance in the ward.

A "court visitor" is required to file a report about the appropriateness of the guardianship which is to include information about the availability of less restrictive means of intervention and the limitations on the powers to be granted to the guardian.

Each year the guardian is required to file a report on the well-being of the ward including his or her current mental, physical, and social condition, and the medical, educational, vocational, and other services provided to the ward. The report is supposed to list the assets of the ward's estate being controlled by the guardian as well as the receipts, disbursements and distributions during the year and must include the amount of reimbursement for services rendered to the ward that the guardian received during the previous year that were not reimbursed by county contract. The ward and interested persons of record with the court *must* be provided with a copy of the report and may dispute statements or conclusions regarding the condition of the ward that are contained in the report and may petition the court for an order that is in the best interests of the ward. Every year the guardian is required to send to the ward a notice of the right to request termination or modification of the guardianship.

The 2011 revision of the law contains a *Bill of Rights for Wards and Protected Persons* in Statute 524.5-120. The rights specified in the law include the right to treatment with dignity and respect as well as the right to timely and appropriate health care and medical treatment, and services "individually suited" to the ward's conditions and needs.

Decisions made by guardians are supposed to give due consideration to the ward's current and previously stated personal desires, medical treatment preferences and religious beliefs. The ward is to be allowed to exercise control of all aspects of life not specifically delegated by court order to the guardian. The ward has the right to petition the court to initiate or prevent a change in abode. The ward has the right to receive, among other things, rehabilitation care and services "within available resources."

The ward is supposed to be consulted regarding the disposition of his or her property and has the right to object to a guardian's plans regarding such property. The ward has the right to execute both health care instructions and the appointment of a health care agent, unless the court has granted a guardian those powers or duties. The Bill of Rights does not indicate whether or not the court has the right to abrogate any health care directives or appointment of health care agent made prior to the person becoming a ward of the state. I later learned that the State House of Representatives House Research Department had addressed this very point and ruled that earlier arrangements could not be superseded by appointment of a guardian (although, like other laws, the court could just ignore them). The ward has the right to be represented by an attorney in any proceeding or for the purpose of petitioning the court. I would take this to mean that a court-appointed attorney would not be allowed to arbitrarily deny services to a ward who wants to petition the court.

Of course the *Bill of Rights for Wards and Protected Persons*, like the *Bill of Rights for Institutionalized Persons* and the *U.S. Bill of Rights*, can be ignored by those who think they are above the law. All it takes is for the judges and the lawyers to keep the defendant in the dark and avoid asking the kind of questions that would bring up embarrassing issues regarding "rights." Cindi Fisher told me of a case in which she and a friend acted as audience-based witnesses at a guardianship hearing in Oregon recently. The 77 year old woman, who lived on a small farm in southern Oregon, was transported by her guardian to a group home some 300 miles away from her support system of family and friends while her farm and possessions were sold off and the proceeds placed under the control of the guardian. Cindi learned that the guardian had 112 clients, charged $100/hour for her services and grossed $349,000 last year. In her business, the guardian used the same $300/hour law firm (touting themselves as specializing in the protection and safety of the elderly) for all her wards and often used the same judge. Cindi had also heard of a person who was charging $4800/month for housing Alzheimer patients in the converted second story of his barn in rural Colorado. Thus, it is apparent that there can be a lot of financial incentives for guardians to get and keep wards in the system.

In 1987 a group of Associated Press reporters reviewed 2200 case files for a six-part investigative series on guardianships. They found that judges were forcing people into guardianships without giving them access to attorneys or legal hearings and often simply because they were old and alleged to be spending money foolishly. And often there were no measures taken to prevent guardians from abusing and stealing from the people they were supposed to protect. The newspaper series lead to congressional hearings, legislative reforms, and new laws which were supposed to ensure due process and closer monitoring by the courts. Judges were supposed to rely on person's actual competencies to handle tasks of daily life rather than easily bandied about labels like senile and incompetent.

Despite the cosmetic changes, monitoring of guardianships remained lax and reports filed by guardians received little real examination if they were read at all. In November of 2001 elder law specialists from the American Bar Association, the National Academy of Elder Law Attorneys, ARRP and the National College of Probate Judges met to recommend changes in state laws and courtroom practices and guardian qualifications and requirements. For example, long time reformer Sally Hurme of AARP proclaimed that guardians and conservators were supposed to implement the wishes, preferences and values of the ward. "They are not supposed to play God. They are not supposed to impose their wishes or preferences on the individual."

However these recommendations were never widely put into effect. An article in the August 17, 2011 issue of the Minneapolis Star Tribune by Brad Schrade and Lora Pabst indicated that Minnesota treats neglect of a vulnerable adult as a misdemeanor and is one of only five states that do not have a felony level penalty for such crimes. In six cases of the 50 since 2004 that the authors reviewed, the victims died and many other "outrageous" cases which they cited resulted in injury and hospitalization.

The extent to which the guardianship system can be perverted is evident in a 2010 study by the General Accounting Office. Between 1990 and 2010 they received hundreds of reported allegations of physical abuse, neglect and financial exploitation by guardians in 45 states and the District of Columbia. Their informants included 16 advocacy groups, news reports, family members, concerned citizens, and legal professionals such as prosecutors, attorneys and investigators. In 20 closed cases, they found that guardians from diverse professional backgrounds had improperly obtained $5.4 million in assets from 158 incapacitated victims, many of whom were senior citizens. In 60% of the cases the courts failed to monitor guardians once they were appointed and in 30% of the cases individuals with criminal convictions or significant financial problems were not identified in the screening process. Abuse and exploitation was allowed to continue in 55% of the cases because the courts did not communicate effectively with federal agencies. In none of the four states where GAO used fictitious identities to apply for guardianship certification did the courts or state certification agencies bother to check credit history or validate Social Security numbers of the phony applicants.

The cases reported by the GAO sound strangely similar to the nursing home abuses of the 1980's and 1990's, the primary difference being that the guardians' financial exploitation and misappropriation of assets is small-time compared to the big-time corporate fraud of the nursing homes. Public guardians caring for an 88-year-old California woman sold her properties below market value to a relative of the guardian and a city employee. Family members had to have the police help track her down because the guardians surreptitiously moved her into various nursing homes. By the time they found her, the woman's leg had to be amputated at the hip because of infected bed sores.

In New York, a lawyer serving as a court appointed guardian stole $4 million from 23 seniors suffering from mental and physical impairments and from children suffering from cerebral palsy due to medical malpractice.

An elderly Texas couple were both declared incompetent and placed in a nursing home after the husband broke his hip. The court-appointed guardians allowed the couple to have a TV set and $60 per month allowance but no personal belongings. They let the couple's house go into foreclosure, let their car be repossessed and let their credit rating go into the sewer.

A Texas probate judge was appointed guardian for a 91 year old woman in 2001 and, after 40 years with the same will, she was convinced to change it so as to give the judge, his personal accountant and the court-appointed attorney $250,000.

A former case manager in the public guardian's office in Nevada decided to start her own guardianship business and was accused of lifting $200,000 from her wards to support her gambling habit.

Guardian, Inc. had three of their officials sentenced to prison in 1999 and 2000 for embezzlement and fraud with hundreds of clients. They once sold a house in a historic neighborhood for $500 to a mother of one of the company officers and collected fees as high as 70% from wards' small Social Security checks.

At least two organizations are now crusading to reduce guardianship abuse. *Boomers Against Elder Abuse* has a presence on Facebook and tries to raise awareness of the problem in the general public. They list, at current count, 180 cases of abuse that interested parties can read and validate.

The *National Association to Stop Guardianship Abuse* (stopguardianabuse.org), started by a group of concerned citizens with first hand experience with the horrors of the system (coordinated by Linda Kincaid), considers guardianship abuse the worst form of elder abuse. They are advocating for reform and a *Guardianship Bill of Rights*. They are asking government representatives (and the public) such questions as: "Why is it legal to abuse and rob the elderly in guardianships? Why is it legal to force an 'alleged' incapacitated person into a guardianship with an emergency or some other hearing without due process of the law where the ward is not present and/or not represented by counsel? Why are our constitutional due process rights under the 14th amendment not protected in guardianships? Why is it legal to isolate a ward, to over-medicate, to chemically restrain, to sterilize, and even authorize an early death through hospice in guardianships? Why do the advance directives of these dear elderly citizens appear to mean nothing? The designation of a pre-need guardian, a power of attorney, or health care surrogate are routinely ignored in the incapacity process. Why is it legal for one person (a judge) to give one human being to another private citizen (the guardian), then walk away, and let that person have their way with the incapacitated person and their estate? Why are there no jury trials?"

NASGA asserts that hundreds of family members suffer from litigation abuse, character assassination, defamation, slander and liable if they try to fight the court appointed guardian. The court will claim that the family members or friends "have no standing" meaning that they have no legitimate "interest" in the case. The court may even deny them the right to visit their loved ones. They think that many family members and friends of a loved one have post-traumatic stress disorder as a result of the abuse they suffer at the hands of the court. Others live with a silent rage or suffer physically and emotionally. In addition, once the guardian has bled their ward's estate dry, they dump the ward on the state so that the government picks up the tab for their care.

The U.S. Census Bureau projects that the number of Americans 65 years old and older will increase by 60% by the year 2025. That will increase the number of physically and mentally impaired seniors, and particularly those who live alone, who require help in carrying out some of the everyday tasks in living, in handling their finances and in managing their property. Thus, it is important to construct systems to adequately protect these individuals from exploitation and abuse.

Amy Klobuchar, Senator from Minnesota, was attempting to craft legislation to curb guardianship abuses in 2011 when she was chair of the now defunct Oversight and the Courts Subcommittee of the Senate Judiciary Committee. Back when she was Hennepin County Attorney, she had prosecuted Roland Amundson, a judge with the state Court of Appeals, who stole hundreds of thousands of dollars from the estate of a developmentally impaired woman. As subcommittee chairman she was trying to get states to run criminal background searches on guardians and people who were applying to become guardians. She believed that adding some simple changes, like better financial oversight and required training for new guardians, would help to keep guardians from "ripping people off of hundreds of millions of dollars." She sponsored Senate Bill S-1744 *The Guardianship Accountability and Senior Protection Act* which died in committee in July 2012.

Zimbledon informed Bill that his hearing would be on Monday, October 24. I talked with Bill a few days ahead of time and he knew it was important and seemed to be planning appropriately, as far as I could tell. I told Jake, "Bill sounds good and is well focused, so he might be able to make a good showing in court if he doesn't lose his cool and insult the judge (even though the bastard deserves it!)."

Zimbledon didn't bother to tell Bill the time of the hearing and Bill was unable to reach him by phone, so he called the Rice County Court to determine the time. They had nothing scheduled for him on October 24th but did have a hearing on Restoration of Capacity scheduled for the 1st of November. I imagined they were putting the question of disposition of his property off until after the guardianship matter was settled. I told Bill to expect a question about how he would take care of his property once the guardianship was gone. Actually, I thought the court should pay for it since they caused it to begin with, but I knew that getting them to take responsibility for their actions was next to impossible.

Bill asked me about what Brian Landers, his attorney for the eviction, had said after his former landlady bamboozled the court into removing his belongings from his apartment. Brian had said that he was going to send information to Bill about how he could file suit for damages due to his eviction and I presumed he meant Bill Zimbledon. I thought Bill Tollefson might want to file suit at this time but when he asked Whimp if he had the information, he was told no, that he had never received anything. And, apparently, Whimp wasn't about to put himself out by calling his colleague to find out what the information contained. I then called Brian's office and was told that he had sent it to Bill Tollefson, not Bill Zimbledon, while he was in the state hospital. Not surprisingly, Bill never received it. Things seemed to have a strange habit of disappearing in state institutions and nursing homes. Brian said Bill could receive a copy by calling his office and requesting it.

As November 1st approached, neither Bill nor I had received an official notification of the hearing from the prosecuting attorney, as we usually did. Bill was unable to get hold of Zimbledon and Wimp ignored his lawyers code of ethics yet again by not calling Bill back. I sent Zimbledon an email stating that Bill was awaiting his return call regarding the hearing on the first of the month and gave him his phone number in case he had misplaced it. Wimp never did return the call. Bill finally called the court and was told the hearing was at 1:30. Jake had wanted to be there but had an appointment for a biopsy on that day.

Bill still felt like he was sitting on hot coals and wished that he could get his old cushion back from out of storage. He managed to get another appointment with his doctor in Faribault, who wrapped his legs in Ace bandages as a temporary measure to try to help get rid of fluids. I thought he needed treatment in a hyperbaric chamber like Jake's friend's brother, who benefited greatly from the treatment, but the battle Bill had with Dr. High probably put the kibosh to that. The Faribault doctor also promised to arrange to get Bill into Mayo Clinic for his other problems.

Supposedly, the social worker at Golden Liver was getting Bill squared away with Hennepin County Social Services so he could order a new cushion. However, either he was dragging his feet or there was some back stage dispute going on between Rice and Hennepin Counties about the status of Bill's residence. I had just that day received a call from St. Joseph's hospital asking for Bill's mailing address and I thought it was from the billing office. My suspicion was that they had been turned down by Rice County when they tried to bill them for Bill's hospital stay several months earlier. When Bill had tried to get Rice County Social Services to order him a new cushion, they had refused, claiming that Bill was no longer a resident of Rice County. It reminded me of the old "dumping syndrome" back a couple of decades ago when counties would buy a mental patient a bus ticket just to get him or her out of their jurisdiction, off their budget, and into someone else's area of responsibility. Recent news reports indicate that this old tactic for counties to avoid financial responsibility was back in vogue.

Bill said there were a half dozen visitors from Health and Social Services at the nursing home before he left for Faribault. They were interviewing him but he had to go off for his doctor's appointment before they were through. I asked if he thought they were sent by the governor's office but he didn't know. They told him they would be back, so he was going to see if he could find out their mission if they ever reappeared. They never did return. However, I much later figured out who they were from reading the account of their inspection via *Pro Publica*. It is reported in the final chapter of this book.

In a couple of days, Jake received a call from Bill. Zimbledon had called him with the news that the hearing had been canceled because Rice County had "officially objected to the hearing." Wimp told Bill he would call back with details but, of course, he never did.

I talked with Bill and learned more news, which I relayed to Jake. "Today the ward nurse told Bill he couldn't see his doctor in Faribault as long as he had the 'guardians.' Then he talked with Zimbledon and was told the next hearing wouldn't be until December 5 - almost a year after this all began! So, his plan to get to the Mayo Clinic is kaput and his plan to move his things into cheaper storage than his brother can provide is out the window because the guy providing the storage is going to Florida the first of the next week. Bill is really mad and depressed as they fuck him over once again!

"Zimbledon apparently did not know the reasons for the delay and why there were the previous delays without any notification of Bill.

"These guys are sadistic, without a doubt!"

Jake responded with as much disgust and pessimism as I was feeling. "Bud, who knows what these guardians are after or why they do anything. Maybe they think he should find a G.P. in Hennepin County or St. Louis Park. Or maybe the nurse is just lying so they don't have to give him any more rides. And Rice County may have realized that they screwed up big time with Bill and might get their asses hauled into court themselves. Bill needs a lawyer who will work on commission. They're hard to find. And I'm sure Gary is in the mix. When I bumped into him six weeks ago or so he told me that he had heard good info that Bill will never be out of a nursing home. Probably heard that from the guardians. The whole thing stinks. But like Jane said, she wouldn't sign the petition because it made Bill look like a 'victim.' Jane must have lost her dictionary!"

Bill was convinced the guardians would be released on December 5th and he made preliminary arrangements to store his belongings with someone he had dealt with before in a rural community not far from Northfield. Jake was not so sure Rice County would let the guardians go because it would be like admitting they "screwed up big time a year ago when this whole thing began." I thought he was probably right. Zimbledon told Bill that the county had objected "to the whole thing" and that was presumably why the hearing time was reset. But I suspected that the delay was in order to give them time to dig up dirt on Bill, probably from their co-conspirators at Golden Liver.

I wrote to Jake, "Some vindictive hate-filled sadist has to be behind this rescheduling. I can't believe it is just a fluke. Rice County Social Services denied help to Bill because he is not currently a resident of the county. If that is the case, they should have no "standing" in court (i. e., whether he is let go or not shouldn't affect them one way or the other). That leaves the "guardians" with the only skin in the game - they have something to lose if Bill goes free. That's my current analysis of the situation anyway."

Up to this point Bill had been very clear-headed. He said he was trying to do what he could with the pair of idiots he had to deal with (the social worker and the nurse) without going off on them. He knew the politics. He knew the motivations that kept them doing what they were doing. He knew he and we didn't have much power in the situation. He also knew he needed to keep his motivation up and maintain a positive outlook if he was to make a good showing in court. Yet his continuing physical problems were wearing on him. His legs weren't getting any better and the nursing home wasn't providing any treatment. They still had not fixed his bed so he could elevate his legs and it is doubtful that he was getting any antibiotics. He was afraid they would keep doing nothing until it was too late and he would need to get his ankle fused. From past experience, he believed that he needed to start with exercise in the water in order to get his ankle flexible before trying any land-based exercise equipment. But they hadn't killed him yet and he was still trying to keep going psychologically and physically, so I was somewhat encouraged. Of course, none of his relatives did anything to help.

Finally, Bill's spirit began to weaken. "I'm worried about these delays in the hearing and what they are up to. I think they are cooking up a new 'Plan For Bill's Life' and don't give a shit what I think or feel about it."

I allowed as how that was probably the case. Just who was doing the plotting and why was a good question but, at this point, I couldn't imagine it to involve anyone who had Bill's best interests in mind. Bill thought his brother Gary was probably involved because Zimbledon had told him he had talked with Gary about Bill's property. I didn't know how that could be ethical and what kind of story line Whimp would buy from the despised brother.

I sent Zimbledon an email about how Bill was being adversely affected by the delays in the hearings and asked him if he thought the information from Brian Landers, the attorney that represented Bill in the eviction matter and storage of his belongings, was relevant to the upcoming hearing. I didn't hear anything from Zimbledon and figured I probably wouldn't, given his MO. I suggested to Bill that he call him just so it was on record that he had done so. I reminded him that maintaining communication with a client and responding to phone calls was one of the requirements in the *Lawyers Ethical Standards*, not that any of these bottom-feeders ever bothered to consult the standards they had pledged to uphold.

A few days later, at least some of the plotters of the "Plan For Bill's Life" were revealed. Bill said he had a meeting with the social worker and the nurse and some person from Rice County Social Services. Bill did not catch what her position was but he said that she had been "in the background" for years. There was talk of placing him at the Valley View facility in Northfield, the very same one that had rejected him a short time before. Bill was very anxious to get out of Golden Liver but didn't want to get his hopes up only to have them dashed again. I was suspicious because Rice County had claimed he wasn't a resident of the county before and I couldn't imagine them doing this out of the goodness of their black hearts. Either someone was afraid of getting into trouble or someone had already started pushing them to do something to get Bill out of Golden Liver.

After not hearing from Bill in several days, I called and learned he was depressed and distrustful of most everyone involved in his situation, as he should have been, but he was thinking clearly. "I woke up this morning with a nightmare that Golden Liver is selling me down the river with false reports they are sending to Rice County." I thought it a reasonable suspicion but presented the alternative argument that they might simply be trying to get him out of there. If they were trying to keep him there in Golden Liver for their financial gain, why would the woman from Rice County Social Services bother to come up there? It didn't make sense unless they were conspiring to keep him out of the way so he didn't start suing everybody.

I asked Bill if he had talked with Zimbledon and he hadn't. I told him, "Even though you don't trust the son-of-a-bitch, you should call him and ask him if he knows what is going on with Rice County and what his plan is for representing you in the upcoming hearing on December 5th. If he doesn't respond to your call or doesn't answer those questions, then you can document that fact and hold it over his head in the future. Either of those alternatives would be a violation of the lawyers code of ethics." It hadn't occurred to me, at that time, that the lawyers code of ethics was just a joke within their fraternity.

In an email, I updated Jake regarding a recent conversation I had with Bill. "He had a terrible day and was in a terrible mood - angry, depressed and "despondent" (his term). His bed is above a heat vent and they can't move it because the room is too small, so he sweats all night until his clothes are sopping wet. He said he felt like he was being baked. He has to wait until the staff is ready in order for him to get a shower and they play games so they don't have to do it. The big task on their part is to roll him down to the room where the shower is and come back 20 minutes later to get him. Since they don't like to do it (or any extra work, it seems), they put it off until Bill gives up and then they tell him it is too late to do it. His bed is still broken and his roommate bitches whenever Bill turns on the light. He has received no money this month at all whereas he usually gets some on the 3rd or 4th of the month. They won't let him go anywhere - no shopping, no outings of any sort. He is fighting to try to get out of the foul mood he is in and tries to be 'upbeat,' but doesn't seem to be succeeding. He says he just keeps looking at the calendar and counting the days until December 5th. He worries about what will happen in court - what they are cooking up for him - and keeps praying that the lies and misinformation his adversaries propound will be made obvious by some kind of divine intervention."

I had earlier determined that Jake's lawyer friend was not up to taking on a case like Bill's but I had asked if the lawyer's lawyer friend in Minneapolis might be willing to give it a shot. The word came back that he had no interest in doing so. The reasons he gave for turning it down were that it would be expensive and time-consuming. He'd have to hire an investigator to get all the relevant facts documented and he'd have to hire an accountant to get all the numbers figured out, which together would come to about $10,000. Since Bill didn't have much income, there wouldn't be much monetary loss to sue over and any punitive damages would have to be figured after the compensatory damages were calculated. Getting court documents would cost a small fortune at $6.60 per page and there would probably be expenses to get medical and other records as well. So, as indicated in a previous chapter, "suing the bastards" was just not feasible either financially or because it would be impossible to get an attorney to represent him.

Once again, it was apparent that justice is just for the rich in this state and probably in this country. Unless you have a barrel of cash, there is no justice for people like Bill and not many people really care. Certainly, the politicians don't - the crazy people in the world don't constitute a voting block and can safely be ignored. Incompetent lawyers, courts, psychiatrists, "guardians," and nursing homes can milk Medicare for all they can get and it is in their interests to keep control of the system. The regulators don't regulate, the elected officials buy the crap the regulators and institutions feed them, and the voters are kept dumb by most of the media that prefer to cover the latest Kardashian debacle. This is not a democracy, it is an "*Idiocracy*" as the movie of that name so hilariously dramatized.

Jake said that his lawyer friend had seen some of these "guardian cases" before. He said the guardians consider a guy like Bill to be merely a "cash cow" and will do and say anything not to lose him. Thus, the purpose of requesting another continuance would be a stalling tactic to get time to make more money off of Bill. Bill's lawyer would have to object to the continuance and, according to Jake's lawyer friend, most judges would not grant a continuance without a really good reason, especially since they already got one 60 days ago. Jake continued, "But if the lawyer is just a lazy bum he probably won't object. Bill has to tell his lawyer "No more continuances!"

Bill continued to have difficulties with getting adequate nursing care. He had asked one aide to unwrap his Ace bandages and was told that he couldn't do it because he would "get in trouble" if he did. Over the phone, I overheard him asking one of the good nurses if she would get that taken care of and she agreed she would. But then, he got chewed out by some nurse who objected to a nurse on another shift setting an appointment for him to take a shower on her shift. He hadn't had a shower since a week ago Friday, about ten days, and he said some skin was coming off his forehead. I'm sure this must be a violation of some nursing home regulation and I thought, if Bill gets stuck in there after the 5th, I think I'll file some complaints about the place.

Jake noted that Bill still needed nursing home care and wondered what would happen if the guardians were dismissed and Golden Liver decided to dump Bill out on the street. I didn't think they could do that without getting themselves into a passel of trouble but I also wasn't sure just how much nursing care Bill needed. I told Jake, "About the only thing he gets at Golden Liver is that someone puts a salve on his back side every now and then to keep him from rotting away. And they wrap and unwrap his Ace bandages when they feel like it. Other than that, I haven't heard of any nursing care. They do feed him regularly and give him meds so he doesn't have to remember that for himself, but I think he could do both of those things if he had to."

Both Jake and Bill were excited about the upcoming hearing. Jake was all ready to bring boxes over to help Bill vacate the place and stash some of his stuff in Jake's basement. He was anticipating Bill getting into Valley View and going off to the Senior Citizen's Center pool to work on his legs. Bill was getting increasingly anxious about the hearing and tried not to think about it so he could get some sleep. He was afraid that the prosecution and their henchmen would again lie and distort information and that he wouldn't be able to counteract their claims. Unfortunately, I thought that was a realistic fear. He was taking Xanax, an anti-anxiety drug, which mellowed him out somewhat and kept him from going over the edge. Unfortunately, he may have been given more medication than was necessary and it took a tole on his ability to think clearly and stay on track.

I was worried that Bill had done nothing to prepare for the hearing. When I would bring up possible issues, he would tune me out, saying that it just made him too anxious to think about it. I had told him repeatedly to call Zimbledon and find out what his plan was to defend and argue for Bill's rights. Whimp was supposed to do that, according to his *Lawyer's Ethical Standards,* and he should have been preparing Bill for how to respond to different contingencies. I doubted that any of that was going on.

Jake emailed me on the 4th of December to let me know that Bill had called him and everything was a "go." Jake said that Bill didn't sound too well – confused, nervous and unable to concentrate. He hoped he would feel better on the 5th and said he would call Lucy to make sure she would be there with him as witnesses to the probably predetermined court proceedings. He said he would let me know the results as soon as he returned home.

The first report I got was from Lucy, who was driving back to Minneapolis from Faribault after she left the court, before the very end of the proceedings. The reception from her cell phone was very poor and I could only guess at much of what she was saying. However, she was very positive and thought things had gone well. She said that she thought Zimbledon had done an OK job and that Bill had presented himself well. She thought the person from Rice County Social Services was really trying to help Bill find a residence in his home town.

Jake's rendition of the proceedings was quite different, without the rose-colored glasses of a super-enthusiastic personality type, who prefers to see the positive possibilities, imposed between her and the data.

"It lasted from 1:30 to 4:30 with a half hour break at 2:30. Bill's tangential thinking was in great form. After almost every question from Zimbledon and the other lawyer, Bill was off and running with foot in mouth. Most people, including the judge, would consider Bill's answers no more than incoherent rambling blather. He had to be told to answer the question about 3 or 4 times including by the judge. A simple yes or no answer would take Bill two minutes or more to answer. And half the time he'd end up by saying I don't remember. Lucy was there and during break she told Bill that he was doing a great job and to keep it up. That was not good advice for someone who already had their neck in a noose.

"Zimbledon knew that Bill's goose was cooked and the judge was not going to can the guardians. Zimbledon had met with Bill for about 20 minutes before it all began and I'm sure he told Bill to keep his answers short and to the point. Not Bill---he wanted to expand his answers and tried to do so. It didn't work and made everyone start to think the guy was half nuts and needed guardians. It was finally agreed in the end to give Bill a 180 day continuance during which time Rice County Social Services would try to find him a better place to live. It was also agreed that Rice County would give Bill a ride to Northfield to meet with a guardian and go through his stuff at Gary's for a period of no more than 3 hours. One of the lawyers said that Gary was charging Bill $90/Mo. for storage in a unit that would normally rent for about $200/Mo. After Bill decides to junk a great deal of his stuff, Gary will haul it to the dump and move Bill into a much smaller unit. (But I bet the rent will stay the same!). Rice County agreed to find a place for Bill that has pool therapy available. I think they will probably give Valley View another try. Apparently, nursing homes like people who have guardians. And by law, guardians have to issue statements only annually. Bill told the judge that his income was about $400-600/Mo and all from S.S. Disability payments. He didn't know what nursing homes charge and never saw a statement from Golden. He said he was taking about a dozen pills per day but didn't know what they were or who prescribed them."

Nursing homes and assisted living places like to have a hold on their clients so that they cannot just decide they don't like the place and go elsewhere. That is why they like their residents to have guardians, a coercive legal device to keep their residents under control and in bondage. The practice was discussed during the hearing and the judge made no objection, instead deferring to the demands of the facilities rather than asserting that this was a type of discrimination against potential residents who are competent. Yes, they are in effect saying to applicants, "If you are sane and capable of handling your own finances, you cannot be admitted." So all the "experts" in the courtroom thought Bill would have a better chance of getting into a facility if he had a guardian. I consider acceptance of this absurdity to be a further corruption of the system and an additional violation of a patient's civil rights

Jake had talked to his lawyer friend and he had told him that Bill had a hearing to get rid of the guardians. "He asked how it went and I mentioned that old jabber-jaw Bill didn't do too well. When I said jabber-jaw he said he knew exactly what I meant as he lost a couple of cases because his clients wouldn't just shut up when in court. He also mentioned that the first thing they teach you in law school about appearing in court is to very carefully instruct your client to answer only 'Yes,' 'No,' 'I don't know,' or 'I don't remember.' And if they have to expand their answer, to keep it as short and direct as possible. Judges hate clients who ramble on and on, taking up court time. And juries can't remember what's being said."

Bill did have a tendency to prattle on when he was anxious and felt under attack. Even when he was relatively calm, he had a hard time keeping his mouth shut. And when what you said to him made him feel anxious, he would shut you out or tell you "I can't deal with that right now." That might be true enough but, in any event, he would use it as a coping method when it might be better to deal with the issue head on. My wife suggested telling him, as a way of getting through to him on this issue using one of his favorite metaphors, "A fish would never get caught if he kept his mouth shut."

I suspected that in the last week alone he had gone over in his mind all the crap that had happened to him during the past year a million times, and that it just came tumbling out of his mouth without any frontal lobe control at all, especially if he was overdosed on Xanax. Of course, the major problem was Zimbledon and his lackadaisical approach to lawyering. He had done nothing to prepare Bill for responding to questions and arguing on his own behalf.

I contented myself with the fact that at least they were working to remove Bill to a better place to live back in his home town. Of course he could do a kind of water therapy on his own at the Senior Center in Northfield if they didn't bother to get him treatment by a certified water therapist. Both Jake and I thought he should apply to Northfield

Retirement Center because our experience was that it was a pretty good place and it would be good for Bill because he should know a lot of the people living there. Each of our mothers had lived there before they died and they were well taken care of insofar as we could determine. There were a lot of volunteers from St. Olaf College coming in all the time for recreation, entertainment and learning opportunities. Bill should have been able to get in there, we thought, since his dad had given them $3000 to get the place going back in their initial funding drive. Jake had made a gift to them too, in the name of Squint Howard, one of the town's two well-known derelicts, but it was never publicly acknowledged. Bill was not so sure he would be admitted.

Jake added another observation from the hearing. "The opposing lawyer knew how to get Bill's goat. One of his questions, after looking over some medical report he had, was, "How long have you been an alcoholic and a drug user?" Bill's face turned bright red and, if he could have jumped out of his chair and belted the guy, I'm sure he would have done so. It sounds like he's taking too many meds. It would be nice to get a list of what he was taking and check them all out."

I responded that Bill had been taking one of the benzodiazapans like Xanax to control his anxiety level and he may have talked the nursing home staff into giving him more than usual because he was very anxious the night before the hearing. That may have impaired his ability to stay focused during the hearing, although he tends to have a problem with that even on a good day.

Jake answered, "I thought Zimbledon should have objected to that question since it has never been established that Bill is an alcoholic--WHICH HE IS NOT!! Bill just has one too many once in a while. But after glaring at the cross examiner for a while, Bill told him, 'Sir, I am not an alcoholic or a druggie.' He then explained that two Thanksgivings ago, he was visiting a young friend who lit up a joint and Bill had a couple puffs on it. Bill also mentioned that he has never paid for or possessed marijuana."

I woke up that morning too thinking that Zimbledon should have objected to that question. For one thing, it was one of those "When did you stop beating your wife?" type questions that can't be answered without self-incrimination. Another thing was that the prosecutor had not established himself as an addictions expert. He should have called an expert witness and asked him the relevant questions, which he did not do. In fact, it appeared that he was posing the question simply as a ploy to try to rattle the defendant. This, of course, raises the question about Bill's right as a ward of the state to be treated with "dignity and respect."

Besides his disclaimer of not being an addict, Bill was never observed to demonstrate any withdrawal symptoms, such as delirium tremens (DT's), at any hospital or anyplace else. Zimbledon should have at least asked the prosecutor, "What evidence do you have that Mr. Tollefson is addicted to either drugs or alcohol?" My suspicion was that the source of the prosecutor's information was Jane, who had tried to convince the doctors in the hospital that Bill was a drunk. Dr. Smart, after talking with Jane, commented to me, "She certainly isn't trying to do anything to help Bill, is she?"

Jake mentioned that there was also talk, during the hearing, of diagnoses that Bill had been labeled with back when this whole sordid affair began, the same erroneous diagnoses that had been discredited by Dr. Smart and his team, the same ones that Jake and I knew were ludicrous from our knowledge of Bill over six decades. As has been observed many times, once a psychiatric diagnosis gets in your record, it stays with you (and adversely affects you) forever. In the VA, a patient could file a complaint and have misinformation rescinded from his record. However, I saw it happen on only one occasion when a patient who had been an activist after the Vietnam War had gone through all the steps to make it happen. Even then, some of the doctors were reluctant to admit that they could be wrong and resisted as much as they could.

Another matter that came up during the hearing was of interest to Jake. "Bill mentioned that he was not allowed to leave the Golden campus due to someone's orders. The Rice County social worker, and the lawyer representing Rice County and the guardians and indirectly Golden Liver, all claimed that this was news to them and they knew nothing about such orders. Someone here is either lying or Golden is making up their own rules. Golden even put a tracking device on his wheelchair once."

Bill had told me about the tracking devices that Golden had attached to his wheelchair on three different occasions. Bill had removed them each time. I have already described the attempt by Golden to prevent Bill from leaving the grounds, witnessed by my wife and myself. He had also been prevented from making several shopping trips, which were available to other nursing home residents. So, yes, someone was lying through their teeth.

It was about a week after the hearing before I had a chance to talk with Bill and get his impressions of the proceedings. The following was my update of that conversation in an email to Jake.

"I talked with Bill this afternoon. He is REALLY pissed! He referred to everyone at the court as a bunch of 'dirty rotten bastards' and said the

whole thing was and continues to be 'a nightmare.' He called Zimbledon
a SOB and complained that he (Zimbledon) asked Bill 'Who needs that
kind of information?' when Bill asked him to get the court records. He
refused to get them for his client unless he came up with $6.50 per page.
He said that the prosecutor claimed no one had ever said Bill needed
water therapy even though I have an email from Dr. Smart stating that
the social workers at Anoka *and* Golden Liver would make 'vigorous
attempts' to obtain same. He said no one is doing anything with his legs
other than wrapping them in ACE bandages. He said, 'I'm dead unless
there is some miracle in Northfield that can be pulled off.' He said
everyone is trying to cover up what goes on at Golden Liver and they
claimed that they never tried to restrict his movements. I know different
and my wife and I can testify to it. Bill said he has received no money for
the last 3 months. One of the workers at Golden Liver managed to lose
Bill's clothes that he wore to court by throwing them in with a bunch of
towels after Bill warned him not to do so. Bill's clothes will be difficult
to replace because of their size. I asked the guy's name and Bill would
not give it to me because he is afraid of retaliation.

"Bill said, 'I can't dream any more. Nothing is going to happen.
Nobody is going to do anything!' He said they claimed in court that he
didn't give his meds list to his doctor in Faribault because he was a
druggie and was trying to hide his drug usage but the real reason was that
Golden Liver did not send a list of meds down to Faribault with Bill
when he went there, and he had asked them to do so. He said that the
only thing the lawyers asked in court was when they were going to get
paid and the judge reassured them, 'Don't worry boys, you'll get paid.'

"Well, that's Bill's understanding of the hearing and he is probably
mostly right. He didn't mention anything about having verbal diarrhea
during the hearing and how that probably went against him. But, in spite
of that, he has been and continues to be screwed over by a bunch of
incompetent assholes. Zimbledon told him he might be able to get the
records if he sent a petition to the judge but when Bill asked him if he
would file the petition, Zimbledon refused, saying, 'You expect me to do
that for free?' If you remember, you said you had heard that comment
yourself. Maybe I can do it if I can figure out what the procedure is."

The lawyers comments about getting paid, the judge's reassurance to
them and Zimbledon's mock outrage at Bill asking him to file a petition
to get court records "for free" rekindled my suspicion that Rice County
Court was trying to balance its budget by dispensing cut-rate justice -
curtailing appeals, neglecting due process and ignoring the just enacted
Bill of Rights for Wards and Protected Persons. As far as I could tell,

Bill's rights had been violated on nearly every item specified in the law. I asked Jake if he could find out if the court was having budget problems or how the funding of the court was accomplished.

The next day Jake sent me a copy of an article in the *Northfield News*. It indicated that, in the last three years the court had laid off 15 percent of their staff of law clerks and administrative employees, while salaries were frozen and courthouse windows were open only part-time. State public defenders had been reduced by one-third.

Jake talked with his lawyer friend in a different county and learned that the same kind of thing had happened all over the state. Some of the counties in northern Minnesota were either bankrupt or on the verge of it and half the residents were on relief. His lawyer friend said that, "It doesn't matter much what the 'law' may say about it---it just isn't going to happen" if the funds are not in the budget. In other words, if the state does not make the funds available to the courts, the civil rights and protections written into law, such as the *Patient's Bill of Rights* and the *Bill of Rights for Wards and Protected Persons*, aren't worth the contents of a brass spittoon. Now that's something to ponder for our democracy.

Jake told me he had just watched a Norwegian movie about a man, Hamsun, who thought the Germans were going to win WWII and encouraged his countrymen not to oppose the invasion as it would be fruitless and cause a lot of death and injury. After the war he was considered a traitor and put into an insane asylum for observation. After a few months they decided he wasn't crazy and let him go with a fine. But he said to a psychiatrist that, when locked up in a nut house, it was more important to have courage than to be happy. "This reminded me of Bill, who's had great courage for almost a year. I hope he can keep it up a while longer."

I wrote back, "I hope so too. It has been a long haul and I think he has a touch of *Continuing* Traumatic Stress Disorder and should be compensated for the disability it causes. Vets I have seen get a percentage of service connection for their *Post* Traumatic Stress Disorder, depending upon the severity. Bill has been on the front lines for longer than most of the vets I saw, who received service connected disability for engagements that lasted from a few hours to a few days to a few months. People may not have been shooting at him with live ammunition but they sure have been with sadistic and punitive actions and derogatory comments, including "friendly fire" from his siblings.

11 <u>THE GREAT ESCAPE</u>

Jake said he would ask his lawyer friend about getting a copy of the transcript through a court order or a petition to the judge.

"He'll know what to do but he once told me that getting transcript copies is like pulling teeth. The counties he's dealt with in Minnesota know that, for legal work, transcript copies are needed for all court proceedings and they charge a small fortune. It's a gigantic rip-off. I remember Zimbledon told Bill, 'You want me to do all this work for free?' I don't know why he even keeps his name on the list of lawyers for use by the county. Zimbledon said that the court reporters only type up transcripts if there's a request for one. Otherwise they just file their shorthand notes in the history file. I'll have to ask about this also."

Jake learned that, in the county where his friend practiced, they rarely used court reporters and just tape recorded the trial or hearing. The tape then became part of the permanent record and wasn't typed out unless someone requested a copy and paid about $6 per page.

"He didn't know what kind of luck Bill would have in getting a free transcript of his hearing. A lawyer – Zimbledon - would have to spend about an hour typing up a one page petition to the court to give Bill a free transcript since it was established in the hearing that Bill is indigent. My friend didn't know if courts would usually do that or not. Zimbledon gets $50 an hour for his work scheduled by the county with Bill, but that wouldn't cover requesting a transcript. Unless Zimbledon is a crook he shouldn't charge more than about $100 to $150 for doing the job, not a penny more. After all, he's not an O.J. lawyer. Think I'll give him a buzz tomorrow and get a ballpark figure of his charge for that work. I'll tell him I'll just pay him cash for doing it."

After Jake called Zimbledon a few times, he reported back, "He never answers the phone or calls me back. I told him I'd pay whatever his charges might be for the petition---probably about 1 hours work, according to my lawyer friend." Zimbledon being Zimbledon, he never did return Jake's calls.

I wrote Jake, "I am doubtful that there is any justice for the poor. Zimbledon sounds like an even worse asshole than I thought, just as bad as the Pecor! This whole thing is just so not right, I can't believe it! Cindi Fisher told me she was almost afraid to ask what had happened to Bill because she has heard so much bad news lately. You would think there would be someone someplace we could light a fire under."

Bill asked me to wish Jake and Big Jim a good holiday if he wasn't able to get hold of them on Christmas. But he was in a very bad mood, getting to the point where he just didn't care about anything. He described his captors as "a bunch of dirty bastards...sick fuckers." The social worker from Rice County and his guardian had a meeting with him on Monday but still had not gotten anything going in terms of finding him a home. The woman from Rice County finally seemed to understand that Bill needed water therapy, saying to him "You're kind of like a fish out of water." In spite of this empathic-appearing remark, Bill still perceived his situation as being hopeless. "It is delusional to think that you can make some yardage in this game."

Golden Liver cut the wires to the phone in the group room he had been using, so he had to use the mobile phone from his own room. The nursing home was in a constant state of disruption because of new very disturbed residents being mixed in with the ones who weren't so bad off. He had a hard time getting any sleep or any peace because of the constant noise and yelling. He said, "I can't talk about it because it is so bad and I can't live in it. Dear God, please take me home. It's over for me. I'm done. Put a fork in me."

Bill believed, probably correctly, that the lawyers were working against him even when they smiled and stared at him. He knew that it takes money to buy justice in this country, especially in Minnesota, and money was a commodity in short supply for him. "Welcome to Christmas in the ASS -sylum," he yelled, his words dripping with sarcasm.

I finished up my email to the two old friends with, "So, there you have it. The bastards aren't really doing much, if anything, to help him although they go through the motions in order to keep their jobs. The nursing home really isn't any different from what it was when it was called the Beverly Corporation and was found guilty of

Medicare/Medicaid fraud. Bill feels sorry for the poor bastards that are confined there, even the disruptive ones, but there is nothing he can do about it and none of us who do care have any power to change anything. This is really a cluster fuck for poor old Bill!"

About that time I read an article in the Health Sciences Institute Newsletter warning readers that the misuse of anti-psychotic medications in nursing homes might be putting many lives at risk. Elderly patients in nursing homes, according to Inspector General of Health and Human Services Daniel Levinson, are often unnecessarily given anti-psychotic drugs in ways that violate government black box warnings (i. e., too high dosages and for too long a time period). Elderly patients diagnosed with dementia face an increased risk of death with these medications and 88% of the time they are the ones for whom the drugs are prescribed. Several drug companies were found to have marketed their antipsychotic drugs for unapproved uses. Eli Lilly, for example, pleaded guilty to criminal charges for illegal marketing of Zyprexa to doctors practicing in nursing homes. Johnson & Johnson was charged with paying millions in kickbacks to foster use of Risperdal in treating nursing home patients. It should also be remembered that the adverse effects of these drugs, or interaction of these drugs with other drugs, can mimic dementia. Another study found that nursing home patients administered anti-psychotic medications were dying at a rate 65-70% higher than those patients who did not receive the medications. (Patients with a psychotic diagnosis fed these medications have been reported to die on average about 25 years younger than those who don't take the medications).

Oh, great. One more thing to worry about! Although Bill was careful about what drugs he would take, he didn't know all of the medications he was taking and it would be possible for them to sneak in an anti-psychotic without his knowledge. However, if they were doing so, he or I probably would have noticed it by its effect upon him.

After being unable to get anyone to answer the phone earlier in the day, Jake managed to get through to Bill just as he was about to hit the sack. Bill told him that a nurse from Valley View was in to see him, along with the Rice County social worker and it sounded like Valley View might be ready to accept him as a resident. Jake reassured Bill that being in a wheelchair would not be a problem since he had seen at least a dozen people in wheelchairs at the place and saw one woman who was so old and weak that she could only go about 4 inches at a time before stopping to rest. He also had learned that a new bus service was starting up in town that might overcome the problems Bill had with the previous service. We were both hopeful that Bill might actually get out of Golden

Liver before his luck ran out.

Jake suggested that he stop by to see Bill's social worker to ask whether a date had been set to go through Bill's possessions that were in storage and then swing by Valley View to see if Bill's name was being processed. While Jake thought a gentle push was needed to get government employees into action, Bill was afraid that might upset the apple cart. "No, no, no don't do that. I don't want to upset anyone down there or push them to move. I just want to wait and let this play out to see what happens."

I responded to Jake, "I used to think agency workers had to be pushed to get them off their duffs to do something. I pushed them to check in on Bill when this all first started to make sure he was all right and look what happened with that! If there is any way they can screw things up, they can probably find it! If they don't do anything, at least they don't do anything wrong!"

I talked with Bill just before the New Year and he was still angry but not as intensely as before. They were still not giving him any significant medical treatment that I could determine, and now they had decided to give him thyroid medication - without bothering to take a measure of his thyroid level beforehand. I filled him in on the 2011 *Bill of Rights for Wards and Protected Persons* and pointed out that it appeared his rights had been violated. He said, "Yeah, tell me about it!" He still hadn't heard anything about getting moved out of there. His bed was still situated over the heating register and they hadn't done anything to help his legs. I mentioned that Jake had called Whimp Zimbledon and left a message but he hadn't heard anything back from him. He wasn't surprised and called him a son-of-a-bitch.

I updated Bill and Jake on the progress of my book about Bill's ordeal. I went through all nine chapters that I had roughed out, did some editing and wrote a preface. I changed the title to *The Fisherman Who Got Snagged in a Minnesota Gulag*. My wife thought it was too long and Bill didn't know what a gulag was, so I made up about 50 different titles and finally decided on *Rights Dishonored, Lives Shattered: Minnesota's Continuing Shame*, thinking that if I insulted the whole state I might get someone's attention. Although the book was not yet completed, I wanted to send it out to some people with the hope that I might find someone who could help Bill and allow me to write a final chapter that had a positive outcome. I sent inquiries to the Minnesota senators, Amy Klobuchar and Al Franken and to a writer for the *City Pages,* a popular Minneapolis online newspaper, to see if they had any interest in reading it. I sent an inquiry to the University of Minnesota Human Rights Center.

I sent a copy to the lawyer in Alabama who had referred me to another lawyer, who in turn referred me to another lawyer, who wanted $5,000 to represent Bill. He had connections with the Southern Poverty Law Center which was the big push behind the civil rights movement back in the 60's. I also sent copies to the author in Panama, the president of the International Society for Ethical Psychiatry and Psychology, to Bonnie Nelson of Mindfreedom in Alaska, to the head of Mindfreedom in Florida, Frank Blankenship, and to Cindi Fisher of MOMS in Washington state. Jim Gottstein, the lawyer in Alaska who heads Psychrights, responded by saying "Don't get your hopes up but we have to keep knocking at their doors." Most of the people who were already fighting for human rights responded favorably, but I got no response from the senators, most lawyers, the university or the journalist.

Jake sent a copy to a friend of his who was a reader for a major publishing house and personally knew Bill. I didn't think that a big publishing house would be interested in it because the potential market was probably fairly small, but I was willing to be pleasantly surprised. A fictionalized version of the book, in which Bill's old-fart friends rescue him from the state hospital in a cunning stealth raid, would probably appeal to a wider audience. Members of my writers group had all gone through the routine of sending off inquiry letters, sample pages or chapters, etc. to potential publishers without much luck. Most people who have tried this route now say it isn't worth the time and effort and are turning to self-publishing and self-promoting. Most of the publishers are themselves either going belly-up or turning to electronic publishing. The member of our writers group with over 20 books published, thought agents were all scoundrels and not worth spit. Some people in our group were thinking of going together to promote our books with blogs, Facebook pages, and other kinds of online marketing. Although marketing is a necessary part of do-it-yourself publishing, I had to admit that the prospect did not really excite me.

Jake wrote, "I doubt if anything serious is being done to find Bill a new living place. The nursing homes might believe all the reports and figure the guy is nuts. That original court psychologist from Mankato should be in jail. Her hack job report started the whole ball rolling down hill for Bill. And now her report is still in his file and might never be removed."

Jake had been scheduled for a biopsy of his tongue but decided he didn't trust the oral surgeon who had suggested it and sought a second opinion from an ENT. He was told there wasn't anything wrong with his tongue by this second doctor and he was relieved to have saved himself a lot of money and pain. However, the scare had triggered some unpleasant memories. He remembered that about 15 years ago his wife's aunt, who was in a state operated nursing home near Brainerd, developed bed sores on her legs that were so bad that they both had to be amputated and she died a month later. Then he promised to tell me sometime how Northfield Hospital had killed his mother. The revelation didn't surprise me and I reminded him of what had happened with Bill's campaign manager.

My wife alerted me to an article in the *Minneapolis Star Tribune* of January 11, 2012 by Paul Walsh which reported on the death of a resident in the Golden Living Center in Hopkins, MN, my wife's home town.

"State Health Department findings said staff at the Golden Living Center neglected the man's fluid and nutritional needs and failed to detect that he had lost 30 pounds within several weeks early last year...Because there were many staff members involved in his care, investigators chose to hold the nursing home responsible for the maltreatment, citing 'a breakdown in facility systems'. Those breakdowns, the report noted, included failure to evaluate the man's weight loss and intake of solids and liquids, as well as failing to notify his doctor and other medical personnel about the weight loss."

This facility was just a few miles from the one where Bill resided and was actually rated more favorably on the Medicare nursing home web site than the one Bill was in. The story had links to stories about deaths due to neglect in two different state operated group homes and the fact that the state facility at St. Peter, MN was placed on two years probation for patient abuse. I was not encouraged by those reports.

On the 27th of January, 2012 Bird Brain, Bill's guardian, showed up with no advance warning, again showing her disrespect for her ward. "She dropped a bomb on me. I can't get into the Valley View assisted-living place. She said they gave no specific reasons. If I can't get back in the water, then I am care-center fodder.

"I cut my left foot in the shower because there was a section of missing grout between the tiles on the floor. Because of the cut on my foot, it is hard to get into bed. Bird Brain claims they have exhausted all the things they can do. I'm too tapped-out and too drained to do much. There is a window air conditioner but I can't reach the controls and if somebody else messes with it, it's not right. The food is lousy, so getting sick is the only thing to do. They're just going to drop me off and hope I'm dead.

"I don't like to think that people you depend on for help are really that way, but that's the way it is. My tank's run out – I have to work at maintaining my positive attitude. The temperature is hot. I need to adjust the window so I won't freeze or roast. My foot and shoulder hurt but I need my bandaged foot because the other ankle is weak.

"I can't expect any civil treatment from them. I can't get where I need to be from here. No one has looked at my legs – they're swollen and discolored. It hurts when they grab my legs to wrap them with Ace bandages. It hurts like hell. I need to go to Mayo. The nurse practitioner just bandages my foot and leaves. She doesn't think I have an infection in my legs, so she doesn't do any tests.

"Bird Brain gave me $100 today after giving me nothing for 4 months. She brought an old cushion that someone gave me a while ago. It is just a foam cushion, too small, without the special features of my $550 cushion. Either someone stole that cushion or they threw it out because it had urine on it. I also need a special custom made wheelchair. They want to see me with bedsores and half dead. Just feed me and park me! How long can a person take a nightmare like this? I just completely lost hope when they did the thing with the court dates. I pray I can survive this somehow. I need a doctor to push for water therapy. I see mice in the hallway. They go from room to room and they found my stash of almonds and sunflower seeds in my backpack."

Jake thought Bill should go through Golden Living Center's physical therapy program, for which they could bill Medicare. Golden Living Center had no water facilities themselves and Bill resisted because he didn't think they knew anything about aquatic physical therapy. Jake asked me, "What harm would it do? It won't do any good most likely, but that would be evidence for his need for water therapy and they couldn't accuse him of refusing treatment. I'm trying to stay optimistic about his future since he's gone thru so much BS already. But it's not easy as at every turn I seem to see bad things arising."

The next report I got from Bill was that they wanted to put him in a group home in Elysian, a tiny rural community west of Faribault. The Rice County social worker told him he couldn't get into Valley View because of his weight. Bird Brain just told him they couldn't serve his needs. "If I don't have an appeal ready by April 2, then I'm sunk. I went to pee and I came back and they had thrown my supper away. They gave me a grilled cheese sandwich instead. I have to raise the bed to get away from the heat register and open the window to cool down. My wheelchair was two inches too short which was why I slipped out of the chair on Dec 7, 2010. The place I got the chair from disregarded the measurements I gave them. I need a custom chair. I told them what was wrong right after I got it and they claimed, 'No, that's what you gave us.'"

Bill had a long talk with his girlfriend and they made plans to celebrate his birthday, but not on the actual date, since she had business to take care of. Bill said she told him "I love you baby!" They had known each other for 45 years, from 1965 when they were both fishing on the river and she fell out of a tree. She was 16 years old at the time.

Bill's doctor never showed up for his scheduled appointment. Bill called his bank and was told that he could not get his bank records. He reminded me that a package of papers 2 ¾ inches thick from the prosecuting attorney was stolen from his room at United Hospital a year ago. He had never opened the package. His watch was also stolen at that time. When he was admitted to St. Joseph's Hospital from the Golden Liver place in St. Paul, the security agents relieved him of his baseball cap and 40 bus tokens. The hospital subsequently paid him $65 for the stolen tokens. So, it seems, some hospital personnel routinely consider poor people like Bill to be easy victims for their plundering ways.

Bill reported that his legs had been weak and swelling for the last three days and he thought he had cellulitis again. The swelling was in a 4-5 inch wide area on his legs and was sore to the touch. His hernia was increasing in size which he thought was due to the gassy foods they served at the nursing home. He figured he had gained weight. On February 3, 2012, Bird Brain showed up again, unannounced. He was trying to do exercises in bed and while standing. He asked her if he could go see the super bowl at a friend's grandson's place on February 5th. He promised to come back by taxi afterward. He was not allowed to go, so instead he watched the game on a TV set on the 2nd floor. When he came back to his room, about 4:00 pm he was told the police had been in his room. No one would tell him what was wrong. Apparently the police were called when the staff couldn't find him. They didn't bother to check on the 2nd floor. The laundry lost his one good pair of pants and a shirt was also missing.

When I next talked with Bill he sounded somewhat better. His hate for the obstructionist staff, especially the big nurse, had not subsided. But he had had a pleasant interchange with Penny, the good nurse who was always very respectful and helpful to me when I talked with her on the phone. They still hadn't done anything about placement or getting him into aquatic therapy. He was having a lot of pain in his shoulders which required that he change ears on the phone frequently. His backside was somewhat better due to his use of a non-prescription aloe based lotion that Penny administered.

Bill reported an interesting dream. In it, he was over by the police station in Northfield and Mickey Schraft was yelling at him, "Hey Bill, you're running!" He looked down and he was running and he looked back and saw his wheelchair had been smashed by a semi on the highway. I took the dream to mean that he really would like to get out of that wheelchair and run away! I would too if I were him. Bill thought that Mickey Schraft, the benevolent figure in the dream and known all his life as a sensitive, caring and helpful person, should have been selected as the police chief but someone else got the job.

I told Bill of my idea about there being a "silent conspiracy" in court and he thought that it all made sense, i. e., that the members of the court just ignored his rights in order to save the court money and they were all in on it by not raising any questions. I asked him if he had received any preparation from Zimbledon before he appeared in court. "I got none, zero, nothing."

In mid January, I made contact with a former federal attorney, Susan Freiman, who now lives in a foreign country. She expressed an interest in reading my first nine chapters about Bill so I sent them to her by email. I asked her for any comments she might have but was particularly interested in knowing who had jurisdiction for investigating or prosecuting a court if it suppressed legal rights by telling contracted lawyers to hold costs down and they responded by simply not raising such "rights issues" during their proceedings. She seemed to think that proving that might be hard to do, especially since no money changed hands between the parties to the conspiracy. I allowed as to how there could be other motives operating in a conspiracy besides personal pecuniary ones.

Susan emailed me references to court cases, trying to find precedents for a legal argument for Bill. One of them had to do with inadequacy of counsel and another raised the concept of a court "abusing its discretion." A third case had to do with the definition of "dangerousness." In that case the court found, "... at a minimum, the 'danger' referenced in section 6500 must involve conduct that presents the likelihood of serious physical injury. The vagaries of emotional injury, mere apprehension of physical injury, speculation and conjecture is not enough to justify the need for commitment," for it violates a person's fundamental due process rights. I didn't think this was proved in Bill's case and I suspected it had never even been discussed, unless they regarded the false claim of Bill having MRSA as evidence of his "dangerousness." If that were the case, it was then a violation of the Americans with Disabilities Act, since the claim was based on hearsay and not on fact.

Susan thought that I had made an interesting observation that the Minnesota *Bill of Rights for Wards and Protected Persons* stipulated that rehabilitation services are required to be provided, subject to the availability of funds, while this stipulation was not present in any of the other rights specified in that law. Since they mentioned it in that one instance but not in the others, it could be assumed that the law makers were aware that availability of money might be a limiting factor but specifically and deliberately omitted it as a condition in the other rights.

She also thought that Bill might be able to sue his lawyer for malpractice and cited the Maples case in which lawyers that the defendant had believed were representing him had abandoned the case without leave of court, without informing the defendant they could no longer represent him, and without securing any recorded substitution of counsel.

Susan believed the court could be sued under Section 1983 of the 1871 Civil Rights Act, also known as the Ku Klux Klan Act because it was designed to provide a civil remedy for violations of federal law such as those committed by the KKK. The law states that

"Every person who under color of any statute, ordinance, regulation, custom, or usage, of any State or Territory or the District of Columbia, subjects, or causes to be subjected, any citizen of the United States or other person within the jurisdiction thereof to the deprivation of any rights, privileges, or immunities secured by the Constitution and laws, shall be liable to the party injured in an action at law, Suit in equity, or other proper proceeding for redress..."

In 1961 the Supreme Court found that a government official, even if he was acting outside the scope of the authority granted to him by state law, could be held liable for damages.

I did some online research to see if Bill's situation would qualify for such a suit. First off, I found that a state, like the federal government, may not be sued for damages but that local governments, including county governments, are considered "persons" and are subject to suit for damages and for prospective relief. Local governments have no immunity from damages due to their constitutional violations, and may not use the "good faith" of its agents as a defense. Therefore, Minnesota state laws granting immunity from liability to officers of the court do not apply under Section 1983.

Acting "under the color of state law" means that the wrongdoer possessed and exercised power only by virtue of state law. In Bill's case, his commitment was an action governed by Minnesota state laws and, although the defendants violated some state laws in exercising their power, they were still liable for the harm they caused.

The harm that resulted must be causally related to the action on the part of the government entity that implemented or executed a policy statement, ordinance, regulation, or decision officially adopted and promulgated by that body's officers, or the result of the entity's custom. In Bill's case, the action by the court - civil commitment - directly caused his loss of liberty and additional harms secondarily suffered due to his loss of liberty.

Section 1983 provides a means for the vindication of rights that are specified elsewhere in the constitution and in federal laws but does not itself specify any new rights. "Due process" is the legal requirement that the State must respect all of the legal rights that are owed to a person. If a government harms a person without following the exact course of the law, this constitutes a due-process violation.

In Bill's case, the due-process violation was composed of the court's failure to advise him of his right to a second opinion by a doctor of his own choosing, their disregard of his request to appeal the decision of the court, and their failure to meet the minimal standards for evidence to be allowed into the proceedings. The test of whether or not the State has failed to provide due process depends on what process it provided to do so, and whether it was constitutionally adequate. As far as I could tell, there were no procedures to guarantee that Bill's rights were honored, no safeguards such as officers of the court going through a check list of defendant rights, and no remedies were available since he was not allowed to appeal. Of course, the court records for the day of his commitment would need to be obtained to verify this assertion.

I talked with Bill and updated him on the contacts with Susan. He was pleased to have some glimmer of hope, although he recognized there was a long way to go before some action might be taken. Jake had provided him with a copy of the book but he was ambivalent about reading it while being in "survival mode" at Golden Liver. He said his dreams lately had a lot of hopelessness in them and he was afraid reading about the many travails since his ordeal started might make him too angry and upset, so that putting up with the everyday hassles of living there would be even harder for him. That was a very rational and proactive stance to take, not what one would expect from a person diagnosed as schizophrenic or demented.

On January 22 I received an email from Cindi Fisher suggesting that I tune in to a program on guardianship issues, scheduled for the next day, that was being presented by Janet Parker of Medical Whistleblowers Advocacy Network. I did so and had an opportunity to tell her about Bill's situation. After she read the first nine chapters of the book, she suggested that I might file for a violation of Title II of the Americans with Disabilities Act and she offered to help me get it properly formulated. She said that violation of the Americans with Disabilities Act is a criminal offence, which would mean that federal agents would do the investigation and "discovery," including getting court and medical records. That would take much of the financial burden off Bill and subsequent claims made for damages would be civil actions. If, on the other hand, claims were made on the basis of civil rights violations, then in most cases it would be a civil action from the start. I wanted to get a look at those court records because I thought there might be more violations than the ones I had already pointed out. For example, I suspected they had never really considered "less restrictive alternatives" to both incarceration and medication yet the law requires them to do so. My bet was that the pros and cons of those matters were never given more than a nod in court and the records would prove that they violated the law.

In preparation for filing federal and/or international complaints, I began to compile a list of everyone involved in Bill's case and their contact information. I also went through all my hundreds of emails related to Bill and created a timeline of events about 25 pages long (eventually, it reached 67 pages in length). I tried to list all the offences that had been committed against Bill and made up documents categorized as 14th Amendment Issues, violations of the Americans with Disability Act, violations of HUD Regulations, violations of Minnesota Civil Commitment laws, violations of the *Minnesota Patient Bill of Rights* (later called the *Health Care Bill of Rights*) and violations of the Minnesota *Bill of Rights for Wards and Protected Persons*. Janet Parker suggested I go through the 25 United Nations *Principles for the Protection of Persons with Mental Illness and the Improvement of Mental Health Care* and identify those that had been violated in Bill's case, which I did. I wasn't sure what level of detail was required and relied on Janet to indicate where improvement was needed.

I ran across the web site for the Human Rights Resource Center at the University of Minnesota. They are connected with the University Law School in some way and I thought they may have some legal help available. I didn't find anything about mental health law or civil commitment on their site but thought that would be in their domain. I sent my inquiry letter referring to the book title that insulted the state of Minnesota, hoping it would peak their curiosity to see what was in it. They didn't bite.

About this time, I got an email from Bonnie Nelson and Jim Gottstein indicating they were thinking about mounting a Mindfreedom demonstration for Bill's case. I wrote back saying I appreciated their thinking of helping Bill in some way but I wanted to remind them that he was worried about retaliation. I had no doubt that it might occur if we didn't proceed cautiously and I wanted to get his okay first before anything was initiated. Jim Gottstein responded, "Retaliation is always a possibility, even a probability. I always talk to people about various downsides to going public." We decided to put that option on the back burner for the time being.

Jake met with his attorney friend again and was told about a well-known professional wrestler from Minnesota that had been living in a nursing home but got into a scuffle with another patient. He pushed the guy, who fell down and subsequently died. The wrestler then got identified as a "troublesome patient," was booted from the nursing home and ended up living with a daughter. He couldn't get into another nursing home because they are, according to Jake's friend, "deathly afraid of someone with that label." Jake wondered if Bill had gotten that label and opined that, if he had, he wouldn't be going anywhere else. His lawyer friend also said that getting false information removed from one's medical record is almost impossible and that the first report from the court psychologist could be with Bill forever no matter how negligent or inaccurate it was. I replied that it was difficult but not impossible and that the HIPAA law specified procedures for correction of medical information as well as access to it.

Bill contacted an old friend who knew of an apartment complex near the Senior Center in Northfield. His friend was going to check to see if they had any vacancies. If it was appropriate for Bill, it would have the advantage that he could wheelchair over nearly every day and spend time in the pool at the Senior Center and get a free meal at the same time. Bill estimated that it would take between 12 and 16 months to get his legs back into shape if he had aquatic therapy four or five times a week. Another possibility was the Northfield Retirement Center, which provided transportation to the Senior Center every day. Jake was going to check that out. And Bill found another possibility at a nursing home near where Jake lived. However, Jake checked it out and found it did not have a deep water pool, so the therapy would be nothing more than splashing around in a shallow pool, and the aquatic therapists would have been supplied by Aegis Corporation, a subsidiary of Golden Living Centers.

In February, a federal court awarded a former inmate at the Dona Ana County Detention Center in New Mexico, Stephen R. Slevin, $22 million for violations of his civil rights. Dona Ana County is where I live and there was extensive coverage of the case in local newspapers. The majority of "Sound Off" and editorial comments in the local newspaper,

even from former insiders, was in favor of the inmate, who had been
arrested for possession of a stolen vehicle, DWI, driving with a
suspended license and possession of an open container of alcohol in a
vehicle. He had a history of mental illness and was placed in solitary
confinement for 22 months before the case ever went to a judge. It was
contended that his detention was "virtual false imprisonment" and when
seen at the New Mexico Behavioral Health Institute in Las Vegas, NM he
was described as malnourished, smelled, was disheveled and had an
overgrown beard and hair, untreated dental problems, bedsores, a skin
fungus and toenails so long they curled under his feet. He was prescribed
psychotropic medications without ever being seen by a doctor. In
December 2008 Slevin filed a complaint in U.S. district court against
Doña Ana County, alleging violations of his due process rights; his right
to humane treatment during confinement; his right to equal treatment —
in spite of his mental illness — a right guaranteed by the Americans with
Disabilities Act. He also alleged false imprisonment because of his
prolonged solitary confinement and negligent maintenance of a building,
stemming from improperly housing Slevin in solitary confinement, rather
than with the jail's general population. The court decided that, at that
facility, the mentally ill were "deprived of adequate medical care and
humane conditions of incarceration ... (which) amounts to deliberate
indifference." I saw the case as being a lot like that of Bill except that
Bill was falsely imprisoned in a mental hospital and he had never
committed any crime. His due process rights were violated and he did
not receive humane treatment either in the hospital or in the nursing
homes.

I wrote to "Beany Boy," the social worker at Golden Liver, asking for
the names of Bill's doctor and nurse practitioner and contact information
for each of them. I included copies of the documents supplied to me by
Mayo Clinic indicating my positions as Bill's durable power of attorney
and health care representative. When I didn't receive a reply, I called
several times and left messages on his voice mail. Finally he got back to
me by email, excusing his failure to respond as being due to his being out
of the office and claiming the earlier emails had been wrongly addressed.
That claim was false and Bill had seen him at the facility one of the days
I had called, so clearly, he was dissimulating (lying). He asked me to
resend the Mayo Clinic documents and said he would have to check with
"the State courts to see how your status fits in with his guardian's status."
As it turned out, the Advanced Directives document that Mayo had sent
me ommitted a page with the notary stamp on it and I had to get Mayo to
send it to him. They would not send it to me, which I found peculiar,

since it specified my position with respect to the patient.

That night, Beany Boy made a raid on Bill's room, claiming that his chart was missing. Then he provided a letter to Bill stating, "You have accumulated an excessive amount of personal items, including food, that pose a safety risk to both staff and yourself. Numerous mice have been reported as originating from your room. In an effort to rid the mice from this unit, a deep clean of the room WILL take place on Wednesday 2/15/12. Staff will aide you in removing all personal belongings from your room. This may include you having to spend the night in another bed on another unit to ensure the problem is properly dealt with."

Bill asked him to send a copy of the letter to me because he thought it presumptuous, insulting and accusatory. In the accompanying email, Beany Boy said that it was a "generic" letter sent to all the residents on that floor.

I responded, "Yes, Mr. Tollefson told me about your pest control problem when he first moved in. It is well documented."

Bill's 72nd birthday was coming up in a few days and he wanted to celebrate it in his old home town. His plan was to get a ride to Northfield on Wednesday morning, check into a motel that had a pool and spend some time exercising in it, go out to where his belongings were stored and make an inventory, get some new pants, have an appointment with one of his former doctors, see an optometrist, and visit some of his old haunts downtown. Then he would get a ride back to Golden Liver on Sunday, the 19th.

He was told that Golden Liver had a three-day rule for any leave of absence and the resident had to say where he was going, who he would be with and the phone numbers and addresses where he could be reached. Bill arranged a meeting with his Rice County social worker, his guardian, and Beany Boy. He wanted Jake and Lucy to be in attendence with me being present on the phone. Jake didn't think the caretakers would allow Bill to go anywhere, but we all gathered at the appointed time. I called the apporpriate number and was shunted off to voice mail a couple of times before I finally got through. Apparently, Beany Boy was not happy to have me participate in the meeting.

Bill had not prepared well for the meeting even though I had talked with him about what to expect the night before. He was "psyched" about going home and thought he could "finesse" his way through the meeting. He appeared to be caught off guard and ended up giving what sounded like tangential answers to some of the questions posed, e.g., the time of his doctor appointments. Actually, he had not made appointments and just planned to wait in the doctors' offices until he was seen. The medical doctor was in a walk-in urgent care facility and the optometrist worked on a first-come, first-served basis, so this was not so unusual. But Bill knew it sounded like he was lying about his appointments and tried to quickly move on to other matters.

When asked where he would stay in Northfield, rather than telling the truth, that his sister had used her credit card to make a reservation for a handicapped room at the motel, he went on about all the people he knew in Northfield and that he'd have no trouble finding a place to stay. Then he said he didn't know where he would stay and might sleep in a snow bank if it was necessary. Jake later asked him why he didn't just tell them where he planned to stay but Bill gave him the finger over the lips sign, as if it was some important secret. I could tell he was trying to skirt the issue but wasn't sure why, so I didn't say anything. Later, when I asked Bill about it, he said, "Then they would ask how I was going to pay for it, and if I said 'Some anonymous donor,' then they would ask who it was and I didn't want to get into that." So, he dissimulated and everyone knew it but they didn't want to press him on it, for some reason. I told him I didn't think they could object to him staying at a motel.

My birthday was two days before Bill's and he took the opportunity to lead everyone in singing the happy birthday song, in the meantime diverting attention from his lack of clear-cut plans. Jake asked the guardian why Bill couldn't get into Valley View and if it was because of his weight. She said no, his weight didn't matter, but the problem was that Valley View was not a "locked facility" and the residents could come and go at their pleasure.

Jake was taken aback and later asked me, "What kind of shit is this? Do the dip-shit guardians think the guy is some kind of dangerous psycho that needs to be locked up? They've probably looked only at his original write up from the 'lets pretend' court-appointed psychologist. I mentioned for all to hear in the meeting that at Bills last court appearance, the judge, two lawyers, a representative from Rice County social services and one from the Owatona guardians, all agreed that they knew of no reason why Bill could not come and go as he felt. No restrictions were in place. Me thinks something is rotten in Rice County, Owatona, and St.Louis Park."

Nothing was settled during the meeting and, since I got off the phone after Beany Boy said that it was over, I did not hear any of the subsequent conversation. Beany Boy said he would check with the doctor to see if it was okay for Bill to leave for a few days. Actually, Bill had never seen this doctor but only a nurse-practitioner working under her direction. He also told Bill that he had an appointment with someone from Fairview Hospital the following day who might be able to help get Bill moved to Northfield. Fairview did have an aquatic therapy program, so I hoped that was the connection, but I considered that it might just be another obstacle they were putting in his way.

Jake accompanied Bill to his room, helped him look for his swimming suit, and filled two boxes and one duffel bag full of clothes which he subsequently stored in his basement. "Hanging around in Bills room for three hours just about did me in. However, one Xanax and two beers later I feel recovered."

The following day, I got a call from Bill just as I was walking out the door for a meeting at which I was the guest of honor. He said his request for leave was turned down and he was told he had to have someone with him 24/7 in order to go anywhere. He wanted me to call his guardian right then and there to see what right she had to do that. I couldn't at that time and he was mad. I didn't know that that would have done any good anyway. I thought we needed to call the court and see what the order was regarding restraining Bill's movements. If they do not have the court's authority to do it, then I think it could be regarded as kidnapping and we should call the police. Bill said that his guardian knew about this 24/7 rule during the previous day's meeting and did not say a word about it.

I also thought we needed to get the medical records to see what the doctor was looking at. We might be wrong that it was because they thought he was crazy that they wouldn't let him out. It might be for physical reasons that they were telling no one, even Bill (who had the right to know). It could be that they were afraid he would drop dead while he was away because they had neglected to treat his legs properly. I couldn't believe that they thought wrapping his legs up in Ace bandages constituted "treatment" for whatever was wrong. If he was likely to die, I thought, he should be allowed to die someplace other than at Golden Liver!

Getting medical records might require obtaining a lawyer to demand that they provide the records to Bill. He had the legal right to look at his medical records in his doctor's office and he had asked to do so but had been denied. There could be a clause about not giving the patient information that might be of harm to him, and they might try to use that, but that could be appealed. He could file a HIPAA complaint with the Office of Civil Rights. The cost would not be as much as with getting court records since HIPPA puts a cap on what institutions or doctors can charge for copies of records (limited to the cost of copying, labor in doing so and supplies). A patient also has the right, under HIPPA, to file to get his records corrected where they are in error. If the provider refuses to make the corrections, then the patient can force them to attach an amendment to his record with his claims on it.

I called Golden Liver to speak to Bill about getting his medical records and was told that he was no longer in his usual building. What! Where the hell is he?

I called the main number and asked where he was and after a while I was forwarded to Beany Boy's voice mail. I left a message but didn't expect to get an answer. I wondered if they had sent him to Hennepin County Medical Center.

To my surprise, Beany Boy did call back. He said that Bill had discharged from Golden Liver AMA (against medical advice) and he thought he had gone to a motel in Northfield. I wondered why they would just allow him to discharge if he was such a danger that on the previous day he required a chaperone 24/7. It didn't make any sense for them to expose a presumably vulnerable patient to the vicissitudes of freedom unless they didn't really believe he was incapable of taking care of himself. Obviously, they had no legal right to hold him or they would have exercised it.

I figured Bill had gone to the motel where he had his reservation and called. Yes, he was registered there, the receptionist answered before she transferred me to his room. Bill said he checked out from Golden Liver about 3:00, angry about the denial of his leave of absence and not being able to stand living in those conditions for even one more day. He traveled to Northfield by R&S Transport, checked into the motel, had a pizza and wheeled around town for about two and one half hours. While I was on the phone, his guardian and Rice County Social Worker showed up and harassed him for about one half hour, telling him he was going to die because he didn't take his medications with him in his rush to leave. He asked them if they would help with that and they refused, i. e., they would prefer he die rather than try to help him. This was consistent with Golden Liver repeatedly refusing to tell him what medications he was taking or to give him a list of the pills they were giving him. They quizzed him about how he was going to pay for his room and he told them "anonymous donors." Exasperated with their hostile, accusatory attitude, he finally told them to get out of his room and they left.

Bill said the police had paid him a visit in the morning, just checking to see if he was alright, probably sent by Beany Boy. They left when he said he wanted to file a theft complaint regarding his property, claiming they were too busy for that. He planned to call a friend who worked at a local pharmacy to see how he might go about getting his medications. I suggested he go to the urgent care place in town and get new prescriptions for what he needed but he wanted to get someone else to pay for them. He planed to try out the motel pool after he called the pharmacy. I told him that the social worker and guardian would probably be back with the police. He figured that was likely and supposed they would try to get him thrown back into the loony bin because he didn't plan sufficiently in advance about his medications. But at the time he left, he said, his ride was waiting for him and if he didn't take it then, he would have been stuck at Golden Liver. Over the phone, he sounded good - clear thinking, joking, and happy to be free, if it was only to be for a short time.

About 2:30 the next day I called Bill at the motel. The receptionist told me that Bill couldn't get out of the pool and the police were called to assist. I left a message for him to call me when he could. About 5:45 I got a call from Bill saying that he was in the District 1 Hospital in Faribault. I called the number he left and was told he was in X-ray. I thought, "Well, at least he's not in Northfield Hospital and that should increase his chances of survival."

When I finally talked with Bill he told me the X-rays did not indicate any broken bones. They pronounced him physically OK but thought he was "nuts," based mainly on past records from Golden Liver. I talked with a nurse practitioner at the hospital and told her I thought his records were filled with erroneous information, that his commitment was rescinded and that the diagnoses (paranoid schizophrenia, schizoid personality and brain damage) had all been discredited. She couldn't do anything to determine the truth (of course she couldn't trust what I was saying), she said, so she wanted to send him to a psychiatric facility for an evaluation. But his social worker from Rice County wanted to send him to Faribault Care Center, a 55 bed nursing home that was only 72% filled and garnered a "minus one star" rating from Medicare ("Below Average").

The nurse-practitioner said that the EMTs from Northfield claimed he was urinating and defecating in the motel pool. As I later learned from Bill, he had been in the pool for 19 hours because his knee would not support him when he tried to get out. Because he has no problem floating due to the amount of water he displaces, he decided to sleep in the pool and worry about getting out the next day. He had voided his bowels before he got into the pool but admitted that he had emitted a small turd, which he disposed of in a towel, after being in the water for that long. How they managed to discern his urine from that of all the other motel patrons who used the pool was a mystery to me.

Bill claimed that 18 police came to get him out of the pool after a doctor from Golden Liver signed to get a court order to pick him up. He said the police made a video of the whole thing and he could get a copy. Jake visited the motel the next day and noted that a family with children was splashing around in the pool. Neither police, EMTs, social worker, guardian nor the motel staff regarded any pool contamination to be so significant as to require any corrective action or reporting to the state health department. But it sure made for an inflammatory entry in Bill's medical records.

Jake and I thought that Bill had cooked his goose this time. They had him on the good old 72-hour emergency hold (even though there was no emergency) and all his records from Golden Liver had followed him to the doctors at District 1, so they probably classified him as a paranoid schizophrenic with brain damage. His impulsive actions had again gotten him into a mess that would make it harder to argue that he wasn't a lunatic. We expected that they would probably end up sending him back to Anoka. That probably would have been marginally better and safer than retaining him at Golden Liver.

Jake went down to Faribault Care Center to see Bill but he wasn't there. He had an FCC employee call District 1 Hospital and she was told that Bill was in lock-down and could have absolutely no visitors. Jake drove over to the hospital anyway, planning to tell them he was Bill's attorney if they tried to prevent him from seeing him. At the front desk he was told what room Bill was in and a cleaning lady lead him there. He was not in lock-down at all and could have all the visitors he wanted. Whether the FCC employee told the "big fat lie" or it was a clerk at the District 1 Hospital is impossible to determine but it does illustrate the wanton dispensation of false information by staff in these institutions. Bill was in a single room watching NASCAR races on TV and was outfitted with cardiac monitors, which was apparently standard procedure. Jake observed to Bill that his legs and feet looked better than he had seen them for years and Bill ascribed the effect to his pool exercise and wheeling around town for several hours.

Bill was very happy with the treatment he was getting at District 1 Hospital. I advised him that if the psychologist who evaluated him the first time showed up to interview him that he should say he didn't want to speak to her and request that they get someone else. I also told him the Golden Rules for the interview: be modest, no big long answers, no digressions, etc. He said, "Yeah but when they push my buttons I feel I got to tell them everything." I said that that hadn't worked for him in the past. He thought he was in the hands of God now and that nothing bad was going to happen to him. I hoped he was right.

Bill said they tried to give him an anti depressant and he rejected it, saying the only time he needed them was when he was locked up. It was interesting that the same night on "60 Minutes" Leslie Stahl did a piece on antidepressants and how they weren't any better than placebos for most everyone except those who are severely depressed and, even then, the gain was not that great (about 14% improvement in depression scores). In the UK, the website antidepaware.co.uk/1600-inquests/ provided a list of 1650 deaths linked to use of antidepressants over the last 10 years in England and Wales and the compiler regarded it as "the tip of the iceberg" because it did not include inquests where the toxicology report was excluded from the report.

I got a call from the doctor Bill had seen in Faribault. On the phone she appeared to be a very nice woman who had an appreciation for what Bill is like. I told her what I thought - that the diagnoses were all crap and that this whole thing was a big miscarriage of justice. I told her I was working with a former federal attorney and an advocacy organization to get matters straightened out. I said that, at worst, Bill could probably be labeled with a personality disorder diagnosis with some compulsive traits, but he was not psychotic and had no significant brain damage. I told her he was an obstinate, bull-headed, self-centered jerk at times, that he had a sense of entitlement and defended loudly what he thinks are his rights. She seemed to understand that but also called him a "colorful character."

The doctor told me that Bill had been sent to Faribault Care Center (formerly Faribault Commons) and that he was being "not cooperative." They were telling him that he had diabetes (which he doesn't) and that he had MRSA (which he doesn't), so he told them to get out of his room and this disagreement with their attributions was taken as evidence of his lack of cooperation. The doctor thought it would be best if he went to St. Mary's in Rochester for a psychological evaluation and possibly to get some medical care, which I agreed would be a good idea. She asked if I would call Bill and get him to go along with it. I did and, of course, Bill was already in favor of it.

When I talked with Bill after he arrived at St. Mary's, he was being on his good behavior, not talking on the phone too long so as to avoid making anyone mad at him. I figured if he behaved himself and didn't get on his high horse, he might be able to convince people that he was harmless and not too crazy to run around loose. If he tried to baffle them with bullshit, he was sunk.

It didn't take long to find out which way it was going to go. Bill called while I was up on the roof of my house putting more elastomeric goop on some spots I had missed on my previous foray. He had been happy and looking forward to some decent medical care. Then about an hour later, he called and was yelling "Emergency, emergency! They are sending me to a care center." Then the message broke up and couldn't be understood. My wife called back and the sound was the same - unintelligible. Then she called the main switchboard and they told her his cell phone was being charged up. I suspected his guardian didn't like his doctor sending him to St. Mary's where he was supposed to get a new evaluation and she tried to head it off at the pass.

While he was at St. Mary's, Bill was given a short test requiring him to remember 3 things and answer some questions after looking at some geometric figures. I thought it probably was a screening test for organicity and wanted to get a look at it, since it might provide data to discredit their claims that he had significant brain damage. (Much later, I found the results of a similar test administered by a state nursing home inspector and it had turned out just as I had expected - no signs of organicity). After the test, they decided he didn't need to be there and sent him off to Faribault Care Center. Bill was mad. His doctor had wanted him to have a psychological evaluation and get some medical treatment, but that didn't happen. But Bill did get to talk over the phone with his former orthopedist and another doctor who had worked with him. They told Bill they wanted to see him again, but since he was jerked back to Faribault Care Center so rapidly, that would probably not happen either.

So Bill was back in bondage at the Faribault Care Center. When he had been there previously after his surgeries, he had met a male nurse who had a penchant for helping suicidal people, over the internet, to carry out their intentions. Bill had liked him and learned that now, after his trial and a brief amount of jail time, he was a truck driver. It sounded to me like FCC did not exercise very good judgment in their hiring practices.

12 <u>OUT OF THE FRYING PAN...</u>

I wanted to get the results of the test that was given to Bill when he was at Mayo Clinic, the one that I thought might contradict the claim that he had significant brain damage. I was pretty sure I had a right to get the records since I was Bill's durable power of attorney and designated health care representative. Anoka had checked that out while Bill was in the hospital the first time and was ready to send me whatever I wanted, for the price of reproduction. That was before Bill had a guardian who could control the flow of information and, at the time, I thought whatever they had was a bunch of crap and wouldn't be of any help in freeing him. Now I wished I had requested some of it.

Jake called his lawyer friend and asked him what rights a person had to receive copies of his medical records and who had more authority, a person's power of attorney or his court appointed guardian. He did not like the answers he received. His friend told him that once someone has a court appointed guardian, any power of attorney documents were invalid and meaningless. Guardians could even have any power of attorney and living will forms removed from all files. Only the guardian could make any life or death decisions for the client. Also, a patient could only get copies of his medical records with the guardian's approval and nursing homes and hospital were aware of this fact, according to the attorney.

Since the papers appointing me power of attorney and health care representative were filled out at Mayo Clinic a few years ago when Bill was a medical patient there, I called them and asked if they could resend copies of the documents to me by U.S. Mail since they had inadvertently omitted the last page from the Advanced Directives when they sent them initially. The person I talked with said she would have to check something. When I called back, she refused to send the documents, claiming that she had talked with Mr. Tollefson's court-appointed guardian, who apparently did not want me to have access to the documentation of my status as attorney-in-fact and health care representative for Bill. I then decided to file a HIPAA complaint, explaining the situation and stating that

I believe there is a considerable amount of erroneous information in Mr. Tollefson's medical record that has significant legal and health care implications for the patient. I think that the guardian and the representative from Mayo Clinic have conspired to obstruct my access, not only to the records of my legal status vis-a-vis Mr. Tollefson, but also to his medical records at Mayo Clinic and elsewhere. I conclude from their obstructionism that their intention is to prevent me from assisting Mr. Tollefson in correcting errors or having disputatious information appended to his records. I believe this is a violation of HIPAA Rules, a violation of Mr. Tollefson's civil rights, and also a violation of my legal rights as Mr. Tollefson's durable power of attorney and designated health care representative.

While I was waiting for their reply, serendipity struck in the form of an article turned up in a Google search for something else. It was a report from the Minnesota House of Representatives Research Department dated April 30, 2009 related to a bill that established a *Bill of Rights for Wards and Protected Persons*. The part that interested me specified limitations on the rights of guardians. The report stated that the law:

Prohibits a guardian from revoking a health care directive of a ward or protected person without a court order. The appointment of an agent for a health care directive may not be revoked unless the agent was appointed within the previous 60 days, multiple agents have been appointed, or a court has determined that the ward lacks the capacity to appoint an agent and has expressly given the guardian authority to make health care decisions for the ward.

The decisions of a health care agent takes precedence over the decisions of a guardian, unless the health care directive is revoked.

Since I had not been served with any court-order and had been appointed more than 60 days prior to the appointment of a guardian, I figured this applied to my situation. I sent a copy of the document to the place where I submitted my HIPAA complaint. I subsequently talked with Dr. Parker who echoed Jake's lawyer friend's pessimism. She didn't think I should have filed the HIPAA complaint because the Office of Civil Rights would be likely to deny jurisdiction in cases of guardianships. Not only that, but the guardian could put some kind of restraining order on me so that I couldn't have any contact with Bill. Basically, she thought the guardians could commit and get away with murder. They could deny access to all medical information, including to the patient, so all their wrongdoing could be nicely covered up. She told me of a case in Pennsylvania where two judges made millions getting kickbacks for sentencing teen offenders to jail and then routing them into some kind of guardianship set up.

Eventually, I got a response from HIPAA indicating that they had provisionally decided to investigate the case, that it would be handled by the Chicago office, and that someone would be contacting me soon. I was pleased that they had decided to investigate the case and thought I might be able to talk with them about other aspects of the case once contact had been established. But, after a couple of months had passed without anyone contacting me, I wrote to ask them what they meant by "soon." I got no reply.

Bill's new residence was Faribault Care Center, previously known as Faribault Commons. The 104,500 square foot building was constructed in 1965 on 2.4 acres. In 2001 it was sold by Nationwide Health Partners to Minnesota Associates, LLC for $2,121,527.00 but by 2012 it had an estimated market value of only $1,225,500 for tax purposes. Deseret Health Group, a family owned company, acquired the property sometime after 2006 when it came into existence. Deseret has 25 relatively small nursing homes in the Midwest and now in Utah, where it is headquartered. It bills itself as a long-term senior care management company with "a proven record for converting distressed senior centers into successful, functioning facilities with high-quality senior and rehabilitative care" and "demonstrated significant success at reducing costs, improving quality of care and increasing revenue." In other words, they search out and buy up old, run-down nursing homes and convert them into profitable businesses by cutting costs the same way Beverly Corporation did. The company more than doubled the number of homes it owned, with a corresponding increase in its revenue, since August of 2010.

The company has more than 1000 employees and boasts that its leadership team "is almost all 'homegrown,' nurtured and taught within the firm." Jon H. Robertson founded the company in 2006 but the company website says little about his past professional experience other than that he had been a senior vice president of Life Care Centers of America, a privately owned operator of more than 225 retirement and health care centers in 28 states with 2011 revenues of $2.65 billion. However, a couple of Los Angeles Times articles, dated October 23, 1997, reveal a person with a flamboyant past.

Born in 1958 in Utah, his father was a social worker and he had 10 siblings. After high school, he entered the nursing home business following the example of an older brother and did well in the business aspect of that industry even though he had no training or college degree. He worked for several different companies and was described in one of the newspaper articles as "smart, impeccably groomed and impossibly charming and persuasive." By the time he was 34 years old he had risen to be a vice president of Life Care Centers of America. However, company officials fired him when they learned that Robertson was setting up his own new business, Phoenix Health Group Inc., while at the same time being paid by Life Care. In California, he bought nursing homes in Reseda, Costa Mesa, Alta Loma, Long Beach and Kern County and he expanded to buy another in Phoenix, Arizona.

As Medicare and Medi-Cal money rolled in, he began to spend conspicuously, buying a custom clothier named Jonathan Behr Bespoke Clothing and himself modeling for its print ads. According to a former employee, "His car isn't a Mercedes, it's a $90,000 Mercedes. It isn't a tie, it's a $75 tie. It isn't a watch, it's a $10,000 watch. Everything had a price tag." He bought a $1.3 million house near Scottsdale and another in Deer Valley, Utah. But, by the end of 1996, his empire began to unravel. He was $60,000 in arrears on the lease for his Phoenix facility, three nursing homes were closed down on short notice and two others were being overseen by a trustee for a U.S. Bankruptcy Court. California was investigating his use of Medicare and Medi-Cal funds. He was said to have entered treatment for cocain addiction at a Phoenix rehab center.

Ten years later, Jon Robertson resurfaced as the founder of Deseret Health Group with two sons as members of the executive team. The current CEO of Deseret Health Group is Garett Robertson, a 2007 graduate of the University of Utah who claims 10 years of experience in the long-term care industry, which would suggest that he dates the start of his career to when he was still in high school. Another son, Skyler Robertson, with a Bachelor's Degree in Business Management from Utah Valley University, manages day-to-day operations of the North Region and human resources programs for the entire company. To me, red flags began to pop up – it was beginning to sound like Beverly-Golden Liver all over again.

Bill's reintroduction to Faribault Care Center was anything but encouraging. When I talked with him on February 27th he said that the previous night the nurses aides had taken away his pain medications and moved his bedside table, containing his drinking water, urinal and call button, out of reach. They told him they were the only two people working that night, so apparently they didn't want him to page them. The next day when the day shift came in they asked Bill why there were a couple of rubber pads on the floor. He told them he didn't know but I suggested, half in jest, that it may have been in order to deaden the sound if he fell out of bed.

A couple of days later at 4:00 am, Bill was taken to the hospital ER with lightning-like shooting pains in his right knee. He thought they felt like the ones he had had years before when he had been paralyzed for six months. At that time, he said, his doctor had erroneously gotten his coumadin (blood thinner) levels too high and he had started to bleed into his abdomen. That caused pressure on his spinal cord and paralyzed one or both legs. This time, the ER doctor decided he was having muscle spasms in his knee, gave him two Tylenol 3s and .5 mg of Ativan. Bill had wanted to go to Mayo Clinic for evaluation and treatment but instead they sent him back to the nursing home.

The next day I got a notice from the prosecutor regarding the appointment of Bill's guardian. As I understood it, they were proposing to take away all of Bill's rights and were relying on all the erroneous information that was used in the original hearing. They claimed he had no mental capacity to make any judgments, assumed he was still on Abilify and there was no mention at all of Dr. Smart's statement that Bill was not crazy and didn't belong in a mental hospital.

Holy cow! If this is allowed to stand, Bill will be totally screwed, I thought.

I hoped we could get something going to stop or reverse this action. I sent an email to Janet Parker and she called back on the phone, asking me to send whatever I had compiled so far to her so she could get the federal prosecutor involved as soon as possible. I sent her 13 pages of violations of state laws and violations of the *Americans with Disabilities Act* along with a copy of the notice I got from the prosecutor and copies of the psychologist's report and prepetition report. She thought it would be a good idea for me to file an ethics complaint against the psychologist who did Bill's assessment. The ethics complaint process all had to be done by U.S. Mail for confidentiality reasons, so I expected it would take a while. I sent off the initial contact letter two days later, telling them who the complaint was about and the nature of the ethical violations.

Jake told Bill he would be down to see him in a couple of days because he had to go to the county court house to get his mother's death certificate. He believed that nurses at Northfield Hospital had overdosed his mother with morphine by mistake when family members inquired about her level of pain. He thought the nurses had taken their inquiry as an implicit message that the children wanted to put their mother out of her misery when, actually, they were just inquiring if she was in any pain. I suggested that, while he was at the court house, he might ask if there was any way to find out what powers the court had given to Bill's guardian. I also wanted him to get Bill's signature and thumb print on a form indicating his willingness to have Dr. Parker represent him in actions to be taken at federal and possibly international agencies.

After his trip to Faribault, Jake sent me an email. "Got a slightly smudged fingerprint and signature. Probably good enough. Bill is in a room by himself with a TV, bathroom, and a leaky window which keeps the room nice and cool compared to GLC. However, Bills assessment was, 'This is the worst place I've ever been in.' At least no one was wetting the floor all over the place. At GLC I went into the bathroom the last time I was there and my shoes almost stuck to the floor.

"Bill was watching the races on TV and moaning about all his pain. I could hardly understand a word he said---too much mumbling, like someone who had a small stroke. I asked him if he was getting his pain meds and he said, 'Yes-that's all ok now.' Then he mumbled something about the Field cops dislocating his shoulder when they pulled him out of the pool. He also has a big sore on his left leg where the skin could not expand as fast as his leg. It was about 3.5 inches long and 1.5 inches wide; very red and raw looking. He said all he needed for it was some ointment. Said he thought he was coming down with the flu & wanted a 12 pack of 7-up which I picked up for him."

I was glad to hear that Bill was back on his pain meds but it sounded like he was still having trouble. That wound on his leg did not sound good. It is just too easy to get a hard to control infection while in a nursing home or hospital.

The next day I got a call from Bill. He was again in the Mayo Clinic. The previous night he had vomited up blood and had blood in his stools. After some time spent dithering, the nursing home sent him to the District 1 Hospital and the doctor he saw there sent him to Mayo. I got a call from his doctor asking for my approval to send a camera down his throat. I told him that Bill had a guardian but that didn't matter to him since Bill had wanted him to call me. He told me what he suspected and that he planned to cauterize the wound if he found an ulcer. He said that the risks were near zero. My wife had had the same procedure, so I said that would be fine. After the camera work, they ended up doing an ultrasound and found ulceration in both esophagus and stomach. He tested positive for H-pilori, the bacteria that causes most stomach ulcers, and was placed on antibiotics.

Bill was very happy to be at Mayo Clinic with its competent care and good food. He was lucid, didn't beat about the bush, memory was good, and he sounded better than I had heard him since he was at the motel (before they hauled him away). About the only time he gets really upset and kind of dysfunctional, I thought, was when some over-controlling assholes start harassing him.

I received the Ethics Complaint Kit from the American Psychological Association (APA) and started getting the nine documents (25 pages) together to send. I was bothered by one item in the packet that I received from the APA: it was required that the complainant sign a statement that he/she would not subpoena records from the APA for purposes of private litigation. While it wouldn't be I who would sue the psychologist - Bill would have that honor – Janet thought the waiver might extend to him because I was his power of attorney. I thought Bill should sue her for malpractice if he ever got the chance, so I didn't want to jeopardize that option. I could resign as his power of attorney and health care agent and then file the ethics complaint and he could then subpoena the records even though APA wouldn't like it. I decided to mull it over for a while.

I reread the notice from the prosecutor. It listed the same old crap about Bill from when he was hospitalized and it sounded like they still considered him to be committed. The notice mentioned that there was a limited time to appeal and I wanted to do so because most of the assertions could not be substantiated, i. e., diagnoses of MRSA, alcoholism, cannabis addiction, Cognitive Disorder, NOS, paranoia, delusions, etc. I knew the kangaroo court would probably ignore anything I had to say, but I wanted to get it on the record anyway. I would be willing to pay a lawyer to read it to the court. So I called the prosecutor's office, as the notice suggested the recipient do, to find out when the deadline was. His secretary said he told her he couldn't talk with me. I said all I wanted from them was the date of the deadline. She said she couldn't provide even that. I called the court house and the clerk said, "Get a lawyer." I called Zimbledon and left a message for him to call back. He didn't. I called Bill and told him he needed to call Zimbledon and find out the deadline, the format for an appeal and the date it would need to be presented in court. Bill thought the matter was already in appeal.

By the end of the day I had reached the limit of my frustration tolerance. My mind rebelled against exerting any more effort. "To hell with it, I'm done. I quite. Let the fuckers kill him. That's what they are going to do anyway and he won't do anything to get himself out of the line of fire. He won't take any directions, he'll just blab his way into the pot and they'll boil his ass for the rest of his days."

After my wrath had dissipated, I found an interesting item during a Google search: the *State Integrity Investigation,* a project by three journalistic groups – the Center for Public Integrity, Global Integrity and

Public Radio International
(http://www.stateintegrity.org/state_integrity_invesitgation_overview_sto
ry). Rather than relying on corruption conviction data, this project
assessed, for each of the 50 states, 330 "Integrity Indicators" across 14
categories of state government: public access to information, political
financing, executive accountability, legislative accountability, judicial
accountability, state budget processes, civil service management,
procurement, internal auditing, lobbying disclosure, pension fund
management, ethics enforcement, insurance commissions, and
redistricting. An overall "Corruption Risk Grade" was computed from
the category grades at the conclusion of the months long project.

None of the states excelled in all aspects of integrity and none
achieved an overall grade of A. The problems were many. According to
the report, "Open records laws with hundreds of exemptions. Crucial
budgeting decisions made behind closed doors by a handful of power
brokers. Citizen' lawmakers voting on bills that would benefit them
directly. Scores of legislators turning into lobbyists seemingly overnight.
Disclosure laws without much disclosure. Ethics panels that haven't met
in years.

"State officials make lofty promises when it comes to ethics in
government. They tout the transparency of legislative processes,
accessibility of records, and the openness of public meetings. But these
efforts often fall short of providing any real transparency or legitimate
hope of rooting out corruption."

Minnesota achieved an overall grade of D+ with F's in Judicial
Accountability (the judiciary is politicized and subject to financial
conflict of interests), Ethics Enforcement Agencies (there is no
enforcement agency and no fines for violating ethics laws), Lobbying
Disclosure (lacks timeliness and essential information) and Redistricting
Openness. Along with the temptation to cut corners during bad economic
times by cutting funding for oversight agencies and short-changing
defendants on their civil and legal rights, this laxness about matters of
integrity might account for many of Bill's problems over the last 18
months.

Bill said that his appointment with his orthopedist at Mayo Clinic on
March 15 went well. His blood tests all turned out favorably and his legs
were almost their normal size, so he thought he might be able to get back
into his shoes. He said he was finding a few people that he regarded as
"good" at FCC and mentioned one woman who went from a nasty
disposition at first to a more amenable one after they started talking
about religion. He was happy about having a private room and a TV that
he didn't have to share with anyone and seemed to be somewhat content

with the place.

The patient phone at the nursing home was another test of frustration tolerance. Many times, no one would answer even after 50 rings. If you did get past that hurdle, someone had to take the phone to Bill's room, where reception was hit and miss. I would start to talk with him but his voice would be drowned out by static. Then the phone would go dead. I would hit redial, talk for about 15 seconds and again lose the connection. In order to talk for a minute it might take 10 redials. The facility administrators apparently had no interest in providing phone service for their residents, even though that function is required according to the *Patient Bill of Rights*.

One day, I called and the person who answered said Bill had been moved to a city-run apartment complex nearby. I looked up on the Internet the name I was given and it looked like a nice place where Bill could be more independent. I was getting my hopes up that things might change for the better for old Bill. I called the two phone numbers associated with the name of the apartment, which turned out to be city offices, but no one answered. The next day I spent about 4 hours trying to get through to him. The first person who answered again told me he had moved. I called the nurses station to verify what I had been told, and it turned out to be incorrect. He was still at the nursing home. The nurse said he was busy doing something and to call back in half an hour. When I did, the guy who answered said the phone needed to be charged up and to call back in a half hour. When I called after a half hour, the phone rang for about 50 rings and disconnected. That happened three times and I gave up. I was getting mighty sick of their phone system!

Cindi Fisher notified me that a ruling had been made in the long-running civil rights case of Daniel Gross, an elderly man from Long Island who had become ill while visiting his daughter in Connecticut. His children fought over his care and who should control his finances, so a judge approved an involuntary conservatorship without the patient being told of the hearing and without his court-appointed lawyer objecting to him being placed in a locked ward with a violent roommate at a nursing home.

Gross' daughter filed a federal civil rights lawsuit against the judge, the lawyer, the conservator and the nursing home. The judge could not be sued but the justices ruled that court-appointed lawyers do not have immunity from lawsuits if they ignore the wishes of their clients, that conservators appointed by probate have limited immunity, and that nursing homes do not have immunity from lawsuits in probate cases. In other words, lawyers and conservators must be held accountable in probate court, at least in Connecticut. This might be a good precedent if it were ever to come to court in Minnesota, although defenders of the status quo might just argue that findings in other states didn't matter.

Bill's scheduled "evidentiary hearing" was in just a couple of days. I tried calling him and was told the phone in the commons area didn't reach to his room and the portable phone needed to be charged up. So, they said they would give him a message to call me. It sounded like what he would need to do was get out of bed and wheel down to the common area to use the phone there. He hadn't done so and I was wondering if he had gone into another one of his "I'll show you" funk periods.

Jake found out that Bill ate all his meals in bed and didn't wheel down to the food room any more. Jake had checked the meal room and thought it was very nice – clean and big, nicely decorated with fresh flowers. He said that, by comparison, the one at GLC was a dive. "If Bill doesn't start climbing into his wheelchair and scooting around the place," Jake commented, "his health (and legs) are all going to go to pot quickly." It was my belief that Bill would not need to be in a nursing home if he were to get aquatic therapy, as Dr. Smart had indicated was on the agenda, but that if he was just vegetating in bed and was in a willful, cantankerous mood, he would make their case for them and things would not go well in court.

On the appointed day, Jake called the court scheduler and was told there wasn't anything listed for Bill Tollefson. I called Bill and he said no one told him the hearing was canceled or bothered to prep him for the event. Good old Zimbledon, I said to myself, violating his professional ethics yet again.

Bill was not doing well, confined to bed and unable to get to the working phone in the commons area. Luckily, a good-hearted nurse let him use her cell phone. He said he had been asking for pain medications for 1.25 hours before they brought him any. The previous night a woman was supposed to come back and wash him, help him do a bowel movement in his commode and put ointment on his bed sores (which had developed in the spots worn sore from his unfitted wheelchair). She never showed up. He asked to receive physical therapy but no one came to see him about it. At that point, he felt too weak to even do aquatic therapy. He had not had a shower for 11 days and before that he had gone 30 days without a shower.

I was pissed. I downloaded a complaint form from the Office of Health Facilities Complaints and made complaints about the delays in providing him pain medication, about the night they moved the table with his urinal, water and call buzzer out of reach, the failure to provide physical therapy, the failure to provide showers and attend to his cleanliness, and the poor quality of the phone service.

Presumed Crazy

I talked with Bill but, as usual, the line was filled with static so it was only possible to get a few words at a time. Apparently the OHFC had not yet contacted them regarding my complaint. Bill said it had been since February 17 that he had had a shower and that the staff had skipped the last two scheduled showers. He said that he had bed sores and "skin problems" and his right knee hurt so bad he couldn't put any weight on it. I speculated that if he got one of those nursing home kinds of infections, that would probably be all she wrote for 'ol Bill. (That was what had happened to my sister - she got klebscillia pneumonia either in the nursing home or in the hospital. I wasn't informed about the infection until after they let her die). The nursing home staff had to get a lift device to move him to his commode and back. He said they would only put him on the commode three times per week.

I asked myself, "What the hell is this? I take a shit at least once or twice a day and they're going to put Bill on the commode just three times a week? Where does the rest of the shit go? What kind of place is this?"

Bill said he felt like a basket case and thought they were just going to let him fade out. He was visited by his guardian & social worker during the week but, as usual, they did nothing to help him.

I updated Jake and he responded. "Sounds like Bill is getting worse, not better. If they have to use a crane to get him out of bed he must be going down hill fast. And most physicians don't really give a hoot about patients who are extremely overweight. I used to work with a guy who was close to 400 pounds and had one bad knee. He went to an orthopedic surgeon who told him, 'lose 150 pounds first and then we can talk!'

"This all started when Bill had a reaction to those pills he was taking. He lost his ability to do much of anything for a few weeks including clean up his apartment. His Florida trip was probably a big set back and then the Rice County court psychologist did a complete hatchet job on him. If she had been a psychology college student her report would have earned a big fat red F. Now it looks like Bill might just punch out before anything positive happens to him. And once that happens, I don't think anything can be done to help anybody. After his death maybe one of his siblings will start to see dollar signs and hire some big hot shot lawyer to sue everyone in sight all over the tragic death of their much loved brother."

I reminded Jake that preventing patients from getting bedsores and becoming less mobile and functional than they were when they arrived were some of the federal standards for nursing homes. I downloaded and began to read the *Case Resolution Manual* from the Office of Civil Rights. From what I read, everything that had happened to Bill and every place where it had happened fell under their jurisdiction. So maybe, I thought, we should send them the whole packet of stuff and let them sort it out.

I received a letter from the Office of Health Facility Complaints saying they were requesting a copy of medical records to review with respect to my complaints. I didn't think the people at Faribault Care center were dumb enough to leave tracks of their violations of nursing home standards in the medical records but maybe they would look at the absence of entries (e. g., for showers) and get something that way. More wishful thinking on my part.

I called Kelby Woodard, the Minnesota State Representative for Bill's district, to find out if he knew who was responsible for enforcing the laws I thought had been violated. An aide called back.

"Can you give me a little more information about your request?"

"Yes. I was calling about what agency in Minnesota I should report violations of the following laws: 253B *Civil Commitment*; 144.651 *Health Care Bill of Rights*; and 524.5-120 the *Bill of Rights for Wards and Protected Persons*."

"Maybe you should start with your local authorities, the police."

"What? You've got to be kidding."

"Well maybe if you gave me more information I could talk with someone else to see if we could come up with an answer."

"Well these seem to be like civil rights laws on a state level. There must be someplace in state government to report violations of them, don't you think?"

"Well, maybe you should start with the police or try other state agencies."

"You don't know anything about these laws, do you?"

"No, I'm in education and I haven't studied..."

"I see. Thanks for calling back. I haven't had much luck with any state agencies I have tried so far."

"Maybe I could ask around and see...."

"Thanks for calling back. Bye."

I received an email from the congressman later saying he was searching for an answer to my question. Apparently that was an endless loop for him as he never responded again.

Jake thought it didn't sound right that the nursing home wanted Bill to defecate in his bed. I didn't think so either so I filed another set of complaints with the Office of Health Facility Complaints. The complaints included the practice of having him defecate in his bed, the continuing failure to provide him with a shower, the failure to provide physical therapy, and the fact that they ran out of the medication that he took with his pain medication to prevent him from having nightmares.

214

Presumed Crazy

Shortly thereafter, I received a response from OHFC saying, "although the concerns you identified are significant it is improbable that a violation could be supported." I was incensed at their cavalier indifference and fired back the following letter:

Dear OHFC:

After your first letter when you said you would send for medical records regarding my complaint against Faribault Care Center, I was pretty sure you were not serious about exposing any wrong doing at that facility. They may be dumb but they are not so dumb as to record their violations of nursing standards in their medical records. But, I thought, maybe you could determine that the patient had had only one shower (on March 22, 2012) since he arrived back at the facility from Mayo Clinic about February 21, 2012. Mr. Tollefson reported that he had tried to negotiate a delay in taking a shower on one occasion (when he was feeling especially bad) and the staff had advanced his scheduled date for a shower by one day. They would not make this accommodation for the patient and probably entered in the record that "the patient refused." But surely one shower in over two months does not comply with the federal standard that nursing facilities provide "assistance to retain and/or promote daily functioning and assistance with grooming" and under 483.25 (a) "that the resident's ability to perform activities of daily living do not diminish, unless unavoidable, and those who cannot carry out those activities receive necessary services to maintain good nutrition, grooming, and personal oral hygiene." Mr. Tollefson, as of this date, is still awaiting a second shower. Furthermore, under 483.25e, "that residents who are admitted without limited range of motion do not experience reductions in range of motion unless unavoidable, and that residents with a limited range of motion receive treatment to increase those abilities and prevent further deterioration." When Mr. Tollefson arrived he was wheelchair-bound but was able to transfer and was able to move about the facility. Now he has lost range of motion in his right leg, is bed-ridden and has received no treatment to increase his abilities, even though he has requested it. Although there are other deficiencies in meeting federal nursing home standards, this will suffice for present purposes.

After my second complaint about Faribault Care Center, you responded by saying that "although the concerns you identified are significant it is improbable that a violation could be supported." I took that to mean that you couldn't really prove anything from the records (big surprise!) and that you were unable or unwilling to do any other kind of investigation.

I then reasoned that probably what had happened was that your budget had been cut and you didn't have the resources to really investigate all the complaints you receive, so you are forced to wait until you have a dead body (like at Golden Living Center in Hopkins and at the two state managed group homes) that causes public outrage. Only then will you take any action, slapping the hands of the offenders and telling them to not kill any more of their residents. Of course this non-proactive approach doesn't do much to help the dead victims. In cases where there are not yet any dead bodies, you just go through the motions, sending out letters to the complainers but not doing any real investigations.

I know that yours is not the only governmental agency to have budget problems that filter down to adversely affect your stated missions and the welfare of the people you are supposed to serve. It is that kind of cost-cutting that has, from the very beginning, brought about this whole dreadful case. In the process, these methods of "holding down the costs" end up being false economies, bilking the taxpayers of millions of dollars more than if they hadn't been instituted.

So, I guess I will write you off, OHFC. I'm sorry I don't have a dead body to present to you, but, at the present rate, it may soon be on the horizon. In the meantime, I will see if federal agencies are any more responsive than state ones.

Still fuming over 18 months of frustration in dealing with people and agencies in Minnesota, I decided to send off a packet of information to the APA regarding my ethics complaint against the psychologist who initially evaluated Bill. I figured that Bill would probably never get it together enough to sue her and, by signing the agreement to not seek documentation from them for private litigation, I didn't think I would prevent him from suing her, although it might prevent him from asking for documentation from them. All a lawyer would have to do would be to get her on the stand and ask her if she ever was investigated for an ethics charge. Or they could get me on the stand and I could give them whatever the APA sent me. Jake, Big Jim, Lucy, Bill's younger sister and my wife all agreed to provide verifying testimony, if requested.

13 <u>A SHOWER IS A WONDERFUL THING</u>

On May 10, 2012 Bill told me he had learned two days earlier that nursing home staff had been slipping Wellbutrin, an SSRI antidepressant, into his medications without telling him or asking his permission. Once he learned of this surreptitious act, he refused to take it and his mood improved and he felt "back to normal." About a week later Jake talked with Bill and noted the change. "He sounded like he was getting back to his old self--a lot of dreams for the future." This was the same kind of effect that Bill had when he stopped taking Abilify, i. e., he returned to his usual mental state. I knew it was not right (and probably not legal) for them to administer a psychotropic medication without a court-order but it was not until August, when Bill was finally provided a list of his medications after asking for one for months, that I learned just how careless and potentially dangerous this had been.

Bill related his medications to me. I looked them up on *Drugs.com* to find what conditions they were for and common side-effects as well as possible adverse drug interactions. There was one major adverse interaction, between Tramadol and Wellbutrin, that could increase the chances of precipitating a seizure, especially in the elderly or in patients with other risk factors such as head trauma or metabolic disorders (e. g., metabolic syndrome, diabetes, thyroid deficiency, obesity). Luckily, Bill's seizure threshold had not yet been reduced to the point where he had experienced a seizure, but continued use of the two medications together could have lead to that outcome. Besides that dangerous interaction, there was no evidence that SSRIs actually reduce depressive symptoms and recently there has been a mountain of evidence that they are ineffective for most people and quite dangerous for some. Even psychiatrists admit that there is no scientific evidence that supports the "chemical imbalance theory" claimed to justify the use of such medications. I asked who had prescribed the Wellbutrin and Bill did not know even though he had asked several staff members who had done so and they denied any knowledge of it.

There were twelve two-way drug interactions that were considered "moderate" in the batch that were prescribed to Bill. The interaction calculator on the web site only dealt with two-way interactions, so more complicated effects (e. g., 3- or 4-way interactions) were not determined. I copied the information on the drugs and sent it to Bill for his perusal.

My impression was that nursing home staff and Bill's doctor were not monitoring his prescribed drugs as they should have and that some of the drugs should probably be discontinued or have an alternative substituted. I thought Bill may have been "carried" on some of his medications simply because some previous doctor prescribed it without subsequent doctors questioning if he still needed it (or if he *ever* needed it). Bill said he never had any of the typical symptoms of gout but got that tag when he turned up with a high uric acid level at the Anoka hospital. He was given thyroid medication originally to counteract the side effects of amioderone, but when he stopped taking the amioderone after having a "toxic thyroid" reaction, the thyroid medication was still continued. This occurred even after he was told at one time at the Mayo Clinic that his thyroid had "come back" to normal functioning. When he stopped the amioderone because the interaction with thyroxin was making him sick, it made the doctor at Northfield Hospital so mad that he called Bill non-compliant and crazy.

Bill was also on a number of drugs that cause loss of magnesium which is important for muscle functioning and can lead to teteny (muscle cramping) and carpopedal seizures (cramping in feet and hands). I thought he needed a complete re-evaluation of the need for each and every one of his medications.

Susan Freiman wrote that she had read all the material I had sent to her and her first impression to my lack of due process argument was that, "You'd have a hard row to hoe to get a court to overrule what's been done until now. To start this road, you'd have to file in federal court. But these are very preliminary ideas, as I'm just at the beginning of my research. The issue is very complicated, and the simplest route for a federal court would be to duck the issue by holding that the state institutions did follow due process." Oh great! Now even the feds can be expected to try to duck the issues. Isn't there anyone who wants to see justice done?

Bill had been living in a hospital gown since he returned from Mayo Clinic. His long pants had been lost by the laundry at Golden Living Center and his bib overalls were in need of repair. His extra-large T-shirts had been stolen from his apartment during his hospitalization. The only other clothes he had with him were a pair of gym pants and a pair of cut-off short pants. He still had not had a shower since March. They hoisted him out of bed using a Hoyer lift and placed him on the commode but this occurred only once because, they said, the commode was not of a suitable size. Instead, they would place him in his bed and every three days or so he would defecate there. Afterward they would come in and mop him up, apparently thinking that was sufficient to prevent infection and of adequate dignity for "just an old fart on Medicaid." Bill said he was looking forward to standing and moving a bit but found that his legs below the knee were "numb," i. e., he had no strength in his muscles due to atrophy because he had been in bed for so long. There was another reason that became apparent later.

Bill kept returning to what he considered the only viable option – aquatic physical rehabilitation – the same option that he had been requesting since he was at Anoka and the same option that had been promised to him by Dr. Smart and others. He needed the buoyancy of the water to support him so that he could do physical exercises to regain muscle mass and range of motion in his joints. His favored facility was the Courage Center because of his previous experience there. Sister Kinney Foundation also had an aquatic therapy program but he felt that his relationship with them had been soured by one of his previous social services workers who didn't like him. On May 16 a physical therapist came in and moved his legs as he sat in his chair. They talked about getting him into aquatic therapy at a pool he had used in Faribault a few years ago but the lift at that facility was limited to 250 pounds, unsuitable for his current weight. A few years earlier, I had given Bill a ride down to that facility so that he could use one or both of their pools.

The next day I received a document from the lawyer who was prosecuting Bill's case for Rice County notifying me of a"Hearing on the Conservator's Final Account" and a "Petition for Discharge of Emergency Guardian of the Person and Emergency Conservator of the Estate" to take place on June 18th. I called Bill and asked him if he had received the same notification and he had not. I looked at the list of recipients and found that his address was still listed as the Anoka hospital. I suggested that he call Zimbledon right away and ask what this hearing meant. Knowing Zimbledon's penchant for shirking his ethical duties to his client by not returning phone calls, I sent an email to him requesting that he contact Bill and explain what this action was about. I included Bill's phone number and mailing address and sent copies to Lucy, Jake and Big Jim to serve as witnesses that Zimbledon had been notified.

Of course, Bill, Jake and I all speculated on what this hearing meant and why it was happening at this time. Jake recalled, "I forgot to tell you. At a meeting at Golden Liver, I asked Bird Brain why Bill couldn't get admitted at Valley View and she leaned over and whispered to me, 'Bill has to live in a locked facility,' not that it was because he required too much care or that he was too heavy."

I responded, "That's interesting if now he is safe enough to be let loose! Bill said the social worker from Rice County was the one who told him it was because of his weight. Goes to show you how much of this crap they just make up! Bill said that they have him down as being suicidal too. I doubt that he has ever been suicidal throughout this whole affair but, if he was, it was a condition that they brought upon him."

I calculated that the Ombudsman for Elder Minnesotans had been back from her vacation for four days and decided to email her to see if she had seen Bill yet. I told her,

> The situation has not changed much. He still has not had a shower in over two months and has had to resort to using a fork to straighten out the mats in his hair. They have finally started to use the Hoyer lift to get him into his own electric lift chair which he has slept in because it is more comfortable than his bed. They have apparently had a problem with the quality of their Hoyer lift sling and have ordered a new one, they tell him, but who knows when or if they will get it. He had to defecate in his bed again the other night because they could not get him onto his commode. This is unacceptable and a violation of federal regulations governing nursing homes. If you are unable to make a visit to Mr. Tollefson, please let me know immediately and I will contact other individuals in your ombudsman organization or other agencies who might be able to expedite corrective action.

She responded that she had been out of the office and was scheduled out for the next two weeks, but assured me that she had been working on Mr. Tollefson's situation.

I wrote to Susan Freiman, expressing my frustration and she wrote back with one word, "Surprised?"

"Yes, a little. I guess hope springs eternal! Not that I expected her to actually jump on the nursing home and demand they do something, but I thought she would pay Bill a visit before they killed him! The woman from the agency that referred me to her said they were running about two weeks behind but that was before the ombudslady took her two week vacation! I guess they don't have anyone who takes up the slack when someone goes on vacation and they just let cases pile up. No, I don't begrudge her a vacation, I just think the agency should have some mechanism to keep cases from becoming stale and irrelevant. But, I have to remind myself that MN is the land of "Let's Pretend:" pretend rights laws and pretend rights laws enforcement. The laws sound good on paper but there is virtually no mechanism to enforce them."

Susan contacted a relative who had been a Lutheran minister and had run a nursing home himself. He suggested that I ask for help from Lutheran Social Services(LSS), since Bill was a Lutheran and that agency was generally well-staffed in Minnesota. He also suggested I relate this "deplorable situation" to the office of Al Franken (which I had already done with no response whatsoever).

Bill thought that contacting LSS might be a good idea. I found a phone number for them in Faribault and called the next day. They wanted to turn me over to their Guardianship and Coordination of Care section. I looked up on their web site to see what they did and it looked like it could be useful to Bill in the future. But I was afraid they would contact his guardian right off the bat to try to work through her and was afraid they would get things all fucked up before the guardian was out of the picture. Bill agreed that that would be the likely scenario. I suggested he contact LSS and make an appointment with a counselor to do some planning for when he is no longer under guardianship, i. e., finding a place to live, getting proper medical care, getting equipment he needs and qualifies for, etc. That way, if the judge were to ask him how he was going to manage without a guardian, he would already have a plan or be in a planning process with LSS. He had quite a way to go before he would become mobile enough to live outside a nursing home and would need some support services once he got out, which LSS could help provide.

The next time I talked with Bill, he was fit to be tied. They wouldn't use the Hoyer lift to put him into his electric-lift chair rather than his uncomfortable bed. They told him they didn't know if he was "authorized" to use the chair. He responded that he had been prescribed the chair by Rice County Social Services and had been using it for nine years. Then they said the sling on the Hoyer lift was too small, but it was the same sling they had been using for the last two weeks. Then they told him they didn't have the time to move him, of course in the process using up more time by giving him excuses than it would have taken to lift him

221

into his chair. And one of the nurses aides he considered "evil" had returned to torment him. When he asked for a complaint form, they told him they didn't have one. I gave him the phone number of the corporate office but told him not to expect much if he called there since the family that runs it had a poor track record. He learned that his belongings from Golden Living Center in St. Louis Park had been picked up by his guardian about a week after he left there. She did not tell him a thing about having done so for the last two months.

But, on the positive side, his physical therapy with a woman named Paula was going well and he got along with her fine. She talked about getting him mobile enough to get back into his wheelchair and then going for some type of aquatic therapy. I hoped the higher-ups at the nursing home or his guardian didn't torpedo her efforts. Bill also had a good talk with his adopted son from his first marriage who lives in Faribault. They didn't talk long but it was established that they had lost contact because of the staff at United Hospital in St. Paul when this whole "deplorable situation" had begun.

The Ombudsman for Older Minnesotans showed up on Friday the first of June for a "resident care council." The only beneficial result was that he got his first glass of ice water since he arrived at the nursing home. A female staff member promised to come give him a shower on Monday but then never showed up. The physical therapist showed up for two days and the results made Bill conclude his legs were "really shot." His Rice County social worker, the social services person from the nursing home and the husband of his guardian's partner (whose position was undesignated) had a "care meeting" but, according to Bill, it accomplished nothing. "They just wanted to get out of here as soon as possible." I remarked to Jake that that may have had something to do with him not having had a shower for the last few months!

Bill told his "care givers" that there were things from Golden Liver in St. Louis Park that they had picked up and put into storage, like his dentures that he could use now. They didn't volunteer to get anything for him. He called Rice County Court to find out the time of day that the hearing was to be held on the 18th but they would not tell him. They told him to call the office of the prosecutor. When he did so, he was told that they couldn't talk with him! Same kind of Catch-22 that I ran into when I called to find out when the deadline for an appeal was. He then called his court appointed lawyer, Zimbledon, but, of course, Zimbledon never returned his calls. I sent an email to the unethical attorney asking him to answer four questions Bill had about the hearing (like, when it was to be and who was the judge) and I again gave him Bill's address and phone number, but as usual, he never responded. So it was just the same old BS and the same old incompetence and irresponsibility.

Bill still hadn't received a shower so I called the woman from the Area Agency on Aging. She suggested we have a joint telephone call with the head nurse, and she got her on the phone. The nurse said that Bill had refused showers and, having asked Bill twice about this, I countered that he had refused just one time, when he was in too much pain to be moved and that otherwise he was begging to receive a shower. She agreed to schedule one and on June 13, after more than 2 months, Bill finally got wet from head to toe.

He said it was quite an operation. They Hoyer-lifted him onto a commode with wheels and wheeled him down to the shower. (How they could use this commode for transportation but not for defecation remained a mystery.) But the door wasn't wide enough, so they had to Hoyer him off the commode, move the commode into the shower and lift him up again and then drop him back onto the commode through the open door. It was no wonder they didn't want to do it any more often than they had to. Obviously, this facility was not adequate for patients who were above average size.

I received a call from the ombudslady and, at first, she seemed to be one of those people who was overworked and rushed, wanting to get you off the phone as soon as possible but feeling duty-bound to do what was expected of a person in her position. However, she did express a positive attitude toward Bill and listened as I countered some of the misinformation she had garnered from nursing home staff and from his medical records (i. e., that he was crazy as a loon and demented). She didn't seem to understand the problem with his legs and was talking about the possibility of amputation, something never mentioned to him by his Mayo Clinic orthopedist. She was convinced that he was diabetic, something Bill disputed because his blood sugar levels had been within normal range until recently (his most recent blood sugar level was slightly above the recently lowered cut-off number). However, she seemed genuinely interested in helping Bill and getting him into a better position. We discussed the shower problem and she said that Bill had told her and her aide that he would refuse showers until he got into a pool.

So I confronted Bill with this information. "I talked with the ombudslady and she thought you were a sweet old gent and I didn't disabuse her of that notion. She really wants to help you get better medical care and get into a better nursing home. And, by the way, she said you had told her and her aide that you were refusing any showers until you got into a pool."

"No, I didn't say that."

I said, "Oh, she must have gotten it wrong. I'll have to ask her about that."

"Well, now just a minute. I may have said something *like* that. I said I might have *thought* about doing that, but I never said I *actually did* that. I'd never say anything like that."

"Good thing," I said, "because that would not be a good idea."

I concluded that Bill had been floating one of his desperation strategies to see what kind of response it would garner. Don't budge, be obstinate, outlast your opposition and they will give in. In children a similar ploy is to threaten, "I'll hold my breath until I turn blue and die unless you do what I want." It will often work, but it can leave a bad taste in the mouths of those who have been bamboozled. I thought that was one of the things that his sister hated about him.

I followed up with a thank-you email to both the ombudslady and the person from the area agency on aging, sending a copy of the first nine chapters of this book and hoping they would read it to get a better appreciation of what Bill had been through. I added that I was working with an advocate to develop a case to present to federal investigators, thinking that that information might get dispersed to his care-givers and spur them on to more professional behavior.

I had signed on to Al Franken's mailing list some time back when I had emailed him about Bill's case (to which I had never received a reply). I received one of his announcements that he had gotten himself appointed to some kind of health care committee and he was asking for comments about health care legislation. Although I suspected his email was simply a self-promotional device, I submitted a summary of Bill's case to the senator. I received the automated reply shortly thereafter:

"Thank you for submitting your message to my U.S. Senate office. Each week, several thousand Minnesotans send me their thoughts and suggestions on legislation and important issues facing our nation. This impressive volume is a testament to the Minnesotan traditions of grassroots activism and civic participation that distinguish our state. I closely track the concerns that are expressed in your letters and emails, and will answer them as soon as possible."

I decided not to hold my breath until I received a response.

Bill called Zimbaldon's number again and left a message at 4:30 on 6/12/12 asking if he had received my email and telling him that he wanted to talk to him about his upcoming hearing. My money was on Bill not hearing a thing from Zimbaldon. He probably wouldn't even tell him the time of the hearing. Since Zimbledon, the prosecutor and the

Rice County Court were all non-responsive representatives of the justice system, Bill resorted to asking his guardian when the hearing was to be. She told him he didn't have to be at the hearing. When he said that he wanted to be there, she told him that the county would not pay for his transportation to court, which is in the same little town as the nursing home and wouldn't cost much. In addition, it is one of his rights supposedly guaranteed by the state. Ha! No doubt, she was lying because she didn't want him there to observe her testimony. So, it was just another instance of Rice County denying Bill his legal and civil rights.

Bill mentioned an article in the *Faribault Daily News* where it was pointed out that Rice County was the county in the state with the greatest number of complaints about their social services department and was being threatened with sanctions by the Minnesota Department of Human Services. The county is responsible for processing financial eligibility forms that determine who gets benefits like food stamps and medical assistance and they had been behind schedule for the last year. The County commissioners voted no to hiring four people to cut the delay time for food stamps so it could comply with federal standards.

A later article told of a group called People for a Better Rice County that had been formed to make sure that those eligible for benefits and government support receive it. The group had a rally at a county board meeting and convinced commissioners to hire two financial eligibility workers. But the issues are politically charged, with those pushing for Social Services reform fighting those opposed to increases in government spending or property taxes. There will probably be no significant change until the county is sued in federal court and has to come up with even more money than is currently being requested.

Bill was emotionally "down" from the shenanigans of the court just as he had been after their previous changing of court dates without notifying him. It was a form of psychological abuse – torture - perpetrated by abusers who thought they couldn't be touched by the law, and it looked like that might, indeed, be the case. Combined with the care givers reneging on the promise to get him into aquatic therapy, he didn't see much prospect of ever returning to his normal life.

Susan thought that the term "hamartia" might appropriately be applied to Bill. While the meaning of the term is still disputed in academic circles, in Greek tragedies a hero character with a hamartia manifests an *error in judgment* or makes an *inadvertent mistake* so that, instead of achieving his intended goal, he achieves the opposite with calamitous results. She thought that his impulsivity and "logorrhea" in court (excessive talking) created situations that his adversaries could use against him, which certainly seemed to be the case.

In literature or screen plays, the *fatal flaw* is often a part of the hero's character and brings about his downfall. From the perspective of the Theory of Psychological Type, we all have our fatal flaw which Jung referred to as our "inferior function." For each individual, depending on his or her psychological type, one of the psychological functions (e. g., introverted thinking) is always least well developed and, under conditions of stress, may erupt in ways that are dysfunctional. When the person returns to his normal state, he may be puzzled as to "what got into me," almost as if he had been possessed by an alien spirit. Jung did not see this as a pathology, but simply as the way the mind works under certain circumstances.

Susan day-dreamed about an ideal situation. "What I'd like to have is a lot of money to buy the transcripts, and spend a month or two just learning the case and the law, and preparing applications to the court and complaints. And then, of course, sticking around to represent Bill in court.

"It occurs to me that a federal action might have the additional benefit of getting the court to pay for all the expenses of getting copies of the medical records and getting the transcripts. I think the federal system has provision for such aid to litigants. If I remember right, and if it hasn't been changed, the magic words for doing legal research in that is "pauper petition."

I found that the Office of Civil Rights and the Justice Department had places online where you could submit "complaints," the same as I had submitted my HIPAA complaint. Given the delay in response to that complaint, I wondered just how much of a backlog I would run into. I figured they probably had a lot of cases, given how screwed up the country is. I needed some guidance on whether to keep it focused on one or just a few issues or try to cover the whole range of things involved in the case. I asked Susan and she said "My instinct is usually to focus complaints narrowly on a few major issues and leave marginal stuff out. Marginal issues tend to distract. But I'd have to see the specific document. Do you want to send me a copy of your complaints for my comments?"

About a month and a half earlier I had sent Susan a number of files I had compiled regarding the case. Included were a synopsis of the case, and what I considered violations of HUD regulations, violations of Minnesota Civil Commitment Laws, violations of Minnesota's *Patients Bill of Rights*, violations of Minnesota's *Bill of Rights for Wards and Protected Persons*, violations of the *Americans with Disabilities Act*, violations of the UN *Bill of Rights for Mental Health* and some possible 14th Amendment considerations. I also included my letter to the Joint Commission, my two complaints to the OHFC, and an overall time line of events. Then, on 5/26, I sent some information on Section 1983 of the *Civil Rights Act of 1871* as it related to Bill Tollefson.

I thought maybe she had "spaced out" these files and reminded her of them. I said, "The complaints I have with the courts, hospital and nursing homes are all contained in those documents, except for the most recent one where he was denied attendance at his own hearing. I know it is a lot of information and in a subsequent email you said you couldn't deal with it at that time. At this point, all I need to know is what to concentrate on and what to discard, what would likely get the attention of the Office of Civil Rights and what I shouldn't bother with. The people in that office are the lawyers and they would know this was coming from a non-lawyer, so I don't know how much of the legal stuff I have to point out to them or if I should just assume they will figure it out. I would expect that the initial complaint/inquiry would just be a first step and they would ask me anything else they wanted to know eventually. So the important thing is to get their attention with that first submission."

Susan responded that the huge amount of information had overwhelmed her and she felt she needed to set aside a month to concentrate on nothing else. I wrote back trying to reassure her that a lot of it was reference material and that what I was really concerned about was whether or not she considered the arguments in the "violations" files to be valid and worth presenting to the Office of Civil Rights. I sent her a link to the Integrity Index article where Minnesota achieved grades of 'F' on Judicial Accountability and on Ethics Enforcement. Her reply was, "Shit. Any chance of Bill moving elsewhere?"

About that time, who should appear as a nighttime nurses' aide at Faribault Care Center but the man who accompanied Bill to Florida two years ago, threatened him with violence, and swindled him out of many of his possessions. This was the guy who claimed to be an ordained minister and helped Bill get his motor home going so he could apprentice himself to Bill as a fishing guide but ended up intimidating his mentor, taking his motor home and other possessions and selling them without distributing a portion of the sale price to Bill. I asked Bill if the guy appeared to show any signs of guilt or shame over his previous actions and was told that he has not yet done so. Bill told him to stay out of his room. I wondered how Bill's sleep would fare knowing that he was under the watchful eye of his former friend.

Jake responded to the news with astonishment. "What next," he asked. "Bill had about 12 beer case size boxes of this guys stuff in his apartment. The guardian should have put them all into storage with Bill's stuff at the storage place and she would be the only person who could legally get into the storage. But if there is no more guardian, who is in charge?"

Susan asked about getting a court order of protection to keep the guy away from Bill, on the grounds that he threatened him with violence in the past. I explained that there was no proof that the guy threatened Bill other than Bill's statement that he did and my impression was that Bill tended to forgive everyone who screwed him over, except perhaps his brother, so I thought it unlikely that he would file any charges. However, I did let the ombudslady know of the situation and my concerns about Bill's safety.

I spent about an hour on the phone with Janet Parker, the Medical Whistleblower Advocacy Network lady. Confined to a wheelchair herself, she had some problems with a group she had sued in the past that she thought might be trying to get even with her. Her home was broken into and a number of her files and personal identification had been taken. Somehow the bank messed up her account and she lost her credit cards, Internet connection, and car. The police tried to take away her newly acquired assistive dog so she had to take them to court, where she won her case. Now, in order to carry on her advocacy work, she had to get on the wheelchair-compatible bus, go to the library, download her email and take it back home. It made life much more difficult for her but she was fighting on.

Janet thought Bill had a good case for an ADA complaint where it could be demanded that he be placed in a suitable nursing home with access to aquatic therapy. She said that the people telling him that Medicare would not pay for aquatic therapy, assistive devices, transportation, and so on were in error. What we needed to do was identify a place for him to move, identify a doctor that would be willing to work with him, inform the doctor that Bill was being neglected and that he needed better quality and intensity of care. Medicare would pay for an assistive device to help Bill get into the pool at the therapeutic pool place in Faribault, so they could not deny him on that account. The Courage Center was the preferred place to have him sent, if the court could force them to take him, and they probably could since they received federal funds. Janet's idea was to get a plan all worked up before it was presented to a federal judge. She believed there was some kind of state ADA coordinator that we would work with as well as a Minnesota Independent Living Center where we might be able to get a case manager to help implement the plan.

She also thought the Faribault Care Center was engaging in elder abuse and that his case manager and guardian weren't doing their jobs. She said she had success with similar cases and that social services, through Medicare, must provide "reasonable accommodations" for his disabilities as well as assistive devices such as lift devices to get him into a pool, a properly sized wheelchair, a properly sized commode, and other devices that would increase the quality of his life. It sounded to me like the excuses they had been giving him were not valid.

I told Jake that I had found online and downloaded the forms for requesting a waiver of fees to get court records. These were the ones that Zimbledon would have filled out if he had followed the law and filled them out when Bill requested that he do so or when Jake asked him to do so for pay. I talked with Janet Parker about them and she said that, since the forms required that we have a specific legal action we were planning to take, that we include Section 1983 of the *Civil Rights Act of 1871*, Title III of the *Americans with Disabilities Act*, and Section 504 of the *Rehabilitation Act of 1973*. The forms didn't appear all that difficult but did require that Bill sign in front of a court clerk or probably get his signature notarized. I decided to worry about those details later. Actually, if the Office of Civil Rights got involved we might not have to request the records since they could obtain them themselves.

Jake had talked with his lawyer friend about part time lawyers, like Zimbledon, that worked as defense attorneys in court rooms for $50 an hour. He said that because the counties were short of funds and usually had a backlog of cases, the lawyers were probably told by the court manager or maybe even a judge to keep things moving along fast. "That means forget about a lot of objections that just waste time or filing a lot of paperwork which clogs up the system. Zimbledon was probably afraid that if he did a good job of representing his client, he'd probably get the ax from his nice little part time gravy train job."

Bill's sister, Jane, visited him at the end of the month and talked with the head nurse about the shower situation. That brought about some action since he got a shower the same day. The ombudslady also showed up for some meeting and briefly talked with Bill. He had a visit from his doctor. He asked her if she would write an order for him to go to the Courage Center and she did not object. He told her that I might give her a call to discuss her willingness to handle his primary care if the ADA complaint was resolved in his favor.

I had sent a copy of the first nine chapters of the book to the woman from Mindfreedom Minnesota who had first talked with me about Bill.

She contacted the head of the Minneapolis branch of the Citizens Commission on Human Rights to see if she might want to get involved in Bill's case. That woman wrote, "We would definitely like to know about any human rights violations. Our mission is to investigate and expose psychiatric violations of humans rights. Feel free to contact me and let me know a little about your story."

I sent her a copy of the now first eleven chapters of the book, waited two weeks and then followed up with an inquiry about whether or not she had any continuing interest in the case. She responded quickly, explaining that she had been out of town. She said she had read the first chapter and thought it was "remarkable" and she considered the writing to be "excellent." So far, so good, I thought. Then she remarked, "Stories like these need to be told and heard. What objectives do you have for this story? Are you looking to get press, file a lawsuit, change legislation, etc.?" I wrote back indicating that I was interested in "all of the above."

I also asked if she could recommend a good lawyer in Minnesota who might be able to represent me as durable power of attorney and health care agent for Bill. What I wanted to do was first run by a competent lawyer the ruling by the Minnesota House of Representatives Research Division that I had found indicating that a health care agent had precedence over a guardian when both were present in a case. What I wanted to know was whether or not he thought some kind of cease and desist order could successfully be prosecuted against the guardian. If Jake's lawyer friend was right, the Rice County Court might jump into gear and try to get a court order to eliminate my power of attorney and appointment as health care agent. Then I would have to fight that by forcing them to establish grounds for them doing so, which I didn't think they could do, although it might require getting the matter heard in a higher court. Because I was in New Mexico and the attorney was in Minnesota, I would have to carry out this conversation by phone or the Internet.

About that time, I got an email from the ombudslady stating, "My understanding from a couple of visits ago is that there is not a heated pool in the area that has a lift that would accommodate Bill. His goal was to lose weight and improve walking through therapy in order to be more independent. If he is able to work with a more aggressive therapy regimen, he may be a candidate for Courage Center where he could be accommodated with a warm pool. They would need to do an assessment."

She said she was not aware of the issue of the improperly sized commode because it had not come up before. I told her that I had found that an extra large sized commode on Amazon would run about $170. I cynically considered that maybe they thought that Bill wasn't worth the investment. The ombudslady had asked the social worker at the nursing home to follow through to be sure Bill was able to sit in his recliner regularly. She reported that there had been an incident where he hit an aide when she was bending his leg. Staff were providing a routine transfer, she said, and the two who witnessed the event did not observe the staff who was hit doing anything different from a normal transfer. Bill had related the incident to me earlier and said he was crying with pain at the time the aide grabbed and moved his leg. He said he reflexively "bear-pawed" her on the back to get her to stop her action.

Jake said that he had sent Bill a memo about a new federal law, probably a requirement of the *Americans with Disabilities Act*, that requires all public swimming pools to have a lift installed to help handicap persons in and out of the pool. The lifts would have to be electric for one person operation and cost would probably start at about $10,000. When I was browsing the Internet for potential therapy pools for Bill, I saw one place that had a platform about 6 ft. long where the person could just roll his wheelchair onto it and then it would go down into the pool, wheelchair and all. The person could get off, move around in the water, then get back into the wheelchair and be lifted up.

Jake was concerned that Bill's condition had deteriorated from the time he was at Golden Liver. "When he was there, he could get in and out of bed by himself and had no trouble using the in-room commode. Maybe his health would have gone down hill anyway at Golden or wherever he was. I would like to see him return to his prime of a couple years ago, but now I don't think that will ever happen."

I wrote back that I agreed that his health status had worsened since he arrived at Faribault Care Center, and that it was probably due to both their negligence and his obstinacy. "The big error was in him not getting any exercise, either in his wheelchair or in the water, although the ombudslady said his legs and feet looked better than the previous time she had seen him. He may screw up a lot, but I can't see that being confined to some dump of a nursing home is the way for him to spend his final days. I think he'd rather spend a week on a boat and drop dead with a fishing pole in his hand than spend three years in a nursing home and then drop dead. Unfortunately, his 'caregivers' don't seem to see it that way."

I received a letter from the American Psychological Association Office of Ethics at the end of July stating that my form was complete and it had been assigned to a committee representative. A couple of weeks later, I received another letter saying they needed more information from the accused psychologist and it might take three more months before I heard anything from them. I thought the matter would have all been completed by this time but I guess the wheels of justice, if they turn at all, turn slowly

Bill was visited by his oldest sister, a retired nurse, who talked with the head nurse at the nursing home about scheduling showers for her brother. She had talked with Bill's daughter from Florida and now the daughter professed her love for him. As Bill had suspected, she was in the process of getting a divorce at the time he visited Florida, which was why she didn't want her father around. Bill was also pleasantly surprised to be visited by his adopted son and adopted daughter, who he had not seen in many years. His spirits were buoyed for a while because he finally was getting a little support from some of the members of his family.

I talked with Janet Parker, from the Medical Whistleblower Network who was writing up the ADA complaint. She was quite outraged that Bill's doctor, didn't answer my letter about a rehabilitation program for Bill. Janet said that she knew what was expected of MDs and the laws they had to obey and knew how to force them to do so. Bill thought his doctor had been silenced by Bird Brain, his guardian, which was probably true, but that would not matter if the complaint were accepted.

Janet asked me to send her the names and addresses of everyone involved in Bill's medical care. I had most of them but would have to see if Bill knew any more from Mayo Clinic. Bill's tasks were to get 1) copies of his Medicare/Medicaid cards which had been lost during his many moves over the last 18 months; 2) a copy of his birth certificate; 3) a photo ID or preferably two; 4) his AARP membership number and 5) the name of the nurse practitioner at Faribault Care Center and her contact information. The AARP membership information was important because AARP was fighting guardianships and if Janet wrote them a letter saying what is being done to one of its members, they might get involved.

On July 30 I received a call from Bill and he was quite distraught. He had awakened in the morning and could not move his right foot. He said his legs were "locking up" and that his right ankle and the forward part of his left foot were painful when he was just sitting in his chair. The facility physical therapist told him she could hear "snapping" in his right ankle when she moved it. He feared the joints in his lower extremities were becoming non-functional and he might never be able to walk again unless there was some medical or major aquatic physical therapy intervention soon.

He had requested to see the facility nurse practitioner each week for the last four weeks and she had not responded. He called his county social worker and she did not respond to his voice messages. He did not know if he had the same doctor as previously and she had not responded to an inquiry by me. His court-appointed lawyer, Bill Zimbledon, was very anxious to see him two weeks ago but then never showed up, so Bill Tollefson didn't know what his legal status was or who, if anyone, was in control of his medical care. He said all of this ambiguity was making him crazy and he was losing his patience, conditions that in the past had precipitated impulsive actions on his part.

I wrote to the ombudslady, "This is the kind of heartless and irresponsible treatment I have come to expect for Bill over the last 20 months, but one never gets used to it and it just perpetuates and intensifies his problems. I don't know if you can do anything to encourage these kinds of people to live up to their ethical standards - I haven't seen any indication they even give it a thought. He has been treated in a more civil manner by the care givers he has daily contact with, but the "professionals" don't seem to want to get involved. Perhaps lawsuits are the only way to get their attention, as some lawyers and advocacy groups suggest."

When I was talking with Bill, I mentioned that I wanted him to get me some documents that were needed for filing the ADA complaint. I related the episode to Jake. "He just went off in his panic mode saying he couldn't be bothered with doing any 'paper work' now, that he had to get someone to get him into aquatic therapy right away. I doubted that that was going to happen unless the county was forced into providing it by the ADA complaint. I again got pissed off at Bill for being so obstinate. I told him "Good luck with that" and was ready to throw in the towel, drop the ADA complaint, and even drop being his POA and Health Care Representative.

I wrote to Jake, "Well, damned if he didn't get something accomplished yesterday and today. He met with his nurse practitioner who is connected with the same satellite Mayo System in Faribault that his doctor belonged to. She spent some time with him and listened to him. She was going to get him some GasX for his gas which was causing his hernia to bulge out. She was going to get him a list of his medications, which he had requested several times before. She was going to get his blood sugar level tested. They discovered that there had been a 6-week follow-up order to do a scope of his ulcers that had never been done. She was apparently referring him to a doctor at Mayo

Gastroenterology Department to see how that condition was progressing. He was also being referred to a pain specialist. She thought aquatic therapy would be a good idea but was unable to write an order for it herself. She was going to help him with that somehow. He called his orthopedist at Mayo and asked him to call him back. I added that he should ask one or more of those people about the infection in his leg muscles to see if that is a chronic condition, can be cured, or what and I told him he should make sure they got a hemoglobin A1C analysis when they tested his blood sugar level. I was impressed with what Bill had done even though I continued to be skeptical that anyone would follow through with what was promised."

The objective of the proposed rehabilitation plan I had drawn up for Bill was to provide a living situation for him that improved his overall quality of life, reduced the need for hospitalization and/or institutionalization, and maximized his degree of freedom, independence and integration into the community. I listed his physical, psychological and environmental impediments to independent living and specified the resources needed to reach the objective.

Step 1 involved a number of referrals to medical specialties to evaluate, treat and determine any limitations that were imposed by problems in the areas of: urology, ophthalmology, gastroenterology, neurology, orthopedics, endocrinology, dermatology and podiatry. I added a referral to internal medicine for a complete evaluation of his medication regimen.

Step 2 involved referral to an inpatient aquatic therapy program to address problems of weight loss, reduced range of motion and muscular strengthening. The preferred program was the Transitional Rehabilitation Program (TRP) at the Courage Center in Golden Valley, MN, where Mr. Tollefson had been previously treated in the 1990s. The TRP provides rehabilitative services to assist people with disabilities and/or people recovering from illness, injury or surgery in gaining greater independence. Licensed as a skilled nursing facility, the TRP serves as a transition between acute care and a home or community living setting. Some alternative facilities were mentioned in the event that Bill was not admitted at the Courage Center.

Step 3 was a reassessment of Bill's personal care competencies and determination of the kind of housing needs that would accommodate his disabilities while maximizing his degree of independence: apartment, assisted living or nursing home. If apartment or assisted living was the result, then an appropriate residence would be secured that was:

    a)   affordable (review all state, federal, and social security options

234

from which to obtain income or benefits)

    b)   wheelchair accessible

    c)   in or near Mr. Tollefson's home town

    d)   within range of a swimming pool that Mr. Tollefson could use to maintain his fitness, weight loss and capability to perform his personal care competencies.

Step 4 would involve determining any modifications of the residence that would be needed to make it safe:

    a)   Install hand-held shower head, shower and tub grab bars, and backless bench

    b)   Have large non-skid mats available for use, if needed

    c)   Make sure the sink is at an appropriate height and that there's proper knee clearance

    d)   Make sure shower door accommodates wheelchair

    e)   Install an elevated toilet seat

    f)   Obtain a stable portable toilet for night-time use in the bedroom

    g)   Install a ramp at entrance, if needed.

Step 5 involved obtaining any needed assistive devices:

    a)   Hospital bed with electrical leg elevation (along with regular exercise in water, elevation of his legs is necessary to prevent accumulation of fluids)

    b)   New appropriately sized wheelchair and heavy-duty cushion (current wheelchair is not the appropriately size for Mr. Tollefson)

    c)   Internet access device (Over the last several years, older adults have been the fastest growing segment of the online population. More and more people over the age of 60 are going online and using Facebook, Google, Yahoo and YouTube. They are emailing, texting and blogging—and it is having a positive impact on their lives as they are communicating more frequently with family, reconnecting with old friends, keeping up with community developments and managing their health issues.)

Step 6 was to arrange for necessary services:

    a)   Home health aide, if needed

    b)   Meals on wheels or equivalent, if needed

    c)   A case manager to manage the connections between support services, health care providers and Mr. Tollefson and implement ongoing monitoring and reassessment.

I had sent a copy of the proposed rehabilitation plan to Bill's last known doctor to see if she would be willing to help in implementing it, but she did not respond, no doubt coerced to not do so by Bird Brain, Mr.

Tollefson's guardian.

I talked with Bill on August 8th and he said he had been in bed for the last three days. He had requested to be transferred to his chair but the nursing home staff denied him, saying that they did not have enough people available to do that. In theory, he is supposed to be getting a shower the same day after defecating in his bed. They missed his shower the week before last, he said, so I surmised that the nursing home was back-tracking on their concessions to the ombudslady (and to common decency). Bill had not seen his guardian since about June 18th, the date of the hearing where she told him he did not have to attend. When he expressed his desire to be there, since it involved his welfare, she told him that the county would not pay for his transportation, even though the court was in the same little town as the nursing home and even though the law required it.

The next day I copied and sent to Janet some articles that had appeared in the *Faribault Daily News* regarding problems with Rice County Social Services, a copy of my HIPAA Complaint against Mayo Clinic and the Minnesota House of Representatives Research that showed that a health care agent out-ranks a guardian unless there is a court order dismissing the agent. I also sent a copy of *Conservatorships and Guardianships in Minnesota* that had been written by a panel of three judges. It was a very detailed guide to the law regarding those relationships that was meant to be used as a manual as to what should be their attitudes and actions in various circumstances. I went through the electronic manual and highlighted everything that was relevant to Bill's case, which turned out to be items on 39 of the 74 pages.

I thought a good case could be made that his current guardian had not been acting in Bill's best interests, with his wishes and beliefs being respected, and she had not been able to establish a working relationship with him and hadn't advocated on his behalf, as she was supposed to do. Therefore, she should be removed. Following the procedures the three judges recommended, rather than the erroneous information that was in Bill's chart, I thought it could be established that he would be capable of making all of his decisions even though he may not be able to implement them at present because of his physical limitation. In that case a guardianship, based as it was on claimed mental impairment, would not be necessary at all.

I had an extended telephone conversation with Janet that day because she was in the process of compiling information I had sent her and linking it to federal and international laws that would support our ADA Complaint. The targets of the complaint were to be Rice County Social

Services, the guardian, and Faribault Care Center but maybe would include other individuals and agencies, such as Golden Living Center. She had to get everything into the proper format for the lawyers at the Civil Rights Division and she believed from past experience that they knew that if they didn't accept the complaint, she would send it to international civil rights organizations at the UN and in Ireland who would then put pressure on the U.S.A. I wasn't so sure that the U.S.A., with its concept of itself as being "special," was terribly sensitive to criticism from any UN or foreign governments.

Janet had wanted to send copies of Bill's birth certificate, his Medicare and Medicaid cards and his AARP membership along with the complaint but all of these documents had been lost, stolen or misplaced during the eight or nine moves since his removal from his home. Bill had talked with the nursing home social worker about getting them replaced and she said she would help him but never did so. I reported to the ombudslady that Faribault Care Center had reverted to their old behavior regarding Bill's showers, toileting and movement to his chair and that he needed some help getting documents replaced. She said Bill's guardian was working on the same issues. I responded to her that it was unlikely that his guardian was working on the document problem since she had not seen Bill since about June 18, the day when she denied him his right to be at a scheduled hearing regarding his case.

I was becoming more certain that "Bird Brain" had done a number on Bill in describing him to the ombudslady. Jake volunteered to go to the court house to try to get a copy of Bill's birth certificate and I found the numbers Bill could call to get replacement cards for Medicare and Medicaid. Unfortunately, the county would not provide Jake with a copy of Bill's birth certificate because he was not a relative and couldn't get a notary to come to the nursing home to certify Bill's signature. The Medicare and Medicaid offices told him to go through the nursing home social worker since his was not a permanent address. I discussed the matter with Janet and we decided to submit the complaint without IDs for the patient.

I sent a copy of the conservator / guardianship manual to Jake who, apparently disgusted by the amount of detail in the rules of the manual, responded, "Thank god I never went to law school! Both my lawyer friend in southern Minnesota and another guy I know up here can't stand working as lawyers, wish they had never gone to law school, and can't wait to get out of the business after 30 some years of practice. When my friend was a senior in college, the head of the poly-sci department practically begged him to go to grad school and pick up either a masters or PhD in poly-sci. He told him that he could guarantee him a job at the university. teaching after he graduated. But my friend had his mind made up - he had to go to law school. He says now that that was the biggest mistake he ever made in his life!"

14 <u>WHERE'S HIPPOCRATES WHEN YOU NEED HIM?</u>

Jake visited Bill in early October and observed that his old friend "didn't look too hot." Bill's legs were black to above the knees and every toe was pointing in a different direction. He would slip down in his chair and that would kink his head forward, making it hard for him to breathe. Jake put a shoe on Bill's foot and noted that his skin had thinned out, leading Jake to believe that he would be likely to bleed under the skin from just a light touch. He knew that Bill had suffered from arthritis for years but didn't think he was getting any effective treatment for it. "I would think Mayo would have sent him to see a rheumatologist." Bill reported that he was losing the feeling in the lower part of his legs.

During his visit Jake obtained Mr. Tollefson's signature and thumb print on an authorization form to request assistance from Senator Al Franken's office. Jake mailed the form to me and I added my name, had my signature notarized and sent it to Mr. Franken's St. Paul Office. The request was acknowledged, saying that they received hundreds every week. It was not until January 3rd that I talked with Diane Gerten of Senator Franken's office and explained the problems being experienced with Mr. Tollefson's health care and human rights. I sent her by email a copy of the ADA Complaint, a synopsis of the case, an updated event timeline, a list of involved persons and a list of other documents that were available if she wanted them. Subsequently, I sent her the first 12 chapters of this book and the draft of a petition I had developed to remove Mr. Tollefson's guardian. The latter document was based on the manual *CONSERVATORSHIP AND GUARDIANSHIP IN MINNESOTA*, published by: Minnesota Conference of Chief Judges, Pending, 2003 Amended 2009, 2010. The petition listed multiple failures by the guardian to uphold over 30 specific rules/laws listed in that manual. The document had previously been sent to Bill, Dr. Parker and Jake for comments.

I informed Ms. Gerten that Jake, who has known Mr. Tollefson all his life, was now back from his surgery and could give her first-hand observations of Mr. Anderson in the Faribault Care Center (FCC) as well as before when he was at the Golden Living Centers and the Anoka hospital. He was also present at several of the court hearings and was ready and willing to testify under oath about all of it. I also urged her to contact Dr. Janet Parker of *Medical Whistleblowers Advocacy Network* who had independently submitted a message to Mr. Franken's office. I informed her that Dr. Parker, herself in a wheelchair and recipient of aquatic therapy, said that there is a kind of wheelchair often used by multiple sclerosis patients that could be purchased or rented that would solve any risk of falling out of the chair (if, indeed, that was a genuine risk) so that Mr. Tollefson could get to his appointments. Dr. Parker thought that Mr. Anderson needed a wheelchair evaluation.

I kept Ms. Gerten updated with respect to ongoing travesties as they occurred and sent her magazine and newspaper articles about cases relevant to Mr. Tollefson's case. She was sympathetic but did not indicate to me what, if anything, she was doing about the case. She never contacted Jake, Dr. Parker or anyone else involved in the case, as far as I was able to determine. I realize that any political figure needs to be cautious about what they say for fear that political opponents could and would take advantage of any misstep, but we were left completely in the dark if any help was being provided.

In November, I called regarding the status of the ADA/civil rights complaint submitted by Dr. Parker and myself. I was told that it was "in evaluation," that the reference number was 404-214, and that I could call 202-307-0663 to get an update on the status of the complaint. When I did so a few months later, I was told that it was still in evaluation, that they could give no information regarding the progress of the complaint and that they could provide no date or even an approximate amount of time before we heard anything about it. For all I knew, the complaint could be sitting under a pile of papers on someone's desk.

At the end of October, 2012 I finally got a response from the American Psychological Association about my ethics complaint against the psychologist who evaluated Mr. Tollefson. Their response was a marvel of obfuscation. It was impossible to tell what they did or didn't do other than to close the case. One thing for sure was that they did not "consider all the evidence in the case," as they claimed, since they did not contact a single witness or the victim himself in the matter. I pointed out the inadequacy of their response in a return letter and indicated that my colleagues commented that I should not have expected any better from an organization that endorses the use of torture in prisoner interrogations (a complaint filed to APA against one of the psychologists involved in torture at Guantanamo garnered a nearly identical response from the so-called "ethics" committee).

I called in Chicago about my HIPAA complaint (CU-12-140009) on October 22. The woman I talked with asked some questions about the complaint and said she would put it "on the top of her list" of things to do. I called back 4 weeks later. She returned the call on Nov. 30 but I was unavailable to receive it. I called her back on December third, fourth and fifth and left messages on her voice mail but she never returned the calls, so a request was filed with Senator Tom Udall's office for assistance in the matter. On January 25, 2013, his assistant said he had sent a letter to the woman in the Chicago office and had left a telephone message with her regarding the complaint which had been in process since February of the previous year. In early March, another woman from the Office of Civil Rights called and apologized profusely for the delay and the non-responsiveness of the Chicago office. She said she would send a formal letter to Mayo Clinic and then probably would do a review of their policy and procedures regarding compliance with HIPAA. My request was for them to investigate why I was not allowed to obtain copies of my appointment as Durable Power of Attorney and Health Care Agent for Mr. Tollefson. The question was whether or not these documents constituted protected health care information simply because they were placed in Bill's medical record.

On April 23, 2013 I called the civil rights investigator for Health and Human Services in Chicago, and she indicated that Mayo Clinic was convinced that Mr. Tollefson was *not* impaired and could handle his own medical decisions by himself, according to Minnesota guardianship law. I asked if that meant that they could be subpoenaed to testify to that statement and she said she thought it would mean that. This would be fine for Bill because it would indicate that there was no basis for a guardianship and that the interference with his medical appointments by his guardian and the nursing home were a violation of his legal rights.

Mayo Clinic claimed to the civil rights investigator that they had complied with the request on February 10, 2012 and had supplied Mr. Tollefson with the documents I had requested. I called Mr. Tollefson and asked if he had ever received any appointment documents from Mayo Clinic. He said he had not. It was not until the following day that I checked my records and found that they showed that Mayo Clinic had faxed a copy of the missing page of the Advanced Directives document to the social worker at Golden Living Center so that I could talk with him about Bill's case. But the request I had made for the documents was more than two weeks *after* that date. I sent a letter to the Chicago civil rights office correcting the error made by Mayo Clinic and the civil rights investigator and told them that I was not asking anything further of them but to include my letter in the file where their report was placed.

In October, Bill reported that the husband of the guardian's partner showed up in his room and just stood there. He had been present another time and had said he was there "to see if you have been a good boy," a disparaging remark that violates guardianship standards. Bill said that the man's presence "screwed up my lunch." He told the man he needed some of his belongings that he had when he was at Golden Living Center. The man lied, according to Bill, and said the things were in Bill's closet. However, they were not there and it later turned out that $250 worth of super-sized clothes were missing from his closet. Bill told him his dentures were lost and that other articles had been stolen but the man did not offer to do anything about it. The man did not say what his role was, did not introduce himself and would not explain why he was there at that time.

On November 16, someone new from the guardianship corporation showed up. He did not divulge to Bill his role or purpose for being there. In February the guardian's partner's husband again showed up and told Bill he wanted to "check on him." More than likely, these ancillary employees of the guardianship corporation, who were not appointed to a guardianship position with respect to Bill, were showing up so they could claim to have met legal requirements and make their charges for their "work" with Bill.

In March, Bill received a letter from the guardian's partner informing him of his right to end the guardianship or object to it. He would have to file a written statement (petition) with the court. I had previously downloaded, printed and mailed the form to Bill but he did not act on it. Bill had the right to request an attorney, which was accomplished by checking a box on the form to request termination of the guardianship. Why Bill wouldn't initiate this action falls into the same category as why he wouldn't take action against his two incompetent and unethical lawyers – he avoided confrontation unless he was so enraged that he couldn't contain himself and he feared retaliation for having made a complaint.

Mr. Tollefson had been trying to get his supplemental insurance plan changed back to the plan he had before his return from Florida but his designated financial worker for Rice County refused to send him information about any of the three plans available or to even talk with him. I contacted the director of Social Services for Rice County indicating that Mr. Tollefson was desperate to have information regarding his health insurance options which were due for a decision on December 14, 2012. I said that Mr. Tollefson had made repeated requests for information on his health care insurance options from his financial worker and his current guardian, but they did not respond to his requests. I asked him if he could look into the matter and advise me as to whether or not there was any intention of his agency providing Mr. Tollefson with the information he had requested.

He responded that his office would be communicating any information about health insurance options to the guardian "as the authorized representative in order for them to make any necessary choice on behalf of their ward." This certainly did not sound like the "capability of making his own health care decisions" that Mayo Clinic ascribed to Mr. Tollefson nor was it in line with the directive in Minnesota guardianship law to involve the patient as much as possible in all decisions affecting his welfare. In reply I said, "In other words, he has no choice in the matter in spite of the law regarding the role of guardians in the state of Minnesota. I shall report that to Mr. Tollefson and to other interested parties."

After two weeks the matter had not been resolved so I emailed Mr. Zimbledon, Bill's presumed attorney.

I am again writing to you on behalf of Bill Tollefson as his Power of Attorney and Designated Health Care Agent. Mr. Anderson is concerned about the December 14, 2012 deadline for choosing a health care plan. He has requested information about those plans from his guardian and his financial worker for Rice County so that he can make an informed decision. The plan he subscribes to can have long term consequences since he will not be able to change plans for another two years. The plan he got stuck with the last time did not provide the kind of coverage he had previously. His guardian and financial worker have not provided him any information regarding his options. I contacted Mark Shaw, Director of Social Services, who said that they gave the information to the guardian and she can do whatever she wants with it and make the decision for Mr. Tollefson. As you may know, not allowing a ward to have any input into

243

decisions about his health care is a violation of state law regarding guardianships. Mr. Tollefson has called you to talk with you about this matter and I hope you will have the decency to return his call.

Zimbledon said he would pass my concerns along to the guardians. "I don't get involved in insurance choices. And I really don't have an ongoing role with Bill Tollefson. The court discharges me 60 days after entering its order appointing guardian and conservator. I try to take calls from Bill when I can and I do pass on his concerns. However, I cannot take every call when they come 10 times a day and I cannot micromanage the services of the guardian."

I wrote back, "Thanks. That is very important to know. If Bill had known that, I'm sure he would not be contacting you. State law requires that wards and protected persons have legal representation to petition the court, so I guess he would have to hire his own lawyer to get the state to appoint a lawyer for him. Interesting Catch-22. Thanks for responding and clarifying this matter that should have been clarified long ago." It is interesting that Mr. Zimbledon denied any ongoing relationship with Mr. Tollefson in spite of the fact that as little as two weeks earlier he had discussed with Bill the possibility of representing him in an action against his guardian.

On December 13 I received an email from Bill's guardian. "I have received correspondence from Mr. Zimbledon and Mr. Shaw regarding your concerns. Bill's calls to you are very telling of how unstable his mental health is at this time, because I spoke with him at length about his current plan and what his options were. After that discussion he chose a different health care plan that he wanted to be switched to so that his current dentist and long time friend in Northfield could be utilized for dental services. I made the request in writing to Rice county to change on November 26th and John was aware of this."

I immediately called Bill and asked him about this presumed discussion of his health care options. He remembered talking about wanting to see his former dentist but did not recall any discussion about the alternative health care plans. I also told him about her unwarranted inference about his mental status from her recollection of his recollection of that conversation. He just laughed.

Bill said that Bird Brain did finally bring over to him the brochures for the three medical plans for which he would qualify. She told him the deadline was the 5th of January, although earlier she had said the effective start date was January 1, 2013. He examined them and decided upon Blue Plus, the plan that he had before he returned from Florida, as the one that would best meet his needs. He asked me to pass his selection on to Bird Brain and ask her if she would please convey that information to his Rice County financial worker since she would not accept his telephone calls or call him back.

Bill's oldest sister called me on December 19. She said that she had been talking with her brother's guardian and complained that her brother had ordered and received at the nursing home such things as an outboard motor and buck knives and wondered if there was anything that could be done to stop it and implied that she had been thinking of stopping payment on his telephone in order to pressure him to do so. She hesitated to take that action because she knew how much telephone access meant to him. I said I didn't think anything could be done, not legally anyway.

She went on to say that the guardian told her that Bill refused physical therapy and that was what was needed so he could transfer and use the pool there in Faribault. I told her that her brother's physical therapy had been stopped, not by him but probably by his nurse practitioner. She got off the phone and immediately called the nursing home back and they told her the NP had stopped the PT because her brother wasn't making any progress (even though his physical therapist told him that they were making progress). I told her that Medicare was re-writing the rules on that after a class-action suit in the northeast. With a self-assured snideness, she said, "and how long is that going to take to get through?"

She claimed that her brother was "paranoid" because he thought his care givers were not trying to help him. I disagreed with her inappropriate characterization of her brother and voiced my doubts that his care givers had his best interests in mind. She claimed Bill wasn't telling her the truth and said that all the information I had was from the patient, which is only partly true but sounded strangely like the argument put forth by the guardian. Because of her lingering resentment toward her brother and her desire to make him pay for his past misdeeds, she was inclined to believe every lie and endorse every negative attribution that the guardian told her.

I called Bill and related his sister's comments to him. He said that the antique outboard motor, purchased for all of $50, was brought to the nursing home just so that he could view it and that Jake then took it home to store in his basement. For someone who was a fishing enthusiast from childhood, the motor was quite an historical prize. He said he never received any knives but did indicate that such knives were a complimentary gift for subscribing to a hunters magazine. He called the publisher and they said they had not sent out any knives and probably wouldn't until January or February. He said he had not told anyone in the facility about his magazine subscription or the gift offer, so how they concluded he had obtained a "buck knife" was a mystery. I thought it would more appropriately be called a fabrication based on violating the privacy of his mail, i. e., they had been illegally monitoring his mail.

He was astonished by his sister's suggestion that he was "paranoid." He was unaware of her long-standing resentment that he had received more attention and respect from their mother than did she and that she thought his mother had spoiled him. He had always thought that she was just a more reserved and studious kind of person than he and didn't know that she harbored any grudges.

Bill had seen a pain specialist (appropriately named Dr. Payne), who had recommended that Bill receive therapy for his chronic pain. It would have been logical for it to be physical therapy although Bill was not sure what kind was recommended. A couple of days after Jake's visit, a U Care nurse (Bill's insurance carrier) showed up unannounced with the nurse practitioner from the Faribault Care Center, apparently related to the recommendation Dr. Payne had made. She asked Mr. Tollefson to draw a clock and repeat three things she gave him to remember. He performed both tasks correctly. Having given thousands of such screening tests over the last 40 years, I knew that the results could not be interpreted to mean that Bill had any significant brain damage. I surmised that they were giving him that test at this time in an effort to avoid responsibility for the recommended treatment. Bill made no comment about what they were doing but just stressed his need to go to Mayo for a physical examination and endoscope to follow up on his ulcers. Neither the recommendation for therapy (of any kind) nor the request for taking action on the follow-up on his ulceration (recommended by Mayo Clinic) were acted upon. It seemed obvious to me that the nursing home, probably in collusion with the guardian, were working to thwart any treatment that would improve Bill's condition.

On October 12, Bill talked with his former physical therapist, Paula, and told her he was upset because his physical therapy had been discontinued. She told him she was going to talk with the head of her physical therapy organization to see what was happening. She had previously told Mr. Tollefson that she thought he had been making progress but her judgment had been over-ruled by her superior. Just how she could do that without seeing Mr. Tollefson was another mystery hidden in the bowels of FCC.

About this time, I read an article in the *New York Times* which implied that Mr. Tollefson should have his physical therapy reinstated and that he should have aquatic physiotherapy as well.

In a proposed settlement of a nationwide class-action lawsuit, the

Obama administration had agreed to scrap a decades-old practice that required many beneficiaries to show a likelihood of medical or functional improvement before Medicare would pay for skilled nursing and therapy services. Under the agreement, which amounts to a significant change in Medicare coverage rules, Medicare would pay for such services if they are needed to 'maintain the patient's current condition or prevent or slow further deterioration,' regardless of whether the patient's condition is expected to improve.

Mr. Tollefson's doctor, apparently unaware of the specifications of the Americans with Disabilities Act, also told him that he couldn't have water therapy because no one had a lift that would handle him.

The negligent care provided by Faribault Care Center continued for the next eight months. They would "forget" to give him a shower on the scheduled days and the 3rd shift wouldn't wash him up because they thought it was the other shifts' job. At times he would have to lay in his fecal matter for over an hour before someone would come to clean him up. The plastic mattress cover would cause him to sweat profusely, cause itching on his backside and made his skin deteriorate. At times he would leave blood spots on his sheets and one time left a blood trail down the hallway when he was taken for a shower. They provided him with only a short gown to wear, like a T-shirt, and then they would criticize him for not covering himself up. They would frequently refuse to move him from his dilapidated bed to his electric-lift chair saying they didn't have time or that he was just fine laying in his bed. His toenails had not been cut since 2 weeks after his arrival. When he asked to have them cut, he was refused with the comment that the staff member "did not have the time." He received no exercise of any sort and was not provided with any equipment (e. g., rubber bands) to do resistance exercises while in his bed or chair, thus ensuring the atrophy of his muscles. His prescription for testosterone was stopped, making the problem with controlling his urination even worse. Application of anti-fungal cream to the folds in his skin in order to prevent development of a yeast infection was often skipped. In June of 2013 he developed an upper respiratory infection that lasted more than five weeks. His coughing and spitting up greenish phlegm from his lungs was ignored and the doctor did not bother to see him. He asked for garlic and onion to help treat himself and was refused with the excuse that they didn't have these common kitchen items. When his hearing became affected, he asked for peroxide and an alcohol and vinegar solution which he had used many times before, at the suggestion of a doctor, for his "swimmer's ear" but was again denied. Finally, his sister, there on a visit, bought him the requested items. He asked for complaint forms but none were ever provided to him.

Bill was again surreptitiously given the psychotropic medication Wellbutrin and when he asked staff about it, they denied that he was receiving any psychiatric medications. The medication made Bill depressed, angry and caused memory problems. The medication was recently pulled by the FDA because they had never actually tested the Wellbutrin XL 300 version of the drug and had just assumed it would work like other versions of the medication. It didn't. When he finally got them to admit they were giving it to him, he tried going off it "cold-turkey" but could not tolerate the withdrawal symptoms. He then requested a gradual withdrawal procedure and soon was back to his normal jovial self (except for the aggravations presented daily by the facility personnel).

Bill described his bed as being like "a torture chamber" because his legs hung over the end of the bed by about 10 inches and he was unable to adjust himself when he slid down after raising the back support, the process of sliding down causing him to choke because it bent his neck at an awkward angle. His requests for help in repositioning him on his bed were frequently ignored and staff would not accept his analysis of the nature of the problem with the bed. On one occasion four people came in and yanked away on the mattress, precipitating a big argument about how to move him. They left in a huff without accomplishing the repositioning. The bed also tilted him about 30 degrees to the left which made it difficult to watch TV or write while in bed.

Finally, at the end of January 2013, a state nursing home inspector on a routine visit came by and interviewed Bill. He made several complaints about the facility and specifically about the bed. The inspector measured the length of the bed and the length of Mr. Tollefson and instructed the nursing home to lengthen Mr. Tollefson's bed. Apparently she let them know of his other complaints for the next day the nursing home social worker, showed up and began asking him questions about being mistreated and trying to get him to answer her questions with the "right answer." Then the head of physical therapy, showed up and "hammered on" him with questions about why he wasn't happy. She was so abusive in her "questioning" that he became upset and could hardly eat his lunch. He found all of this harassment to be mentally exhausting and he just wanted them to "shut up and leave me alone." And, of course, he would have to pay for his complaining later. But they did comply with the inspector's demand, lengthening the bed and giving him a mattress that was six inches longer. However, they did not provide a mattress cover to prevent the development of bed sores nor did they fix the left-tilting back support.

Mr. Tollefson had received several stories about the whereabouts of his wheelchair. One person said it was in storage, one said it was somewhere around the Faribault Care Center, and one said it had been taken apart and thrown away. He was not consulted about its disposition in any way. When Jake visited on November 28, he was told that Bill's wheelchair was in such bad shape that they tore it apart and discarded it, without asking Bill's permission.

Mr. Tollefson had been asking to see the nurse practitioner servicing the nursing home for six weeks. She finally showed up shortly after Christmas and told him that she was going to write an order supporting his request to go to the Northfield Eye Clinic. She said it was her opinion that "they" (nursing home staff) could not cancel his medical appointments and transportation to medical appointments. He asked her about going to Mayo Clinic for a follow-up evaluation of his stomach and esophagus and she seemed to be amenable to that too. They discussed whether or not it would be a good idea for him to take blood thinners to prevent development of blood clots.

On January 9th, a nurse came into Mr. Tollefson's room and asked him if he wanted to meet his new doctor. He said, "What new doctor? Nobody told me about a new doctor. What happened to Dr. Judy?" No reason for the change was presented to Mr. Tollefson and his input was not requested. The nurse just asked him, "Didn't the social worker tell you about that?" After a while the social worker came in and said that his guardian had changed his doctor and, "If you don't take this doctor then you will have no doctor at all."

Mr. Tollefson's doctor had not notified him of her termination of her role as his doctor, which would be required of her as part of her medical ethics. When I asked the ombudslady for elder Minnesotans why his doctor had been replaced she said that the Mayo Clinic for which his former doctor worked (as well as the nurse practitioner) would no longer provide services to that nursing home. Another medical clinic had also decided they would not service that particular nursing home. No explanation for the decision was given. Later in the conversation, she admitted that they had had many problems with Deseret Corp. in the past. She said they had failed to pay employees, did not pay the state the taxes they owed and absconded with employee 401K pension funds. They disappeared for a while but then returned with the CEO claiming that he had nothing to do with his relatives' misdeeds. Somehow they got a license to continue to operate. According to the ombudslady, those staff members who were not burned out had a difficult time doing what they thought was proper treatment while trying to deal with an inadequate administration at the same time. I indicated to her that Mr. Tollefson thought that there were a few good staff members at the facility but he also feared that they might soon get socialized into the prevailing negative attitude toward their jobs.

Bill had one front tooth with a large cavity but when he asked to see his regular dentist, the nursing home staff would not allow him to see him. They told him, by way of explanation, that the dentist's office did not have a chair that was large enough for him to sit in. Mr. Tollefson informed them that he had been to the dentist's office before many times, and either sat in the dental chair or sat in his wheelchair (ADA requires that medical providers have appropriate accommodations for patients with disabilities). His visual acuity had deteriorated so much that he found it difficult and painful to read and write. He also had some kind of objects that felt like pebbles under his eyelids but when he asked for eyewash or saline solution , they would not give it to him or claimed that they had none. The nursing home brought in an "eye-guy," apparently neither an optometrist nor ophthalmologist, that they wanted to force on Bill but he wanted a qualified person because of some pressure he was feeling in his eye, suggesting possible glaucoma.

Bill finally decided to make his own appointments with his eye doctor and his podiatrist and arranged for transportation to his appointments. The appointments were summarily canceled by the nursing home social worker after a "secret" meeting with Bill's guardian, who never bothered to see Mr. Tollefson while she was at the nursing home. When Bill called the social worker to find out why the appointments had been canceled, she slammed down the phone on him. He then called the eye clinic and the secretary told him he could have no appointments unless it was with the nurse's approval (apparently referring to his facility NP). This was the second time that the nursing home staff made it impossible for him to get to appointments.

Bill made another appointment to see his eye doctor on Thursday, January 17, 2013 and six days earlier tried to contact the nursing home social worker about his appointment. He wanted to make sure that everything was authorized for his appointment, especially the authorization for transportation. She did not return his call. I then placed a call to the social worker on Bill's behalf. At first I was told that she was "taking a lap" but, after 10 minutes holding on the line, I was told she had gone to lunch. This was at 1:10. I left a message and my telephone number but she never returned my call. On January 14, 2013 Bill again tried to reach the social worker to find out if his transportation had been authorized. She did not respond and he became quite worried that he would again be denied. He wanted to be able to cancel the appointment, if need be, well in advance out of consideration for the doctor's schedule and to maintain a working relationship with people at that clinic (since he had had to cancel twice before). He called me and I sent an email about the problem to the Ombudsman for Elder Minnesotans to request her assistance.

After discussing problems with Faribault Care Center, the ombudslady then proceeded to blame the patient, Mr. Tollefson, for his current difficulties. She said that he was not working at his physical therapy. I reminded her that his physical therapy had been discontinued by his care givers on the pretext that he was not making any progress. And I pointed out to her that this was illegal according to the recently settled class action suit heard in New Hampshire. She said that Mr. Tollefson was not getting out of bed and had no muscle strength in his stomach so that he could not sit in a wheelchair. She cited the incident where he fell out of his chair and I pointed out that he did so after having a "sudden urge" that overcame him and defecating in his chair, thus making the seat slippery. She had not heard that story. I mentioned that Jake had arrived shortly after the incident and was told the story by the person who was cleaning up his wheelchair.

His appointment for his eye doctor, that he was looking forward to because he was unable to read, was canceled for the third time. The ombudslady claimed that Bill was furious about that and I was not surprised since Mr. Tollefson had tried everything in his power to make sure it transpired. The ombudslady said that both his guardian and the social worker had championed giving Mr. Tollefson a try at it but that the physical therapist had vetoed the effort because she could not or would not risk Mr. Tollefson falling from his wheelchair when away from the nursing home.

The ombudslady stated that Bill had a diagnosis of Bipolar Disorder and I asked her who had provided that diagnosis, since it was something new. She did not know. I disputed the accuracy of that diagnosis and said that I had never observed Mr. Tollefson to be psychotic at any time. She agreed that he was not psychotic but wanted to hold onto her belief that he was Bipolar even though that is a psychotic diagnosis. It should be noted that one of the psychologists that helped develop DSM IV now contends that Bipolar Disorder is not a genuine psychiatric disorder. From my experience over 40 years of practice, I think it is an over-used label and often is applied to people in the normal range of personality distributions. I did conceded that Mr. Tollefson was often quite bull-

251

headed (which is not a psychiatric diagnosis) and that this personality trait presented a problem for people who deal with him. He does become obstinate when care givers try to force things on him without listening to his input and she said that when he gets angry at such things that have happened to him, she didn't blame him since those things were often not his fault.

The ombudslady said Mr. Tollefson was being illogical. When I asked what she saw as evidence of that, she said that he wanted to have aquatic physiotherapy but didn't want to accept that he needed to be able to walk a certain distance for that to happen. I indicated that being in a pool where he could exercise and gain muscle strength with the support of the buoyancy provided by the water was a good argument for him getting into a pool. She said that walking and being able to get into a wheelchair were requirements of the facilities that provide aquatic physiotherapy, but she was talking only about the one they had approached, namely one in Faribault. Facilities in other cities might very well have the necessary equipment.

The ombudslady said she was trying to get an evaluation team from Linking Elderly Support (LES) from Wilmar to come in and provide a complete evaluation. She also talked about wanting to get Bill moved into a better facility and maybe getting ARMS workers to help him be able to live in the community. However, she also thought he had to participate more in his treatment by getting out of bed and doing some exercises. I told her I didn't think he could do that on his own and needed some kind of physical therapy to help him improve his level of functioning and that physical therapy had been terminated, illegally, by his care-givers.

Later Bill learned that, even though the ombudslady was at FCC when the decision was made to cancel his appointment, she did not tell Bill that his appointment with the ophthalmologist was canceled. Nor did the social worker or any of the nurses. Bill was waiting patiently, with his backpack filled, ready to get picked up on Thursday morning when two nurses aides working in his room told him he would not be going. What this means is that Bill could not have been "furious" on Wednesday (as the ombudslady claimed) since he still thought he was going to keep the appointment – after all, the social worker had told him so. So, for some unknown reason, the ombudslady was lying. He was dejected to find out the next day that he would not be making his appointment and he believed that the eye clinic would no longer make any appointments for him because he had to cancel three appointments in a row due to screw-ups by the nursing home staff or interference by his guardian.

In contrast to what the ombudslady claimed, Mr. Tollefson was not now seeing a psychiatrist. He was surprised by the allegation of him having bipolar disorder and knew of no one qualified to make such a diagnosis ever having done so. He has had sufficient experience with the condition to know its major features since he has a younger brother who has been given that label. While there are those in the mental health fields that believe it is not a legitimate diagnostic entity, I think that, at the very least, it is an over-used label. In any event, Bill does not meet the criteria required for the diagnosis.

This change in the ombudslady's orientation toward Bill seemed to indicate that she had been coerced or "brainwashed" by someone and, since her new "beliefs" were those spouted by the guardian, the latter was the most likely suspect. However, it could have been superiors in her own organization that had come down on her. Obviously, someone wanted to get this complaining person to shut up before they were embarrassed by their ill treatment of him.

Apparently what the ombudslady was referring to when she talked about a psychiatrist was a plan the nursing home had hatched, with her knowledge but without Bill's, for a mental health worker to see Bill. In February and March a PsyD (not a PhD) psychologist paid three one hour visits to Mr. Tollefson and allowed Bill to tell his story. Bill liked the guy and thought he had a pleasant manner. Obviously he was there not to treat Mr. Tollefson but to do an assessment, since he terminated after just 3 sessions. It was not clear who had requested his services since Bill had not done so nor had he given his approval for someone else to make arrangements. Bill asked his medical doctor who had initiated it and was told that it occurred before the MD had joined the staff and he presumed it was his guardian. Bill thought he had favorably impressed the psychologist but withheld final judgment until he saw what kind of report the psychologist wrote about him.

Bill signed a release of information that would allow me to get copies of whatever documents the psychologist developed with regard to Mr. Tollefson. I immediately sent a request for any and all documents that he generated with Bill as subject, including bills sent to Mr. Tollefson's Medicare/Medicaid account. The PsyD did not show up for his next appointment with Bill, did not call with an explanation and did not respond to a call that Bill had made to his office. The PsyD did not respond to my request for documents and Bill decided that he did not need to talk to someone about his problems that was less than honest and direct. Bill concluded, from the PsyD's failure to respond to my request, that he was not working for him and his best interests but was probably working for the guardian or nursing home. When the psychologist called to schedule another impromptu appointment that day, Bill told him to call in the morning so that he could arrange his schedule. He never called again. So here was yet another health care professional who was unable to live up to his ethical standards. (Or, perhaps, ethical standards were never devised to be lived up to but only to serve as window dressing to lull the public into a false sense of security about the character of those who serve them).

Bill called the eye doctor's office and was assured that any necessary procedures could be done with him on a gurney. He called his dentist and the doctor had told him he thought he could manage to get him into the office. He got a measurement for the width of the gurney (22") which was narrower than his wheelchair. Then, on March 13, 2013 Bill had what he termed his "first sensible meeting" with his guardian and the social worker employed by Faribault Care Center. They promised not to interfere with his eye doctor appointment on March 21st and his plan to see his dentist on that same day. He told them that his legs were feeling better now that his bed had been lengthened and he had a new mattress that is the appropriate size (after sleeping on one that was 6" too short for a year). He told them again that he needed a cover for the mattress that would prevent bedsores and this time they agreed to it. He also mentioned that he had previously been unable to bend his knees but now he was able to bend both and he was eager to do some exercising. The director of the physical therapy company that contracts to FCC did not show up when she said she would, so Mr. Tollefon talked with his guardian and FCC social worker about using a machine called a "New Step" that they have available at FCC and that he could use to help exercise his legs. He had used it before and he believed he could be Hoyer-lifted onto it if the staff would cooperate. They had no objection to that.

He also asked for a "trapeze," a kind of lift bar that would hang from a frame over his bed, that he could use to do pull-ups and other exercises. He needed a truss for his umbilical hernia if he was to use his stomach muscles in exercise and he thought a temporary one could be fashioned from one of the safety belts they use for people who are just learning how to use a walker. He indicated to them that going to the Courage Center was an imperative for him but his guardian claimed she had tried to get him in before but was denied. (I know there was a newspaper article that appeared about that time in which one of the staff members at the Courage Center was interviewed. He indicated that they did not like to take patients who were paid with state funds because they lost money on them. I am sure they receive federal funds, so if Bill were denied on that basis, I think it would be a violation of ADA. At any rate, they should have tried to get him into that facility again or one that is similar to it).

His guardian thought he should go to Mayo Clinic again but didn't seem to have any particular rationale in mind, as far as Bill could discern. He mentioned that his new medical doctor had skipped over him for three weeks even though he was requesting to see him and the social worker volunteered that she would see that the doctor would see him the next time he was at the nursing home.

As if practicing a special brand of torture, just six days later the FCC social worker killed Mr. Tollefson's self-scheduled appointments for the 4th time in a row with the excuse that she didn't think his doctor's office was able to accommodate his size. Bill promptly called the State Health Department nurse but got no response to his message left on her voice mail. He then called Deseret Corp. and talked with someone in Human Resources who was going to run his complaint past her superior and get back to him. Deseret sent a Regional Nurse who twice gave Bill a three word memory test and then told him she wanted to resolve his complaint. Still in a snit because of his dashed hopes, he told her it was too late for that and she left, never to return.

I called my old classmate who founded R&S Medical Transport and discussed the situation with him and asked what they needed to know for the transportation to be successful. He said it was a simple matter of taking a tape measure and measuring the width of hallways and any obstruction and measuring the width and length of the stretcher that would carry Mr. Tollefson. He said his son was now running the business, so I called the office and talked with a very nice young woman named Paige. She told me they had a stipulation on Mr. Tollefson's transport that he could not make his own appointments for rides. I asked if they could do the proper measurements to see if Bill could fit into the doctor's office and she said that someone from their company was already scheduled to do so that evening or the next day (March 22).

In an email letter to Senator Franken's office I said:

It is now April 1 and no one has bothered to tell Bill the outcome of the measurements. He has heard nothing from the corporate nurse and nothing from the ombudsman. He does not have a mattress cover that prevents bedsores and the direct contact with plastic causes him to sweat profusely and he continues to spot blood from his hind quarters. His bed also does not position properly so that he gets choked (which is evident in his speech, at times) and experiences severe pain in his neck. In addition, the bed tilts him about 25 degrees to the left. The physical therapist has made no visible attempts to provide him with exercise equipment (even rubber bands). There is no trapeze and no use of the "New Step" machine. They continued to give him Wellbutrin 300 mg. and when he asked them if they were giving him any psychotropic medications, they denied it. Somehow he got them to place it on a PRN basis and when he stopped taking it, he began to feel like his "old jovial self" again. But shortly he had difficulty with the "cold turkey" withdrawal and had to resume it. It generally is not a good idea to just stop taking such medications all at once. Rather, a gradual reduction in dosage is recommended. However, the staff doesn't seem to be able to effect such a regimen. He is still required to lie in his fecal matter for up to an hour (as he did today) before they come to clean him up. And, of course, there has been no mention of trying to get him into an appropriate facility for aquatic physiotherapy.

So the incompetence and medical neglect is going on with no end in sight. Obviously no one in authority in the State of Minnesota gives a good-goddamn about the state's vulnerable adults, and I am doubtful that the feds are going to do anything either. Even the University of Minnesota, my alma mater, isn't able to act responsibly and ethically in their psychiatric drug trials. I know the problems are widespread as I hear the horror stories from people in other states and their frustrations in getting any help. As Bill says, it is just easier for them to look the other way and pretend the problems don't exist. So maybe it is time to give up trying to wring any shred of decency out of public officials and concentrate my efforts elsewhere.

Bill and most of the staff at FCC seemed to settle into an ongoing war of nerves. The staff didn't like Bill's haughty criticism of them and seemed determined to bring him down a notch or two by delaying response to or ignoring his requests and generally making his life more uncomfortable than it needed to be. Bill was defiant and determined not to let them get him down, to kill his enthusiasm for life, make him depressed, and force him into compliance with what they wanted him to do.

I talked with Bill's younger sister, in Portland and she said that she had received a phone call from someone early in the morning doing a survey about Bill's nursing home. She was not yet awake when he called so she didn't pay attention to who he said he was. He told her he had sent a paper survey earlier but she had not responded so he was following up on the phone. She said she never received a paper survey. She didn't tell the interviewer anything positive about the nursing home, she said and told him about the problems with getting showers and getting moved into his electric-lift chair.

Dr. Parker was busy sending out more letters on Bill's behalf. In December, Jake obtained Bill's signature and thumb print on a release of information form so that she could send a letter to the Special Rapporteur on Disability of the Commission for Social Development, Mr. Shuaib Chalken at the Office of the United Nations High Commissioner for Human Rights (OHCHR) regarding Bill. In the letter, she outlined the problems in getting adequate medical care for Mr. Tollefson and in getting his care givers and guardian to abide by human rights principles. She indicated that we were "...looking for a way to bring this human rights problem more effectively to the US government and would like your input on how to do that."

In January, she sent another letter, this time to Karol Balfe, Mental Health Campaign Coordinator, Amnesty International Irish Section. She again outlined the problems with Mr. Tollefson's health care and the failure of his care givers to respond to his medical needs in an appropriate manner and be respectful of his human rights. She asked, "Could you please as human rights advocates, review the information I have attached to this email and give us your opinion regarding Bill Tollefson's human rights. A letter from you would certainly help move the US Attorney's Office and the court to more expedient action to protect him and restore his human rights and to treat him with dignity."

In April a member of the Minneapolis Chapter of Mindfreedom, the one who had contacted Bill when he was first hospitalized, requested a synopsis of Mr. Tollefson's case so that she could present it to a panel of county commissioners to help try to convince them there was a problem with mental health care in their community. A version with no personally identifying information was sent to her. About that same time, both she and I became aware of the work of Dr. Carl Elliot, an ethics professor at the University of Minnesota who was trying to get the governor to investigate a case of forced drugging of a young man who subsequently nearly decapitated himself with a box cutter and died, at a University of Minnesota psychiatric treatment program. We both had signed his petition to Governor Mark Dayton, the same person I had petitioned earlier with no response whatsoever.

She went to a presentation by Dr. Elliot and was so impressed that she volunteered to try to get other speaking engagements for him to spread the word in the community. I responded to a request for case information to Dr. Elliot. He asked me if I wanted to get a reporter interested in Bill's case and I said I sure would. Shortly thereafter, I received a call from Brad Schrade, a Pulitzer Prize winning reporter from the *Minneapolis Star Tribune*. He quizzed me on various aspects of Bill's case and I sent him a copy of the first twelve chapters for him to review. He said he would be in touch but that was the last I ever heard from him.

Susan Freiman, former federal attorney, sent me an article about the lawsuit going on in New Hampshire based on the ADA and Olmstead rulings that require states to enable people with disabilities to live in the "least restrictive environment." It was a class action lawsuit (Lynn E. v. Lynch) with the New Hampshire Disabilities Rights Center, the Center for Public Representation, the U.S. Justice Department's Civil Rights Division and the Bazelon Center for Mental Health Law joining together with the law firm of Devine-Millimet & Branch against the state of New Hampshire. I thought that was the kind of action that would be necessary for Minnesota to do anything about the problems in their courts, mental health systems and nursing homes.

Mary Lynne Wolfe, director of the Minneapolis branch of the *Citizens Commission on Human Rights,* emailed that she had turned over the first few chapters of the book about Mr. Tollefson's case, now called *Presumed Crazy: A Chronicle of Arrogance, Incompetence and Immorality.* to a volunteer who was enjoying reading it. It remained to be seen if they had any interest in promoting the book.

In March an article appeared in the *Faribault Daily News* about a group that was trying to bring about reform in Rice County Social Services. Bill wanted to contact the group, called "Citizens for a Better Rice County." I emailed the article to Jake to print and give to Bill. It was not until June that he was able to make contact with a member of the group, Mary Carlsen who is head of the Social Work department at St. Olaf College in Northfield. I emailed her a copy of the first 12 chapters of this book and about a week later she responded, saying she would present a description of Bill's plight to her group to see if they had any interest in trying to do anything about it.

15 FIGHTING IGNORANCE AND THE MOB MENTALITY

Occupy Psychiatry was formed by Jim Gottstein, an Alaska attorney and head of The Law Project for Psychiatric Rights (PsychRights®) to bring together those groups and individuals protesting against the abusive power of psychiatry to lock people up, drug and electroshock them against their will, all based on untruths. Besides PsychRights® and unaffiliated individuals, the groups composing Occupy Psychiatry include Mindfreedom International, Voices of the Heart, The Freedom Center, Portland Hearing Voices, Madness Radio, Speak Out Against Psychiatry and the Center for the Human Rights of Users and Survivors of Psychiatry (CHRUSP). Gottstein added an organizing committee in January that was originally aimed at organizing protests against abuse of psychiatric treatment, particularly with respect to forced drugging of children, which Gottstein had established as his priority area. Coming soon after the Sandy Hook shootings in December and the resulting national controversy, the group soon devolved into a general discussion group about various problems in psychiatric treatment, discrimination against individuals with mental problems, mental health laws and their application or lack thereof.

There seemed to be developing what Gottstein called "a mob mentality with the objective of further restricting the rights of people diagnosed with mental illness and forcing them to endure harmful, counterproductive, psychiatric interventions." Some leaders in public mental health policy-making were encouraging expanded involuntary commitment laws (including forced outpatient drugging) and institutionalization under the benign sounding code words of "prevention and early intervention." New York rushed through a law that expanded state and federal criminal databases of people labeled as mentally ill, unconnected to any actual crime or act of violence, and expanded so-called outpatient commitment (forced drugging while the patient resides in the community). The New York governor ordered state officials to confiscate private patient records from psychiatrists, making the standard of "doctor-patient confidentiality" meaningless. In Colorado the governor and Office of Behavioral Health tried to fast-track a number of unconstitutional measures and an outrageous gun-control measure that would allow any mental health professional who was simply "concerned" to put a patient on a "no-buy" list for five years. On the national level, President Obama formed a Task Force on Gun Violence with Vice President Joe Biden as the head (and with not a single representative of the groups targeted for restriction of their liberties on the panel). Psychiatric profiling appeared to be the order of the day. As Gottstein commented, "In essence, society cannot agree to do much, if anything about easy access to guns with great killing power, violent video games and movies, or the other societal factors that go into the extremely high rate of gun violence in this country, so society is focused on pretending to do something by clamping down on people labeled with mental illness with even more psychiatry oppression. We know this is fruitless for its stated purpose. It is scapegoating."

Gottstein sent a letter to the President's Task Force on Gun Violence pointing out that psychiatric diagnosis does not predict violent behavior and that the discussion about gun violence needs to include the role of psychiatric drugs in causing violence. PsychRights was not the only one making these points. To protest the alarming rush to judgment about individuals labeled with a psychiatric diagnosis and causing them even more stigmatization and oppression, Tina Minkowitz – an attorney, head of CHRUSP and herself a survivor of psychiatric abuse - called for and launched the Occupy Psychiatry Event, National Day of Action to Stop Mental Health Profiling, to be held on Martin Luther King Day.

In her response to proposals made in the Biden Committee, Ms. Minkowitz suggested there be congressional hearings on the impact of the NCIS database on stigmatized groups and on alternative approaches to prevention of gun violence, on what constitutes responsible gun ownership and on how it could be monitored in society. She called for a reversal of what now seems to be the federal policy to recruit healthcare providers, families and police to monitor and control those who seek help with mental problems or are labeled with psychiatric diagnoses because it further criminalizes populations that are treated as expendable. She thought the proposed funding initiatives could lead service providers to gloss over the immoral profiling measures in order to promote their own services and shape policy-making.

In March, Ms. Minkowitz and Maxima Kalitventsev went to Geneva to meet with the UN Human Rights Committee and succeeded in getting them to ask the U. S. government to clarify how forced medication in psychiatric institutions could be consistent with their obligations under Article 7 of the *International Covenant on Civil and Political Rights* to ensure that no one is subjected to torture and ill-treatment. The Committee was considering the related question of compulsory psychiatric commitment and treatment as a violation of Article 9 of the *Covenant* – the right to liberty and security of the person.

On March 4, 2013 at the 22nd session of the Human Rights Council, the Special Rapporteur on Torture called for an absolute ban on forced psychiatric interventions including forced drugging, shock and psychosurgery, restraint and solitary confinement (seclusion), and for repeal of laws that allow compulsory mental health treatment and deprivation of liberty based on disability including when it is motivated by "protection of the person or others." All these practices are at least inhuman and degrading treatment and may amount to torture. The Rapporteur said that commitment and forced treatment must be replaced by community services meeting people's expressed needs and respecting their autonomy, emphasizing alternatives to the medical model of mental health.

Ms. Minkowitz then addressed the "reservations, understandings and declarations" (RUDs) attached to the United States' proposed ratification of the UN *Convention on the Rights of Persons with Disabilities*. She argued that the U. S. proposal was a "failure to meaningfully accept the obligations essential to ratification of a human rights treaty, in particular the obligation to conform domestic law to universal standards. Certain RUDs have a discriminatory impact against persons labeled with psychiatric disabilities, and purport to limit the obligations of the United States with respect to core elements of the treaty, in particular the right to legal capacity and the principles of respect for individual autonomy, and equality and non-discrimination." She asserted that, "It is an inherent principle of international human rights law that human rights are universal, and that no state can declare its own law to be the measure of compliance with the treaty," as the U. S. was attempting to do with its RUDs. She pointed out, in letters to the National Council on Disability

261

and to the U. S. Senate, that the Obama Administration's own memorandum of transmittal to the Senate acknowledged that state laws on guardianship violated Article 12 (right to legal capacity) and Article 14 (laws authorizing compulsory treatment and detention) of the CRPD. Why should the U. S. be the only country to have an escape clause to allow it to evade international law?

The dynamic Ms. Minkowitz proposed that June 26 be celebrated as an "International Day of Solidarity with Victims of Torture" and she asked members of the group to express their "opinions, feelings, vision for a future without psychiatric torture or detention, recommendations for what governments and others can do to make this a reality, tell your story and bear witness to the reality of forced psychiatry. This activity is for survivors and resisters of forced psychiatry and also for all human rights defenders to speak up as allies." I submitted a *Synopsis of the Case of Bill Tollefson* and Tina placed it on the CHRUSP website along with several other articles. She suggested that I send the case to the Special Rapporteur but I indicated that Janet Parker had already done so and in addition had sent it to the Irish branch of Amnesty International.

Some members of the group related their own abusive experiences at the hands of mental health systems and their observations of other events, making it clear that Bill Tollefson is not alone in his battles with the courts and the mental health "system," including county social services and nursing homes preying upon Medicaid patients. One member said that in North Carolina all it takes to have someone incarcerated for allegations of psychiatric disturbance is for someone to go to the magistrates office and fill out a form. She said it was often used in domestic disputes. Another member said her son was forced into unneeded hospitalization and she was sent for a mental evaluation after a neighbor made a 911 call without any actual investigation of the allegations. A Virginia resident said that a man who worked out of town had a relative who claimed to be his guardian. She had him committed every time he returned to check on his house even though he had had her removed as his payee on four different occasions. Another patient was said to have been detained whenever she lost her temper. The brother of one member had her detained without having seen her for 20 years after telling a mental health worker that she had been acquitted of murder when actually she had been a witness in a murder trial. Another member who works for an advocacy organization said, "We have women with babies in arms living on the street and our big plan is to ship the metro area folks to a refurbished prison in a rural community with the added perk of free mental health 'care.'" A Connecticut resident said, "The discrimination against people based upon psychiatric labels is widespread and rampant." They have had a lawsuit in court for the last seven years because the state judicial system will not provide reasonable accommodations to people with disabilities even though it is required under Title II of the *Americans with Disabilities Act*. A Colorado advocate said they also had a lawsuit against the state on behalf of 2000 people inappropriately placed in nursing homes, "many of them locked and ALL of them much worse snakepits than either of our institutions. Privately owned and hardly any oversight."

The case of Dan Markingson was brought up. He was a young man who was apparently coerced into a research program (a commercial market promotion drug trial) at the University of Minnesota. His psychiatrists would not listen to the pleas of his mother to remove him from the program because he was getting worse. Finally, the patient committed suicide by nearly decapitating himself with a box cutter. More recent evidence suggests that other research subjects may have been harmed or died because of misconduct at University of Minnesota psychiatric research projects. Eight bioethicists at the University of Minnesota itself had called for an external investigation, yet the university continued to refuse.

Rather than acting with honor and conducting a thorough investigation of the case, the University stonewalled and researchers lied about the extent of their participation in the drug trials. The patient's mother, his friend Mike Howard, and bioethics Professor Carl Elliot persisted for years in their efforts to expose improper goings on in the University's medical research and soon 175 international bioethicists and scholars signed a letter to the UMN president and faculty senate asking for them to take up the matter. The faculty senate did so and voted 67 to 23 for the university to re-examine the suicide and the president finally agreed to the demands, although he still quibbled about their exact terms. A petition to the Governor, Mark Dayton, was also submitted but at this writing the governor has not yet responded.

There was much discussion of evidence suggesting the role of antidepressant medication in precipitating suicidal thoughts or outbursts of irrational violence against others, both when taking the drug and when withdrawing from it. Several cases were cited: Steven Kazmierczak shot five people and wounded twenty-one others while taking Prozac, Xanax and another psychiatric drug; Jeff Weise, shot and killed his grandparents, seven students, a teacher and then himself while taking Prozac; Jason Hoffman, wounded three students and two teachers while taking Celexa and Effexor; Eric Harris who (along with Dylan Klebold)

263

killed twelve students and a teacher at Columbine High School before killing himself was taking Luvox; Kip Kinkel, who murdered his parents and two children at school while wounding twenty-five had just gone off Prozac. The Sandy Hook shooter, was said to be on medication but later reports indicated blood tests were negative for drugs.

The case of Mark Taylor, the Columbine shooting victim who was campaigning against the use of psychiatric drugs because the perpetrators of the shooting were both taking such medications at the time of the shooting, was brought up. He had been locked up and forcibly treated with psychiatric medications in spite of efforts by his mother and our own Dr. Janet Parker (of Medical Whistleblowers Advocacy Network) to have him freed. Interestingly, both Sanjay Gupta and Tom Ridge, in a January 13, 2013 *Natural News* article written by Peter Breggin, MD, warned about the contribution psychiatric drugs may have had in several mass murders, including Columbine. Dr. Breggin has written about the overuse of medications in psychiatry (*Medication Madness*, 2008) and believes the over drugging of soldiers and veterans is bordering on criminal and leads to chronicity, disability and accidents.

One member of the committee asked why there wasn't a public outcry for the 1,247 women murdered by an intimate partner in 2000 when, by comparison, the number killed in mass shootings in 2012 was only 151. Another asked where were the calls for "doctor control" when one is many more times likely to be killed by your doctor than by someone else using a gun. Iotrogenic (physician induced) disease is now the third leading cause of death in the United States. That number includes 106,000 deaths directly attributable to drug effects, 80,000 from hospital caused infections, 12,000 from unnecessary surgeries, 7000 from medication errors and 45,000 from other hospital errors (http://www.yourmedicaldetective.com/public/335.cfm). Some authorities place the figures of harm much higher than these because they do not include non-fatal outcomes and errors made to outpatients. The total number is three times the 43,000 people who are killed each year in auto accidents in the U.S. In any case, risk of death is greater from acceptance of medical treatment than from getting shot by someone else. One is also reminded of the article *Lies, Damned Lies and Medical Science* (http://www.theatlantic.com/magazine/archive/2010/11/lies-damned-lies-and-medical-science/308269/?single_page=true) that suggests that about 80% of the research that doctors rely upon is eventually found to be untrue. Another article in *The Economist* suggested 75% of *all* research is probably false. As indicated earlier, the former editor of the New England Journal of Medicine indicated that she could no longer believe the results of any published clinical research.

In Israel, another member noted, 151,240 people were admitted to the mental health system from 1955 to 2002 and 46,754 died (31%). Reference numbers indicate that 30,000 people were killed in auto accidents from 1955 to 2011 and 26,680 people were killed in all of the country's wars and acts of terror since it was established. Fifty percent of the fatalities were in people under 65 years of age and only 9% of them committed suicide. The Ministry of Health refused to disclose the causes of death citing patient confidentiality, even though the information that was requested did not request individual names. Thus, there appears to be considerable risk of death if one becomes involved with the mental health system in Israel and authorities appear to be covering up that risk.

It was also noted that a recent study (https://www.ncbi.nlm.nih.gov/pmc/articles/PMC3688067/) indicated that about 20% of Medicare patients discharged from a hospital develop an acute medical problem within 30 days that requires readmission. Nearly 70% of the re-admissions were due to conditions other than the initial reason for admission. The authors proposed that there is a "post-hospitalization syndrome" due to stress occurring during the hospitalization itself: sleep deprivation, disruption of normal circadian rhythms, poor nutrition, pain and other discomforts, mentally challenging situations, medications that alter cognition and physical function, and deconditioning by inactivity or bed rest. (Bill was subjected to all of these conditions).The patient surviving hospitalization in a general hospital might get labeled with a psychiatric condition on readmission. The patient initially hospitalized for a psychiatric condition may have his emotional reserves depleted by acquisition of a physical condition.

Members of the committee also had lots of suggestions about what to do. Tina suggested that members express their outrage against disability/mental health profiling in letters to their elected representatives, participate in demonstrations, teach-ins, talk-ins and similar kinds of activities to publicize their message. She suggested that members talk about human rights violations and failures to ratify treaties as social causes of violence and reach out for allies to those concerned about social justice, non-discrimination, trauma, non-violence, children and human well-being. "Educate ourselves about all the ways that people can be profiled and locked up for who they are rather than what they did - besides forced psychiatry, there are the youth detentions including for 'status crimes' like not going to school, racialized enforcement of drug laws and other laws, immigration laws, 'three strikes' laws with mandatory long-term sentences for petty crimes, 'sex offender' laws that penalize a wide range of nonviolent conduct (and use civil commitment) etc."

Since the statistical association between mental illness and perpetuating violence (as opposed to being the victim of it) is essentially zero, another member argued that, if the purpose of increased funding is to reduce violence, it should go not to coercive mental health services or those focused on psychiatric labeling (such as the the White House Project AWARE which seeks to diagnose 750,000 school kids as mentally ill) but to community programs (such as Cure Violence) specifically designed to de-escalate situations and reduce violence using conflict mediation techniques. The American Psychological Association also came out with a report in 2013 that indicated there were no reliable psychological profile or set of warning signs that could be used to predict violence in the general population. Instead, they recommended directing efforts to behavioral threat assessment with a subset of the population that has already communicated threats or planning to commit violent acts.

An advocate suggested we use the funds for "Prevention and Early Intervention" (which she believed was really screening and drug-based treatment) instead for methods that might actually help a person before his/her emotional issues got out of hand, such as building viable families, community supports and nutritious foods.

One member extolled the virtues of the founders of the mental health consumer/survivor movement (later consolidated into the National Coalition for Mental Health Reform) who "understood the only way to gain rights and independence was to come together and unite in a common cause. Meeting in churches, apartments and basements, we discovered the power of sharing our stories, of *being heard and of being understood*, instead of the idea that our labels defined us. We discovered we could shift into a vision of leading independent lives where we become authors rather than victims in our lives. As a result of the example of this early leadership hundreds of self-help groups, consumer-run initiatives, and statewide consumer organizations have been formed all over the country."

While having some local success, these groups found themselves being "spoken for" by other more politically-savvy groups (such as the National Association for Mental Illness or NAMI, which receives the majority of their funding from drug companies) that did not always represent the interests of consumers. Acknowledging that they have proclaimed "Nothing about us without us," she decried the fact that they had not yet organized themselves into a common voice to achieve this goal.

This person advocated for education in ethics and compassion for all public employees at all levels. She believed the key issues were: 1) reliable legal representation - both mental health law and family law; 2) reliable mental health professional court opinions; 3) funding for both of these. She said she was unable to find any community or organization that supports any of the above in her ongoing efforts over the last four years. Some practical steps that she thought could be implemented immediately included developing a list of reliable, honest, experienced and qualified lawyers for referral (since most lawyers say they are "too busy" or "not interested" in these type cases), developing a list of reliable, ethical and sincere professionals who would testify in court, and organizing training sessions using people like Jim Gottstein and Dr. Peter Breggin. She proposed starting a non-profit foundation dedicated to providing funding for legal expenses and expert opinions and trying to change legislation so that a legal voucher system could take the place of court-appointed counsel.

It was reported that PsychSearch.net (http://www.psychsearch.net/psychiatrists/) was now doing a background records search on every psychiatrist in America, including criminal records. In their first sweep they retrieved state disciplinary documents in California, Maryland, New York and Texas. Missouri was next in line.

Several members of the group referred to a front page article that appeared in the New York Times (http://www.nytimes.com/2013/02/03/opinion/sunday/sunday-dialogue-treating-the-mentally-ill.html?pagewanted=1&_r=0) that made a number of astute and interesting observations. I quote from the post in its entirety:

Objective (biological, chemical, physical) tests for diseases are based on the assumption that diseases are somatic phenomena. Accordingly, the claim that mental illnesses are brain diseases is profoundly self-contradictory: a disease of the brain is a brain disease, not a mental disease.

Because there are no objective methods for detecting the presence or establishing the absence of mental diseases, and because psychiatric diagnoses are stigmatizing labels with the potential for causing far-reaching personal injury to the stigmatized person, the "mental patient's" inability to prove his "psychiatric innocence" makes psychiatry one of the greatest dangers to liberty and responsibility in the modern world.

The legal system recognizes the elementary distinction between innocence and guilt. The psychiatric system does not: it proudly rejects the concept of personal responsibility. Crime is a *well-defined act*. Mental illness is an *ill-defined mental state*. Criminal prosecution is defined, and popularly understood, as *adversarial*. Psychiatric treatment, even when forcibly imposed by law, is defined and widely accepted as *nonadversarial*. Those differences, together with the notion of mental illness, are the two great lies and injustices that undergird the psychiatric enterprise.[See Associated Press, "Duke Lacrosse Players File Lawsuit," *New York Times*, Oct. 5, 2007, http://www.nytimes.com/aponline/us/AP-DukeLacrosse.html?hp; Associated Press, "Duke Prosecutor Sentenced to Day in Jail," Sept. 2, 2007, http://www.usatoday.com/news/nation/2007-08-31-nifong-jail_N.htm.]

It is possible to establish that a person accused of a crime is not guilty, that is, has not performed the illegal act attributed to him and is the victim of *malicious prosecution* serving, say, the personal-political ambitions of an unscrupulous district attorney; it is also possible to punish the person responsible for such malicious prosecution. In contrast, it is impossible to establish that a person diagnosed as mentally ill is not mentally ill and is the victim of *malicious psychiatrization* serving, say, the economic-ideological ambitions of the diagnostician; it is not possible to punish the person responsible for the injurious diagnosis that may be *erroneous but, by definition, cannot be malicious*.[See Thomas Szasz, *Law, Liberty and Psychiatry: An Inquiry into the Social Uses of Mental Health Practices*.]

In the Anglo-American adversarial legal system, the accused is presumed innocent until proven otherwise, and the onus of proof of guilt is on the accuser. In the psychiatric-inquisitorial "medical" system, this relationship is reversed: the person diagnosed as mentally ill is presumed insane until proven otherwise, and the onus of disproof of insanity is on the (usually powerless) individual incriminated as "insane." A priori, psychiatrists disqualify such claims of "psychiatric innocence" as evidence of the "insane patient's" denial of his illness.[See Szasz, *Insanity;* and Szasz, *Liberation by Oppression: A Comparative Study of Slavery and Psychiatry.*]

Another member related the new standards on reporting of stories relating to mental illness that appeared in the *Associated Press Stylebook* and reflect a surprisingly advanced ethical position and sensitivity to the effects of word choice on audience perceptions:

Do not describe an individual as mentally ill unless it is clearly pertinent to a story and the diagnosis is properly sourced.

When used, identify the source for the diagnosis. Seek firsthand knowledge; ask how the source knows. Don't rely on hearsay or speculate on a diagnosis. Specify the time frame for the diagnosis and ask about treatment. A person's condition can change over time, so a diagnosis of mental illness might not apply anymore. Avoid anonymous sources. On-the-record sources can be family members, mental health professionals, medical authorities, law enforcement officials and court records. Be sure they have accurate information to make the diagnosis. Provide examples of symptoms.

Do not use derogatory terms, such as insane, crazy/crazed, nuts or deranged, unless they are part of a quotation that is essential to the story.

Do not assume that mental illness is a factor in a violent crime, and verify statements to that effect. A past history of mental illness is not necessarily a reliable indicator. Studies have shown that the vast majority of people with mental illness are not violent, and experts say most people who are violent do not suffer from mental illness.

Avoid unsubstantiated statements by witnesses or first responders attributing violence to mental illness. A first responder often is quoted as saying, without direct knowledge, that a crime was committed by a person with a "history of mental illness." Such comments should always be attributed to someone who has knowledge of the person's history and can authoritatively speak to its relevance to the incident.

Avoid descriptions that connote pity, such as afflicted with, suffers from or victim of. Rather, he has obsessive-compulsive disorder.

Double-check specific symptoms and diagnoses. Avoid interpreting behavior common to many people as symptoms of mental illness. Sadness, anger, exuberance and the occasional desire to be alone are normal emotions experienced by people who have mental illness as well as those who don't.

Wherever possible, rely on people with mental illness to talk about their own diagnoses. Avoid using mental health terms to describe non-health issues. Don't say that an awards show, for example, was schizophrenic.

Use the term mental or psychiatric hospital, not asylum.

The controversy raging over the fifth version of the American Psychiatric Association's *Diagnostic and Statistical Manual*, DSM 5, was not noticed by the mental health initiatives coming out of the White House early in 2013, in spite of all the recently published books and magazine articles on the subject by prominent individuals in the mental health fields, e. g., *Saving Normal* by Allen Frances, chairman of the task force for the fourth version of the manual. Occupy Psychiatry members did not miss the controversy, however, and a subgroup (of which I am a member) began a movement, under the able direction of Jack Carney, PhD (a New York-based retired social worker), called *Boycott DSM 5* that sought signatures on a web-based petition to protest use of the DSM 5 diagnostic scheme.

The petition alleges that the DSM-5 categories are not supported by scientific evidence and will harm rather than bring relief to persons in distress. The "psychiatrist's bible" will expand the scope of mental illness to include many normal behaviors, resulting in many millions of people being unnecessarily diagnosed and treated with potentially harmful psychiatric medications that have not been validated to be effective. Even individuals with some medical problems would also qualify for a psychiatric diagnosis and could therefore be inappropriately prescribed psychiatric medications.

The new manual has removed the multi-axial aspect of diagnosis from earlier versions and has eliminated all references to and consideration of psychosocial, environmental, cultural and spiritual factors in aberrations of behavior. Treatment considerations are reduced to biology and the prescribing of psychoactive medications.

Widespread opposition to the manual by professionals, advocacy groups and the lay public was ignored in three public reviews of the proposed categories. Fourteen thousand people signed an "Open Letter to the DSM 5" requesting independent scientific review of proposed changes but this too was ignored. It appeared to the Boycott DSM 5 Committee that the American Psychiatric Association had "undermined its own credibility, choosing to protect its intellectual property and publishing profits, not the public trust."

The National Institute of Mental Health decided to abandon the DSM 5 for its research studies while developing their own biologically based system. The British Psychological Society as a group lambasted the new psychiatric manual. The Boycott DSM 5 committee was supported by the National Alliance of Professional Psychological Providers of Orange County, California, the Academy of Medical Psychology, the Initiative for Individualized Treatment of France, and the MISS Foundation of Phoenix, Arizona.

Besides the widespread conceptual mistakes existing in DSM 5, Dr. Frances recently argued on his blog (June 11, 2013) that the manual is replete with writing errors because the committee "(1) lacked an experienced text editor; (2) the work groups were free to write criteria sets in their own careless way; (3) DSM-5 was rushed to press prematurely because its deadlines had been missed and publishing profits beckoned. There was no time left for adequate central editing and proof reading." He found "egregious mistakes" on nearly every page that he examined but found 18 errors worthy of note, a sampling of which follow. Criterion A in the Autistic Spectrum Disorder category does not specify how many of its three items were required, making reliability in diagnosis impossible. The definition of ADHD is relaxed so much that there will be excessive diagnosis of children that are going through normal periods of impulsivity, inattention or hyperactivity. In just three pages, four inconsistent age ranges are specified for Disruptive Mood Dysregulation Disorder. There is no longer an Unspecified Mood Disorder category in DSM 5, eliminating cases that do not yet have a clearly evident presentation. Dr. Frances found both depressive and bipolar sections to be unclear and inconsistent. The "Other Unspecified" option has been added to most categories in the manual. This practice encourages "creative diagnosis" that leads to unneeded medications and "mischief in the courtroom." Mild and severe depressions are co-mingled in the new "Persistent Depressive Disorder." The exposure criterion of PTSD does not now require actual experiencing or witnessing of a traumatic event in DSM 5 as it did in DSM IV, making for a mess in forensic situations such as determining compensation. The Intellectual Disability category no longer requires an impaired IQ level, also leading to problems in forensic situations. As indicated above, many people with medical illnesses will be misidentified as having a mental disorder because of the vaguely written criteria for Somatic Symptom Disorder. The author said that, "The wording of Mild Neurocognitive Disorder (p605) is so impossibly vague that it includes me, my wife, and most of our friends. It will cause unnecessary worry and a rush to useless and expensive testing."

This statement has been shown to be true in the much publicized case of Justina Pelletier, the teenager with mitochondrial disease that Boston Children's Hospital claimed was an instance of Somatic Symptom Disorder. The hospital, in collusion with the relevant state agency, managed to wrest custody away from the parents without any evidence to justify it. Litigation over this abomination of the psychiatric – legal system continues at this writing

16 <u>WHEN HE IS FIT AND SEASON'D FOR HIS PASSAGE</u>

Shakespeare

Bill had been bothered by an upper respiratory infection with ear involvement since June 1st, 2013. By June 14 he was so uncomfortable he exclaimed that his ear problems were so bad that, "I'm losing it!" He received no treatment for it from nursing home staff and when he tried to use his standard home remedies that he had used for years for such conditions, the staff would not provide him with the necessary materials of peroxide, vinegar and garlic. A nurse told him she "had to blow him off," and that Dr. Spittal had authorized this action (Bill learned from a cleaning lady that "everyone" at FCC was unhappy with the new doctor).

Finally, his sister bought him the peroxide and vinegar for irrigating his ears when she visited. The staff would not provide him with a syringe so he had to pour the mixture into the cap of one of the bottles and then tilt his head while pouring it into his ears. One of the more responsible aides picked up some garlic for him in a grocery store. These measures moderated his symptoms somewhat but did not cure the problems, which were quite apparent when he spoke over the phone.

Ten days later Bill had turned his emergency light on because he was choking and no one came. He tried calling the nursing station but they did not answer the phone because they had caller-ID and knew it was him that was calling. After an hour, he threw something against the wall to make a noise in order to gain someone's attention. His doctor would not see him but he was finally able to get some antibiotics from the nurse-recorder.

In spite of his discomfort, Bill continued to try to accomplish useful things. A long-time Boy Scout and troop leader, he learned of an old soon-to-be-abandoned light house on Lake Superior and thought it would make an ideal site for scouting activities and training, like what had been accomplished at the old Ft. Snelling with the "Base Camp" project. He contacted the person handling the application to have the facility turned over to a non-profit group, had the form sent to me by email, and then I sent it to Jake Heckler to bring to Bill. After he evaluated the conditions for transfer of the property, he then contacted his old Boy Scout Regional Office and found they were quite interested in the project and would pursue it further.

On July 8, 2013 Bill reported that he felt like he was again being given Wellbutrin or a similar psychiatric medication without his awareness or permission. The cricket noises in his head had returned, he complained of feeling clumsy and having cotton-mouth (a common side effect of psychiatric medications), he was sleeping "way too much" and he was having "miserable" dreams. Objectively, his speech was noticeably slurred when Jake and I talked with him over the phone.

When he asked the morning nurse what medications he was being given, she would "get in a snit" and walk out of his room saying, "You don't need to know that." The staff did not wear name tags and didn't verbally identify themselves, so it was difficult for him to know who to report. Again, it seems, the ethically challenged worker prefers to work in an anonymous environment where he or she can, quite literally, get away with murder and the ethically challenged institution prefers to have inept government inspectors who are willing to be bamboozled and the ethically challenged state prefers to keep everything nebulous so no funds need to be expended and no corrective action needs to be taken.

Bill was supposed to have an appointment with Dr. Payne on July 12 but he got a call from some temporary secretary telling him that it had been canceled. The person who canceled it was someone named "Jenny" who represented herself as Mr. Tollefson's guardian. He called Mayo Clinic Patient Affairs and complained. A short time later a person representing Mayo Clinic's "Patient Experience Division" in Owatonna called Bill to rebut his objection to his appointment being canceled. She told him that his guardian had to arrange all appointments and that he was not cooperating with therapy. He countered that he was receiving no therapy whatsoever even though he was crying out for it.

When I learned of this, I immediately called the person representing Mayo Clinic and informed her that I had, in writing from a federal agency, that Mayo Clinic considers Mr. Tollefson to be capable of making all his own medical decisions and that would include making appointments and arranging for transportation. I informed her that a HIPAA complaint had been filed against Mayo Clinic and that in response Mayo had claimed that Mr. Tollefson was capable of making all his own medical decisions. She said she did not know that and asked if a legal action had been initiated. She was informed that it was "in process." She said she would get back to me but, of course, she never did.

Consequently, I sent letters to the civil rights investigator and her supervisor informing them of the statement made by the person representing Mayo Clinic which contradicted the claim made by Mayo clinic in defense of their denial of the records I had requested. I asked them to reopen my original complaint against Mayo Clinic because of this contradiction and because they had previously investigated the wrong request for information. Weeks later I received a letter informing me that the matter had been turned over to a federal office in Washington State rather than the Chicago office which has jurisdiction over HIPAA matters in Minnesota. No explanation was given for the change of venue. I suspected it was just another time consuming dodge to get me to give up so they wouldn't have to confront the big elephant in the room – Mayo Clinic.

On July 27th three nurses were walking behind Bill as he was being transported on a wheeled commode used as a shower chair. The "skin nurse" said something to the effect that she didn't know what they had been doing with regard to Bill's skin. Bill commented that if he had had the right kind of sheet on his bed and had had his skin debreeded with a moist towel, he wouldn't have the moisture caused skin problems. After he made his comment, the nurses called him "abusive" and stormed off. When asked if he had sworn or made any hostile remarks to them, he denied it. "Just because I want things done a certain way from my side of things, they argue and call me abusive."

Jake visited Bill on August 1st and noted that Bill's bed raised his knees but not his legs. His head would slide down to the joint on the two parts of the bed, causing pressure on the back of his head which would compress his larynx. This, in turn, impaired his breathing and caused choking when Bill would try to eat, so that for the last two days he had been unable to eat anything but yogurt, milk and water. Bill commented,"I'm just laying here dying. This is not healthy."

His phone had been out of order and he asked for two days for nurses and nurses aides to check to make sure that it was plugged in but they wouldn't do so. Finally, the cleaning lady got the maintenance man to check it and he plugged it in so that Bill could again be in contact with the outside world. Bill said that it seemed like every time he would ask for something the staff would become angry and intimidating.

Bill learned from a staff member that the new head of nursing had already left her post and the position was empty. The administrator and the assistant administrator were both scheduled to leave shortly. A nurses aide told him, "If the state came in here now, they'd close the place down" because of lack of staff. This particular nurses aide had been working two straight days and was all alone the previous day on Bill's wing of the facility whereas there were usually three people available to cover that area. Another staff member confided to Bill that she had observed one or more instances of improper staff behavior and would like to report it to someone. Bill gave her the telephone number of Deseret corporate headquarters in Utah, probably a poor choice for any kind of corrective action.

Bill had not seen the doctor for about five weeks and said that he chose to work only through the nurse-recorder and rarely saw patients directly. Mr. Tollefson had not been moved to his chair in several weeks.

On Sunday, August 4th at 8:00 pm Mr. Tollefson was experiencing pain in his right leg and felt what he thought was a swollen muscle, which he assumed might be due to the chronic muscle infection the doctors at Hennepin County Medical Center told him he had. He asked a nurses aide to look at it. She did so, made a face, and exclaimed, "Ee-uh" and proceeded to run out of the room. Bill asked her to send someone in who could do something but no one showed up. After waiting 2 hours, he called the nurses station and a nurse came to evaluate his complaint. She made arrangements to have him transported to Mayo Clinic ER. There, they first did an endoscope to check if his previous ulcers in his esophagus and small intestines had healed (which they were supposed to have done several months earlier) and found that they had. Then they checked for any problems in his lower colon.

Finally, they decided he had a blood clot nearly the whole length of his leg and placed him on blood thinners (which he had been taking up until the time of his ulcer incident). The staff caused him considerable pain by the mechanical method they used to move him and he injured his back by trying to get onto an inappropriately sized bed pan (even though he told the staff member it wasn't right). But he wanted to please them and tried anyway.

About a week later Bill was still experiencing "terrible pain" on his backside. He told the staff he had an injury from sitting on a bedpan years earlier and that the bed pan incident at Mayo had aggravated it. On this day, when he was Hoyer-lifted and transported on the wheeled commode to get a shower, the pain kicked up again. He tried to get as much weight off his backside as possible by adjusting the bed but he had a long night of pain and the bed was still choking him as well as irritating his behind for the following night. "I've been run over too long. How do I last? Show me a way to go home." The "home" he was referring to was his heavenly home, which he considered preferable to continued agony at FCC.

My wife and I visited Bill on August 18 and 19. Pictures were taken of Bill, his teeth, his legs, his bed and his room. He was in constant pain and tried to find a position of the bed where he could get a few seconds of relief, but was unable to do so. I made a sound movie of Mr. Tollefson and his commentary as he tried various combinations of back-rest, leg lift and forward and backward motions of the bed. It was heart-rending. When I got home, I obtained a movie editing program and added subtitles to what Bill was saying so it was easily intelligible, added some still pictures and some narration and made a short DVD which I sent to Senator Al Franken's office as well as to some other individuals that had shown an interest in Bill's plight.

The staff put him in a different bed on Friday, August 23rd. Apparently, it was a new frame but was supplied with the same type of short mattress he had before the time when the nursing home inspector required them to change the bed and use an extra-long mattress. Trying to make-do, they put a bolster and two pillows under his legs and let his feet hang over the edge of the bed as they did before the nursing inspector arrived. One difference was that this bed had some kind of cycling movement programmed into it that caused him a great deal of pain each time it cycled. Although he complained about it for hours, it was not until 12:30 pm that they turned the cycling program off.

Another problem with the bed was that it had a pillow-top cover into which he would sink so that he could not use his urinal properly. The angle of the urinal when set on the soft top was wrong so that his urine ran out onto himself when it was only 1/4th full.

Previously, he was able to get some pain relief by laying out flat but that ceased to work. He continued to get the "pain meds" (actually, muscle relaxants) once about 1:30 pm and then sometime between 2:00 am or 3:00 am at the staff's discretion (as everything seemed to be). The meds continued to cause him to have nightmares.

Bill mentioned the bed problem to staff every day but, he was told, there would be no administrator present at the facility who could make such momentous decisions for at least the next 4-5 days. The recording nurse and substitute for the doctor, said he would try to email corporate headquarters about the bed problem even though FCC staff had claimed they had no email capability the last time he requested they contact corporate headquarters.

On August 27th I talked with Bill on the phone. There was no improvement in his condition. "I'm on the edge of death. If they cremate me there will be no remains and no evidence. All I can tell is if it is daylight or dark and if they put something on the tray in front of me. I've had agonizing dreams ever since they started giving me some kind of medication. It is a substitute for Flexerill because they say my insurance won't pay for Flexerill. I'm praying for the Lord to take me home, praying for mercy." He was moaning all the time and would at times exclaim, "Oh god!" He said, "I'm trying to live through it but it may not be doable."

I talked again with Bill at 10:30 pm and he sounded very drowsy and was becoming anxious that he would be kept awake all night by pain. He said he sometimes had to beg for pain pills up until 4:00 or 5:00 am. He explained that he was "half way out of the well" [meaning only partially alert] but he would have to live with whatever the staff did or did not do to get him ready for the night. He reported having more agony dreams and commented, "I'm just trying to survive." He complained that his eyes were pouring out tears for the last two nights, a problem he had had for several months since he first tried to get to see his eye doctor.

The next day Bill did not get a shower on his usual day for one. He had had no personal care (e. g., washing with a wash rag) for at least 24 hours. He was concerned because of the problem with his scalp, referred to earlier, was worsened by lack of washing. The nursing home staff did empty his urinal and provide him with meals but ignored his inquiries about getting a shower. He started saying something about it at 6:10 pm and finally put his call light on because he was worried it would soon get too late for them to do any thing about it. Two hours and 50 minutes later the light was still on. A charge nurse showed up with his pills and he explained it to her. She left. A male nurse from Somalia showed up and he mentioned it to him.

Someone told Mr. Tollefson that he had said he didn't want a shower but he responded that that statement was a lie. I called the facility and talked with someone named Stephanie who said the person to complain to was a nurse. When I asked for a name, she said "Richard" but did not know his last name. I was unable to contact any Richard. Bill did not receive a shower the next day either but an aide named Angela come in at 5:45 am, awakened him from a sound sleep, roughly grabbed him, washed him up and changed his bed.

On September 1st, the nursing home social worker told him that he was going to the Grace Unit in Hastings, MN for a "second opinion." She was supposed to return to Bill with a description of the place but, of course, she never did. A nurse told him she thought perhaps he should go to the Grace Unit, implying it was an undesirable place, and he perceived this as a threat. I found a web page for the place on the Internet and relayed the information contained to Mr. Tollefson. Their self-description made it sound like it might be a positive step in rehabilitation and a way to get out of the dead-end (literally) of FCC. Bill cautioned, "Yeah, unless it is all bullshit!"

FCC would not reveal to me whether or not Bill was still a patient at their facility and the Grace Unit would not confirm nor deny whether Mr. Tollefson had been admitted there. A call to Bill's sister in Portland resulted in a phone number for the unit but they would not allow me or any of Bill's friends to talk with him. Apparently, he was being held, in violation of the law, like a prisoner at that facility.

On September 17 Bill was returned to FCC and I got the report. "Another dirty rotten run," was Bill's summary statement. Apparently their web site hype was, indeed, all bullshit. Every day he was there he asked to have access to a telephone but was denied, again violating his patient rights under Minnesota law. He did not receive a shower while there. He was so dehydrated that they couldn't draw blood for a blood test. There was tape placed over the nurses call button and when he removed it, he was chewed out because, he was told, it was "just for emergencies."

He resorted to yelling "help" so that visitors to the facility would hear him and it would embarrass the nurses into paying attention to him. He described them as "walkaway nurses" for the way they treated him. He was allowed no radio, no TV and no nurses light. He was placed in an old Lazy Boy chair which was more uncomfortable than his bed at FCC and they would not give him a wheelchair. He said his vision and hearing changed for the worse but his olfactory sense was back to normal.

He was forced to use a catheter while in Hastings even though he said it was stated in his medical records that he should never ever be catheterized again. Although the device performed its function, he did end up getting a urinary tract infection as a result. The psychiatrist, a Dr. Bore, did not examine him but told him he must be crazy because he had been in all the hospitals in his record. He said Dr. Bore "became livid" when he mentioned Christianity and told him "I don't discuss religion or politics."

He received no physical therapy and he said he had more bleeding from his butt than he had before. He felt he was near death's door until they finally gave him pain medication on Wednesday night. He observed people crawling all over the floor and when he inquired about it, he was told it was some type of therapy. He found that odd as did this reporter. They tried to force medicate him and it was unclear if they had succeeded.

When he was being moved by Hoyer lift, he asked them to be careful of his legs and feet because they were sensitive. They managed to slam him into the leg lifts and he felt they had broken his left toe (later confirmed by Jake, who visited 9 days later). On his arrival back at FCC, he found that they had a new administrator and another new director of nursing.

Bill called Jake, Big Jim and me several times on September 25th and seemed to be in a drug-induced euphoria bordering on mania. He was full of ideas about what he wanted to do and began calling people he knew all over the country trying to find resources to get out of FCC and begin to live his life again. He recalled times in the past when he managed to pull off accomplishments that others said were not possible and he did not see why that might not be possible again.

He said he requested a wheelchair and that the social worker was over-joyed and would try to get him one. He wanted to go outside and get some exercise. He talked with the Athletic Activities department at Courage Center and thought everything was a "go" if he could get a doctor to recommend it (no small task since his doctor seldom saw him and Bird Brain was likely to interfere with his plans, no matter what they were). He called and talked with his millionaire TV fisherman friend who said Bill didn't have to pay him back for putting him up at a motel in Florida on that last disastrous trip there, as long as he was still a Christian.

He talked with an old Northfield lawyer and mayor, who referred him to a retired lawyer who apparently liked to 'push' the establishment. In later calls he talked with a friend about the Fraternal Order of Fools, the partying organization in which he was strongly invested in his earlier years. He lamented his relatives not supporting him in his time of need, talked about going to visit Big Jim in Wisconsin, about Pastor Pete The Pizza Delivery Guy in Faribault who was also an ordained minister, about his trip to Norway and the Trombone Orchestra.

He rambled all over the place with slurred speech and sounding breathless at times. He complained that the administrators at the nursing home were hard on employees and the result was that they communicated their frustration to the patients and made them irritable as well. He tended to minimize obstacles to achieving his goals, which might be attributable to his drug-induced heightened sense of self-efficacy.

He was visited by the Ombudsman for Older Minnesotans and her supervisor, and he told them that he could no longer put up with the lack of attention to his needs, that he was not a "system" type of person but rather a "direct" person and it was not in his nature to be patient with bureaucratic methods. He told them, "You people have taken three years out of what will probably be the last decade of my life. I have no time to waste." The sense of urgency about living a life outside of a nursing home while it still might be possible seemed realistic to me but Bill underestimated the resistance he would encounter from his so-called care givers and overestimated his ability to enlist cooperation from those who didn't like him or were unwilling to get out of their comfort zone. How the staff could completely miss the behavior change that was obviously associated with over-medication or wrongly prescribed medication, was another mystery.

The next day Jake visited Bill at the nursing home and confirmed that he had a broken toe on his right foot and one toe nail about ready to fall off, results of his treatment in Hastings. Bill continued to voice plans that were unrealistically optimistic, which Jake attributed to the relief from pain due to the medications. I sent a report of the latest developments to Diane Gerten at Senator Al Franken's office. An automated reply from Franken's office said they were out of business until the government shutdown was over.

Big Jim was quite sure the drug Bill was taking was some kind of morphine and told Jake that he himself had once taken them for back pain and they "turned me into a jabber-jaw just like Bill." He said that he had to stop taking them when he got so goofy that he forgot how to open a can of soup. The three friends agreed that the drug-induced euphoria that Bill demonstrated would allow the nurses to ignore any responsibility to take action by saying, "Well, that's what the doctor ordered." And then when Bill started floating near the ceiling, they could say, "Well, that proves it - he is crazy as a bedbug and needs to be here or in the state hospital." And his guardian could be expected to say, "See, I told you he was a looney!" They were sure Bill didn't want to get off the meds because they were so much better than the excruciating pain he had been experiencing.

On October 8th an expose article appeared in the *Minneapolis Star Tribune* about the laxity of the state nursing board and I sent a link

(http://www.startribune.com/lifestyle/health/226301371.html?
page=all&prepage=1&c=y#continue) to it to Jake, Mary Carlson
(Citizens for a Better Rice County) and Diane Gerten (Senator Al
Franken's office).

Two days later Bill was sent to Mayo Clinic after "going down bad in
the evening" with "scary" vital signs. He said that he was told he had had
pneumonia for a long time and that it was probably being passed around
in the nursing home by the nurses. He complained that the nurses had
removed his phone for some reason and when Jake tried to reach him the
next day it still wasn't working. Jake decided to visit Bill anyway but
when he arrived Bill was gone and someone had cleaned up his room and
tossed out all of Bill's belongings. Even his food table was clear and
clean and the bed was folded up with nothing on it. Jake asked a woman
where he was and she sent him to see the head nurse. Heckler was afraid
Bill might have "bit the big one." The nurse told him that they had to
send Bill to the hospital. He asked if it was Rochester, Hastings, or Rice
County District One. She paused a second and then said
Abbot/Northwestern, and explained that it was due to chest pain. With all
the pain meds Bill was taking, Jake didn't know how he could have any
chest pain, but he remembered that I had said Phill sounded "winded"
when talking last time. Jake couldn't imagine that at his age, weight, and
physical condition, they would do much of anything and thought he
probably wouldn't survive any surgery.

I called Bill's hospital number three times without any response. Big
Jim called me and said he had talked with Bill and learned that he had
pneumonia, which, in retrospect, was not surprising since he had had a
persistent cough for many weeks. Bill later said that his left lung had
been three-fourths filled with fluid as a result of the pneumonia but they
did not feel it necessary to drain it. Big Jim said Bill was on some kind of
drug that was making him loopy, so he didn't make a lot of sense and Jim
couldn't get very detailed information from him.

Two days later Bill asked a nurse to talk with me about his situation.
She got on the phone and asked that I call her back at the nurses station,
apparently not wanting Bill to hear what she said. She said Bill was told
while dinner was being served that he was going to be discharged back to
FCC. When the transportation arrived, he told them he would not go. She
said she had a doctor talk to him on the phone and another talked with
him in person and then a social worker talked with him. He told her he
hadn't received proper warning and didn't remember talking with any of
those people. I told her he probably didn't want to go back to FCC and I
added that it was with good reason – he had developed ulcers and

pneumonia under their care, they interfered with him seeing his doctors, and they halted his PT even though his physical therapist thought they were making progress. I forgot to mention the problem in getting regular showers and his blood clot but I did mention that they had allowed him to go from wheelchair bound to bed bound in his time there and that they kept him in a bed that was 6" too short for him for a full year until a state nursing home inspector forced them to change it. She sympathized but said that was not their concern - he had to go. Afterward, Bill said he did remember talking with one doctor and he knew he had to leave, but he was going to institute a "foot-dragging strategy" to see if he could get any kind of consideration out of them. I told him I thought that was what he was trying to do. He laughed and said, "Bud, you know better than anyone the way I operate.".

Bill was returned to FCC the next day. His legs were still swollen due to water retention and he said he had a new pain in his leg that he had never experienced before. The following day his doctor was supposed to visit him but he never appeared. On the 19th of October he wasn't allowed to sit in his power chair but he did get a shower – the first one in over a month

I called the Department of Justice regarding the ADA complaint that Dr. Parker and myself had submitted on September 11, 2012. I was told they could not give me any information because I was not listed on the complaint. I had called them previously and did not have this problem. So I sent them an email with a copy of the ADA Complaint attached and asked them to read the first sentence which stated that the complaint was being submitted by Dr. Parker and myself as co-complainants and to read the notarized letter to that effect which was included in the paper documentation sent to them. I asked them to correct their records and notify me when they had done so. I said that I would like to know what, if anything had been done with this complaint. It had been over one year since it was filed and, so far as I could tell and so far as the patient reported, nothing had changed for the better in that time. In fact, the conditions leading to the original complaint still existed and additional violations of the patient's rights and neglectful care had occurred. I received their automated reply saying that someone would respond to my inquiry at some indefinite time in the future.

Since the PsyD psychologist had not responded to Bill's request for his records of his visits with Bill, Jake sent Bill's HIPAA Complaint against the PsyD off to the Chicago OCR office as per the instructions. A letter was also sent to Regina Health Center in Hastings for copies of his records from his time there. If they did not respond in the appropriate time frame, a HIPAA Complaint would also be filed against them.

On October 25th when I talked with Bill he wasn't manic like he was when he was on the pain meds but it sounded like they were slipping him some other kind of medication that was making him sleep all the time. When Jake talked with Bill, he noted that the patient was very groggy and was unable to subtract one number from another. The next time I talked with Bill, three days later, we had just a short conversation because some aide was there to clean him up and if he asked for a delay because he was on the phone, it probably would never happen. His speech was greatly slurred and he said he was being "devastated" by the pills they were giving him. He had repeatedly asked for a list of his medications but they would not provided them for him. Bill said he would call back later but he never did, either because he forgot or because he was so far out of it that he couldn't. In describing the conversation to Jake, I commented, "Sounds to me like they are trying to murder him."

An article on US Attorneys.com proclaimed, "Overmedication as Restraint Plagues Nursing Home Residents." It stated that about 20% of nursing home residents are given anti-psychotic medications (like Abilify) and that close to 40% of those suffer from dementia. Since it is no longer legal to physically restrain patients except for extreme cases, understaffed nursing homes rely on chemical restraints to keep patients from talking or moving and from complaining about their inadequate care. For the convenience of the staff, patients might be left in a chemically induced stupor for days or remain asleep most of the time, not allowing them to engage with visitors or participate in activities, even though it violates their basic human rights and is psychologically devastating.

Use of anti-psychotic medication in dementia patients can increase risk of stroke which is why the FDA issued a Black Box Warning and stated there are no approved drugs for treating dementia-induced psychosis. The patients taking these drugs are also at increased risk of falls and of developing respiratory infections (like pneumonia), definitely not the kind of substance that should be foisted off on Bill, especially since he had a recent bout of pneumonia.

I found a site on *Pro Publica* that allows a person to obtain inspection reports on nursing homes all over the country. I downloaded the reports on FCC including the report that described the inspection that found Bill's bed to be 6 inches too short. I sent a copy to Jake, who responded, "I love the report that mentions that on 1/31/13 the SOCIAL WORKER (bird brain?) said that the patient never mentioned his bed problems during a care conference!!! Sounds like a good "save my ass" lie. When I worked at Honeywell as a production coordinator, when things would get screwed up, we used to write "SMA" memos and backdate them a day or two." I corrected his assumption that the social worker was Bird Brain and specified that it was actually the one from FCC There were a number of other "reports" that simply said "no data for this time period," i. e., FCC never sent anything in and the State Health Department never did an on-site inspection. So when I sent in my complaints about the place and the state sent for records, all they got was the lies the staff wrote in the records. Of course, if Bill had said they were putting lies in his chart, they could accuse him of being 'paranoid.' FCC was listed as having 38 deficiencies which is right up there with the worst nursing homes in the state.

On October 31st Minnesota came out with its Draft Olmstead Plan. Although they touted the action as something they came up with themselves, Minnesota actually had ignored the law until they were sued under the Olmstead Act, which was one of the complaints we included in our ADA Complaint. I sent copies of it to Susan Freiman and Janet Parker as well as to Jake. With the new Olmstead Plan, if Bill had had a decent lawyer to begin with or a decent judge, he never would have gone to the state hospital and ended up at FCC. Ms. Freiman, being an attorney, looked at it closely and thought it was a pretty good plan. She asked when Bill would be affected by it but I had to tell her that Bill would be unable to take advantage of it until he became mobile again, and FCC was doing nothing to make that possible.

Bill continued to be pretty much out of it for the first two thirds of November. His speech was slurred and he slept most of the time. He said the staff really had to work hard to wake him up. I told Bill he didn't sound like he was operating on all cylinders and was not mentally alert. He was quite aware of that and said he was operating on only four of eight cylinders.

I thought he was so out of it that he didn't have the energy to kick up a fuss (and that was probably the way the nursing home staff wanted it). He may also have found it a relief to be out of it rather than to clearly experience the shit pot he was in with no hope of ever getting out - just sleep until he dies. I know he didn't really want that but he may have been running out of steam and the drug stupor would make it hard for him to connect one idea with another.

He obtained a list of his medications but he was too anxious to share them with me. He was not in pain but described his felling state as "sloshy" and said his physical situation had gotten "tragic." He asked me,

"At what point do they write you off and don't bother to bring you back?" I had no response to his question but feared that that point may have already been passed months ago.

When Bill noticed that he hadn't seen the recording nurse and intermediary between patients and Dr. Spittel, for some time, he asked about him and was told that he was no longer an employee but was "on call" (although no one had seen him show up). Someone told Bill it was a way of easing him out of his position. I speculated that the nurse-recorder may not have lied enough to suit the management or maybe lied too much and got caught by the board of nursing. Governor Dayton came down hard on the board of nursing the other day after the investigative report came out in the *Star Tribune*, calling them "asleep at the switch." The board may be cracking down on obvious offenders to make a showing of "toughness."

On November 21st Dr. Spittel came to see Bill and asked him a number of questions. Then he said that he thought he might know what the problem with Bill's excessive sleeping might be and implied he thought it was one of his medications (duh, really?). Apparently, the offending medication was discontinued for when I talked with Bill a few days later he sounded pretty much like his usual self. He complained that the volunteer sent by the ombudslady talked about helping him but never did a thing in four different visits. "He was doing his social butterfly thing, trying to be a Masonic Lodge guy," Bill thought, whereas he wanted help to organize his papers which were scattered in piles all over the room.

He still had problems with his bed which he now attributed to a deformation in his upper spine. This gave the staff the opportunity to turn the tables on him and get in a dig: "So it is *your* fault that you have a problem with the bed!"

He said he woke up at 5:00 am and began working on how to solve his financial problems and felt that God had given him inspiration for selling some new products. He also had recovered some of his usual sense of humor, saying that sometimes you just have to laugh at the situation you find yourself in. He reported dreaming a lot about being able to walk again. In his dreams, he was "walking very carefully." He said he needed to start exercising in a pool and was studying nutritional approaches to weight loss.

On the 26th of November Bill complained that two staff members and the charge nurse "manhandled" him when trying to turn him on his side. He said they pushed his face into the side railings of the bed when trying to wash him up and hurt him so much that he was in agony when one of them got on top of him. He yelled and called them bitches, whereupon they left the room saying that if "you're calling us bitches, we're not helping you." He did not receive his shower the previous Saturday and had had a bowel movement in his bed since then. They had taken all his papers and bedside effects off his bed so that he could not reach them. His foot was pressed up against the footboard so he could not straighten it out. He said his heart was "racing" but he had been doing fine until the charge nurse came in and started "flapping her jaws."

Bill called the local police and reported the assault. I overheard the conversation with the officer over the phone. The officer had talked with the nurses prior to coming to the room and already had his mind made up that this was just another crank call. I explained to the officer that this kind of abuse was occurring all over the country and urged him to take Mr. Tollefson's complaints seriously, to ask him about his face being pushed into the side of the bed. The officer stated that he was not naïve about such matters of abuse but said he couldn't see any blood or bruises on the victim, so he was inclined to dismiss it. Bill expected this outcome but he knew that the officer would have to make a record of the incident, which could later be subpoenaed.

The next racing heart event occurred on December 2nd and Bill was rushed to District 1 Hospital in Faribault. He had an administrator call me, as his power of attorney, to let me know that he was there. Bird Brain had lied by claiming she was Bill's power of attorney and telling the nurse that I was not. Bill explained the matter to the nurse and she made the call to me.

Bill said that it felt like a mule had kicked him in the backside and that "it hurts like hell." He said that at one time in the past he had received an accidental double dose of heparin that had caused bleeding in his lower spine and he thought this might be something similar. Bill said that he was missing an eye appointment he had made and I volunteered to call and cancel it since he was in the hospital. When I did so, I was told that Bill did not have an appointment. Bill and I immediately supposed that Bird Brain had canceled the appointment.

Bill asked that I call Jake and Big Jim to let them know he was in the hospital. Whoever he saw at the hospital had given him a nebulizer and told him he thought that he might still have the pneumonia for which he had been treated at Mayo Clinic a short time ago. He said he was waiting for a surgical consult to look at his esophagus because he had vomited up blood the previous day. He made another desperate attempt to get support from the doctors to have him moved to the Northfield Retirement Center rather than return to FCC. However, it seemed to be the case that Bird

287

Brain had blocked that move. With a renewed resolve, Bill asked me to see if I could find the names of the lawyers he had talked with in Hastings because he definitely wanted to get rid of Bird Brain as his guardian.

On December 5th, Bill was returned to his cell at FCC. He said he had the worst ride of his life back on the medical transport vehicle. He had asked for a blanket to cover himself up in the cold Minnesota winter but they claimed they did not have one, didn't bother to get one from the hospital, and took off for FCC. When I talked with him that night he said he was still shivering from that ride. Just prior to this, Bill had a run-in with the charge nurse at District 1 Hospital and he threatened to throw a glass of water on her if she persisted in her haughty and rude behavior toward Bill. When she did not desist, Bill said he told her, "Here it comes" and claimed to have scored a direct hit.

When I talked with Bill the next day, he was having trouble breathing (shortness of breath, an indicator of possible heart problems). A nurse or aide could be heard over the phone urging him to get off the phone so she could wash him up because, she claimed, she would not have time to do it later. This threat was typical from the night-time staff and could be used to justify their avoidance of a task they didn't like. Rather than having him sit in his detritus all night I told Bill I would talk with him the next day.

On December 7th, three years to the day after Bill had been pulled out of his home, taken to Northfield Hospital where he offended a doctor because of his religious views, and was hauled off to St. Paul and then sent to the state hospital at Anoka. the events that started this whole ugly mess, Gary Tollefson called to tell me that Bill had died at FCC. Apparently, he was found unresponsive about 5:00 am. No mention was made of whether or not Bill's emergency light was on or how long it might have been on before he was discovered dead. Past experience, however, suggested that any requests for help were probably ignored because the staff would say they didn't have time to bother with it. The fact that Bill had just recently been in the hospital three times with symptoms of heart problems didn't seem to matter to FCC staff.

The last three years of pain and misery for Bill were a gigantic exercise in arrogant, incompetent and unethical practices of social service workers, doctors, lawyers, judges, and nursing home personnel and, I am afraid, those practices are not likely to end any time soon.

Even though I had been expecting this event for some time because of the way Bill was being treated (or not being treated), I was still shocked by it. My sigh was as if I were a giant helium-filled balloon that had suddenly been deflated. I was reminded of Milton's comment, "Torment, and loud lament, and furious rage" as the anger at all those people and institutions that had failed Bill – the jaded social service workers, his lackadaisical and unethical lawyers, the arrogant and clueless judges, the self-important and incompetent psychologist and psychiatrist, the sadistic guardians and nursing home workers, the useless state and federal government agencies and employees, even his own unsupportive family - all flooded over me along with a profound sadness because Bill never had a chance to live out the remainder of his life in the environment he so cherished – the out of doors - doing the thing he most enjoyed – fishing. There was some consolation in that he was out of his ongoing misery and frustration, but I didn't find that very convincing. Images of Charles Bronson in all of his revenge movies crossed my mind.

If they had wanted to push Bill into heart- attack territory, they could not have done a better job than they did by increasing his physical discomfort; frustrating his attempts to obtain dental, vision and pain treatment at every possible turn; boosting his hopes and then dashing them a few days later; hauling him off for a cockamamie "second opinion" that served only to increase stress; pouring him full of chemicals that made him manic for days on end and then switching to drugs that made him comatose; not helping him obtain treatment that was known to be beneficial to him; subjecting him to H-pylori, blood clots and pneumonia and not treating the diseases caused in an appropriate time frame; and, most importantly, treating him like a non-person whose ideas, wishes and feelings did not matter.

All of the documentation of what had happened, the chasing down of leads for possible lawyers, the writing of complaints to government agencies, the attempts to get help from any source possible, was for naught as far as Bill was concerned. I was able to boost Bill's spirits on occasion and give him some hope from time to time with what appeared to be "good news," but I regretted not having been able to really pull something out of the hat for my old friend. He deserved better.

17 A DEATH SENTENCE

Bill was guilty of being an ENFP with all of the virtues and vices associated with that psychological type. He was guilty of doing what ENFPs do when under stress. But he was not guilty of being schizophrenic or of manifesting any other kind of psychosis. He was not guilty of hallucinating or being delusional. He was not demented or suffering from organic brain dysfunction. He was not dangerous to himself or any other person. After seven months, only one person had the clarity of thought and strength of character to himself examine Bill and find out what all of us who knew him fairly well already knew.

How sliding down in a wheelchair turned into a death sentence three years later for a 70 year old man is an amazing chronicle of arrogance, incompetence and lack of professional ethics. Bill himself had foreseen the end result when he exclaimed to the judge that his commitment would be a death sentence if he did not get the kind of physical help, aquatic physiotherapy, that he needed - and he was right.

Bill played an inadvertent role in bringing about his own demise. He was out of sorts because of the circumstances he found himself in and he made home health care workers mad at him by being a cantankerous old man who rejected their puny efforts to be helpful. County budgets were such that what Bill really needed was not high on their priority list, so rather than acting diplomatically, he turned them away with rudeness and out of a sense of frustration with the system. This was one of the reasons he wanted to get out from under their control by going to Florida to try to rekindle his career as a fishing guide. After that "possibility" crashed and burned, and after he had an adverse reaction to his medications, he was even more intolerant of their futile efforts that he knew would never bring about the changes he needed.

Their corresponding frustration with the independent-minded old man in a wheelchair was such that they refused to have anything to do with him, not exactly a professional stance to take since they should have been trained to expect such reactions from elderly patients as part of their jobs, but their sense of outrage at being spurned is understandable. No doubt they talked among themselves about this "impossible" and verbally abusive patient who did not appreciate their ministrations. So when the opportunity arose for them to get him out of their hair once and for all, they jumped on it, concocting an "indictment" populated only by negative statements made by those who disliked him or statements by others that could be construed to justify calling him insane. No supportive statements were obtained from any of Mr. Tollefson's friends or even his relatives. It's the kind of thing any experienced social agency person knows how to do in order to dump a difficult patient into the laps of some other agency. They know that the patient has no support system that is going to push back and that the courts want to "process the case" as expeditiously and inexpensively as possible, so they will just go along with whatever the agent presents. Some county social service agencies even have their agents give the patient a bus ticket to another state to get them out of the way, justifying themselves by claiming that "it's not part of my job description" or they "don't have time to deal with that shit."

For people without money, county social service departments are the usual entry gate to the mental health gulag. (Folks with money usually have some relative with a lawyer trying to put them away so they can take their assets and use them for themselves). According to the Regional Ombudsman for Mental Health and Developmental Disabilities, Rice County is one of the worst in the 16 county region in terms of complaints about county social services over the last ten years, due largely to an overall lack of human resources. In addition, Rice County crisis mental health services are seriously lacking, and that is combined with a system that isn't friendly to clients that try to engage with it. The most frequent complaint is that a client who is already on assistance, despite having all his papers in order, is not renewed in time and loses his coverage, including medical coverage and medications. There were approximately 150 complaints of this type in the last year and a half. Initial requests for assistance are processed at a slower rate than called for by state guidelines. Clients are frustrated with case managers, especially in the mental health area who tell them that whatever they request is "not my job" whereas they should be helping them to get referred to resources that might be helpful. Case managers limit clients' choices by the options they present to them, and by being dictatorial as opposed to educational and presenting all possible options. Financial workers tell a client to fill out the paperwork on their own and don't provide any information regarding referrals, basically leaving clients to their own devices. Bill experienced all of these problems with Rice County Social Services. The fact that Jake and Bill both ran into other victims of rigid and domineering case workers from Rice County in their travels makes it even more likely that this was not just a fluke or one-time occurrence.

My experience suggests that wide-spread failure to live up to professional standards of ethical behavior when dealing with clients is a problem at the top levels of administration. Agency directors must provide oversight, supervision and in-service training as well as incentives to maintain ethical standards. If they don't, the staff serving under their direction will cut corners, at the client's expense, when they are stressed by a heavy work load. Of course the ability to provide those services that enhance employee skills is dependent upon securing the necessary financial resources, whether by writing grant proposals or by convincing voters to direct funds in their direction, both skills one might want to have in an agency director. And advocacy groups in the county must educate voters to take local government seriously, demand that funds be devoted to social services and act as watchdogs to ensure that the agencies are carrying out their mission.

Some social service positions in the county require only a bachelors level education and it is doubtful that that is sufficient to make the kinds of judgments they are required to make. For example, a vulnerable adult worker is required to make a fair and balanced assessment of the actual functioning of a client, not to run around gathering top-of-the-head comments about a client or searching for data that will support the results she already has in mind. Thus, it might be necessary to elevate the requirements for certain positions so that the occupant not only is familiar with certain psychological concepts but also is capable of rendering an objective judgment, uncontaminated by personal feelings. An even better approach would be having two independent evaluations by two adequately trained social workers who have no previous history with the client in cases of possible commitment.

It is also important, at this initial level, for there to actually be an emergency for a 72-hour hold to be used. And an "emergency" must have tangible evidence of an imminent danger (within the next couple of days), not just some vague feeling that something bad might happen sometime. The law requires this or else a standard legal commitment procedure must be followed. But all too often, for the sake of expediency, the client is rushed to an ill-informed and arrogant doctor who is only too willing to comply with a request from some social service worker with whom he is already acquainted. In Bill Tollefson's case, there was no emergency and the doctor violated the law by claiming that the client's non-compliance with medication use was evidence of his "delusional" status and his praying was taken as evidence of hallucinations. The police told Bill they were concerned about his legs but no treatment was provided either at Northfield Hospital or at United Hospital in St. Paul. Thus, the "emergency" was all a ruse to get around the law and "process" Bill straight-away so that he could be inducted into the mental health gulag and quickly placed on that pathway to oblivion. In order to halt this unethical practice, it is probably necessary to require that the person filling out the form also specify the concrete observational evidence he has to support it and to provide severe penalties to those who abuse the practice.

The next way-station on the route to the gulag is the court proceedings. In Bill's case this was a complete disaster. He was not allowed a second opinion by a doctor of his choosing nor a lawyer's presence when he was examined; he was not allowed to appeal; the standards of evidence were not adhered to; his lawyer did not question the allegations made against him; his lawyer did not object when he was called by the wrong name five times; his lawyer wouldn't help him get a waiver so he could get court records; his lawyers made no attempts to prepare him for his court appearance or even return his phone calls; he was not allowed to appear in court at a hearing that concerned him, and the list goes on. Laws were not followed, lawyers did not follow their code of ethics and judges appeared to be clueless about matters of mental health.

Attempts to obtain a competent lawyer to represent Bill pro bono were all in vain and state agencies and organizations who claimed to provide representation did not, in fact, do so. In addition, the procedures for Rice County were radically different from those of Hennepin County, i. e., there was no uniformity across the state in the manner in which state law was implemented. What this meant was that, in Rice County, Bill's fate was in the hands of one poorly paid court appointed lawyer rather than, if he had lived in Hennepin County, three reasonably compensated lawyers that had received specialized education in mental health. The Rice County Court did indeed seem to function as a rubber-stamp, kangaroo court with the judiciary arrogantly assuming they knew all the facts, knew all of the options and could choose what was best for the defendant and thought so little of people who found themselves in these circumstance that they thought they could skirt the law with no significant consequences. The fact that the county budget was overextended no doubt allowed the court to justify their decision to pervert justice. Apparently, such problems occur all over the country.

Ignorance of the law and of the nature of mental difficulties that exists in the court can, in theory, be corrected by selection and proper education. For voters to elect competent judges, they must know what knowledge and skills the job requires and how well the candidate's background prepares him for the tasks he will be asked to adjudicate. Unfortunately, most voters are unaware of the task demands of a judgeship or of those characteristics of the candidate that are relevant to those task demands, so local elections are largely a crap-shoot based on name recognition. Advocacy groups might take it upon themselves to educate the voters on such matters and quiz the candidates about how they view different aspects of the job they are seeking.

Both lawyers representing the county and lawyers representing the defendant in commitment hearings should be required to have specialized training in mental health law, as should the judges, and this training should be periodically updated. All training should involve instruction about the range of "normal" behavior and experience, not just "abnormal psychology." Some states, like California, have judges colleges that try to teach judges about differences in people and how to make better decisions using this knowledge. Attendance at periodic workshops on professional ethics for lawyers should be required as part of their licensure. The same should be required of sitting judges. All members of the court who observe a violation of professional ethics and are unable to correct it before it harms the defendant, should be required to report the offense to the state bar; if there is a failure to do so, the non-reporting person shall be considered a participant in the violation and be reported to the bar.

While the Court Visitor Program in Rice County did not provide observer-witnesses for commitment hearings, it seems only reasonable that such a program be extended to the probate court to have someone available to report on such violations of due process as occurred in Bill's case. If it is known that someone knowledgeable and with the authority to report inappropriate behavior is watching, participants have a heightened consciousness of what they are doing and are more likely to act professionally. It is like the "trust but verify" maxim in international relations.

At the legislative level there should be a clear designation of responsibility and a specified mechanism for reporting violations of a person's legal and civil rights that occurs in the court to someone at a higher level in the judicial system outside of that court.

Court records should not be a money-making venture for counties to balance their budgets on the backs of poor people, but can and should be made available to the defendant at minimal cost. With current means of recording, there is no need to have typists transcribe records the old fashioned way. Simply run off a CD, DVD, Flash Drive or copy a tape transcript for what it costs. If the user wants the whole or a part of the record transcribed, he can do it himself.

There also should be laws passed that make implementation of commitment laws uniform across the state. It is not fair that people living in one county receive a high quality evaluation and defense while those living in another county are subjected to unmotivated lawyers and cut-rate justice. If a county does not have the volume of cases to justify having three appropriately trained lawyers available for each case, the county can contract with another county for such resources. A regional court system with appropriately trained personnel would be another alternative.

***

Bill's sojourn in the state hospital was, for the most part, an illustration of the practice of *presumptive medicine*. On the ward, Dr. Quack could see no psychotic behavior on Bill's part. But he did not bother to do any further investigation to determine Bill's condition, presuming that what was written about him that he had received from the court must be accurate. After all, how does one end up in a mental hospital if he isn't crazy in some way? And he could not trust what I had written about Bill in my letter to the Attorney General either because I was simply an unknown who was advocating for a crazy friend. He didn't bother to check on my credentials and over 40 years of experience, although it would have been quite easy to do. Instead, he presumed Bill must be psychotic and he engaged in human experimentation, without benefit of oversight review, to see if his drug, Abilify, would have an effect on Bill. It did but the effects were all negative. It was not Dr. Quack, but his supervisor, who eventually stopped the drug.

Other members of the staff followed Dr. Quack's lead and presumed Bill was "in denial" of his addictions. They were functioning under the false belief that the way to break through that denial was to hammer the patient with accusations and interpretations using psychiatric jargon until he accepted responsibility for his excessive use of disliked substances, just like the police, in earlier eras, interrogated suspects under a glaring light bulb until they confessed their misdeeds. Bill never "cracked,"

296

which no doubt made them try even harder to crush his defenses so that he would be properly compliant, like breaking a horse for riding. The nurse harassed him like a mad fishwife when he did not get up in time, even though there was no clock in his room and his own alarm clock and watch had been stolen. She presumed that he could afford to go without breakfast because he was obese and was presumed (inaccurately) to be diabetic. One of the staff even threatened him with continual incarceration if he did not accept *their* delusional thinking and take his psychiatric drugs.

As was indicated previously, once you get cast as a crazy person and it is written down in your "jacket" or case record, people in hospitals treat you as if the words are real, in spite of what they see with their own eyes and hear with their own ears or from friends of the patient. In fact, the stain of madness must affect the friend as well, since he has not abandoned "the crazy one" as any sane person would do. The consulting psychiatrist for the first Golden Liver that Bill was in was convinced that Bill's complaints about his leg were bogus and that he was just having another crazy episode. When he was transferred to St. Joseph and they did indeed find that his leg needed treatment, they still believed what was in the record about his mental status and they did not bother to check out evidence to the contrary.

This mad cycle of self-fulfilling assumptions continued until *one* physician out of the many who saw him decided to find out for himself by direct observation and critical reading of reports (including court reports). Unfortunately, when he left the institution, the staff lapsed into its old customary presumptive practices. This anti-therapeutic hospital culture is common in public institutions where a poorly trained and poorly paid staff are required to process too many patients in too short a time period and the belief system is dominated by the "medical model" rather than a psycho-social one. The practice of presumptive medicine seemed to take place in all of the hospitals to which Bill was sent subsequently. An excellent book in which to read about doctors' thinking errors is *How Doctors Think* by Jerome Groopman.

In principle, it should be easy to change the kind of thinking prevalent in mental hospitals: just gather up all the staff and put them through an educational program to identify how their thinking distorts and restricts their understanding of patients, brings about unintended consequences and thwarts the objectives of their work. In practice it is not so easy because there are an array of special interests that do not desire change. Psychiatrists' claim to occupy the top rung of the status hierarchy in mental hospitals is dependent upon everyone believing that defects in biology are the keys to mental "illness" and that drugs or other operations on the body will fix the defects. They have the biology market cornered with their MD degree and prescription pads. But if that were to change, anyone might be able to occupy that top rung – psychologists, social workers, nurses, pastors, anyone who could be shown to have a knack for bringing about change in patients.

Drug companies have a vested interest in maintaining the status quo because psychiatrists are the intermediaries who push their products. The more patients are taking medications, the better is their business. Third party payers, while they might like to get rid of high-priced psychiatrists and expensive drugs, like to have rigid, clear-cut categories upon which their actuaries can calculate probabilities for rates of return on investment. Since they are already set up to handle existing categories, they don't want some period of upheaval where they won't know how they are going to come out financially.

What might bring about a change in hospital culture and practices is a change in public understanding and attitudes fueled by research showing that there is no biological deficit in most (but not all) mental conditions (other than those caused by drug treatment itself) and that other modes of treatment are as effective or more effective than drug treatment and without the adverse side-effects. Disclosures of drug companies fraudulent research, insidious marketing schemes and attempts to suppress disclosures also weakens their ability to deceive the public. Such information is being disbursed online and by various advocacy groups more and more in just the last few years. Petitions asking for investigations of institutions that support such research, often spurred by tragic incidents such as in the Dan Markingson case at the University of Minnesota, are more frequent too. Once the public starts to demand change, and it becomes politically popular to support it, it will probably come about.

Violations of patient rights occur as a matter of course in hospital and nursing home settings. While many states, including Minnesota, have legislation that specifies a *Patient Bill of Rights* or the *Rights of Wards and Protected Persons,* they are simply not enforced. Most people I contacted, including a state legislator, did not know who was responsible for this duty. My own complaints filed against the state hospital first found their way to some kind of Medicare watchdog agency, who could not take any action unless the violations were so severe as to require closure of the whole facility. (They referred me to the Joint Commission on Accreditation of Hospitals which took the information and confronted the hospital with it, but it is unknown if that had any effect on Bill's treatment, although they did stop the Abilify). But there is no reason that a violation cannot be investigated without being so severe that the whole institution must be shut down. And "let's pretend" investigations (like sending for patient records) just don't cut it. Why not supply the state health department with enough personnel that all complaints can be thoroughly evaluated for each institution? The cost would probably be less than the settlement for one lost civil rights trial.

An article in the *Minneapolis Star Tribune* for March 3, 2014 by Cris Serres proclaims, "Public care for the mentally ill in Minnesota is deeply flawed, with patients cycling in and out of county jails and hospital ERs because of a severe shortage of psychiatric beds and community treatment, according to a stark new review by the state agency in charge of those services." The Department of Human Services found that Anoka Metro-Regional Treatment Center, where Bill was sent, retains up to 40 percent of its patients only because they have nowhere else to go and that those patients therefore receive $13,800,000 of unnecessary "treatment." This bottleneck prevents other patients sitting in emergency rooms from gaining admittance, which Anoka claims is because they receive "resistance from group homes or other facilities that may be reluctant to accept a psychologically complex patient," because of community fears associated with the stigma still attached to mental illness, and because patients are not getting adequate follow-up treatment in their communities.

While the Office of the Ombudsman for Mental Health and Mental Retardation doesn't seem capable of providing any help to individual patients, they are able to jawbone the rest of state government about mental health matters They have known since at least 2003 that Minnesota's mental health system is dysfunctional. In a document titled "Mental Health - A System in Crisis" (available on their website http://mn.gov/omhdd/images/system-in-crisis-report.pdf) they stated, "What we have is a revolving door system that provides crisis treatment and stabilization and very little service or huge gaps in services in-between crisis periods. ...a system beginning to fall apart and in desperate need of fundamental reform." They see the problem as due to both increased demands and a shortage of services and they think many current laws are not enforced and some need to be changed or removed. "The current maze of services often defies common sense."

The major cause of bottlenecks in the system start at the local hospital level. There are a lack of available beds for patients who are in a significant crisis due to local hospitals having closed down their mental health units (if they ever had them) because reimbursement rates are insufficient. These rates are driven by Medicaid rates which are set by the Legislature at the lowest possible level. So these hospitals transfer patients hundreds of miles away from home where there is no family or community support available. There is also an abuse of Hold Orders (e. g., 72-hour holds) in order to get law enforcement to provide transportation of patients and a misuse of the commitment act in order to guarantee payment (because court ordered treatment meets the criteria for being "medically necessary"). On the other hand, some patients may wait until they deteriorate to the level where civil commitment is seen as necessary by concerned relatives and then the experience is likely to be so abusive that they will not seek help in the future. Nursing shortages may also force closure of a unit if staffing is not adequate because of how their contracts are written. While the patient is in the local hospital, there is a delay in initiating treatment because he or she is expected to be transferred to a different facility and treatment professional where the whole process starts from square one again;

At the state hospital level there is a backlog of patients ready to discharge to the community because some providers fear lawsuits and liability issues if they release patients too quickly and they end up harming themselves or others. There is also an unavailability of transitional or permanent housing and needed community services which, in turn, causes expensive hospital beds to be filled with patients who are provided services they don't need. This is due to the failure of county and state agencies to develop adequate resources and services for the number of persons who require them (as specified in the *State Mental Health Act*). Counties do not provide sufficient numbers of case managers to deal with the demand for their services, so neither state nor county hold them accountable to the requirements of the state's case management rules. No agency monitors the case plans and no one steps in when there is a failure to provide for the services specified in the plan or to include some important element in it.

There is also an over reliance on medication and what is referred to as the "Medical/Insurance Model" for expedient solutions rather than providing effective long term social support and rehabilitation. And mental health providers may use data privacy laws (HIPAA) in order to avoid dealing with families, friends, community providers and primary care physicians "in ways that defy common sense, are not helpful to the client and are not even consistent with intent of the law." Many physicians are never trained how to interface with these "outsiders" so as to use their knowledge and skills to contribute to a patient's care. They feel safe and secure only within their well defined domain of hospital or office.

Most of the fixes the Ombudsman proposes involve expanding resources in some way. Make it feasible for local hospitals to have mental health units by increasing reimbursement rates to reflect the actual cost of care. Start a capital improvement grant fund for local hospitals all over the state but especially in smaller communities, to increase number of beds for persons with mental disorders. Develop housing options ranging from total independent living to assisted living using incentives or tax credits to landlords and developers who will actively recruit mentally ill residents. Develop post discharge housing with staff available on the site. Encourage primary care clinics to include mental health services using psychologists and consulting psychiatrists as providers. Develop short stay crisis intervention facilities for stabilization, assessment, and treatment plan development that divert people away from high cost hospital emergency rooms. Locate State Operated Services (beds and intensive quality services) in smaller community settings, near to the client's home where he or she can receive social and community support, rather than having to travel to a distant institutional setting far from friends and families. Provide an incentive for private providers of psychosocial rehabilitation to get involved by increasing reimbursement rates and allow State Operated Services to provide such services where the private sector provider is not available. Use federal funds from the President's New Freedom Initiative to help develop community based options to increase client independence. Prevent the loss of housing while persons are hospitalized by adequately funding programs to address such needs. Expand and fund Community Mental Health Centers to help the mentally ill stay out of hospitals, which was their original intention. Allow more flexibility in funding so case managers need not fit patients into existing programs but are able to do what is appropriate for the particular client.

Some proposals sought to use cheaper mental health providers. For example, Psychiatric Clinical Nurse Specialists (CNS) and Advance Practice Nurses (APN) could be used for medication management, follow-up care and "physician extenders" who allow more patients to be seen by a psychiatrist by relieving him of some minor duties. These providers could be enlisted into the manpower pool more rapidly because of less extensive training and financial incentives could be provided to get nurses to pursue such certification. However, you tend to get what you pay for and having more hands rather than more skilled and inventive practitioners might be yet only one more short-term solution.

One significant proposal would involve redesigning the court system for patients with mental problems: "Establish Regional Mental Health Courts with common understandings, standards, forms and consistent time lines so that all parties will be operating with clear knowledge of expectations, standards and time lines. Have costs associated with the civil commitment process handled by this court. This should improve efficiency and shorten delays in access to treatment which will also be most cost effective."

While the ombudsman's focus is on consistency and efficiency, if properly designed, a regional court might also prevent the use of unmotivated and untrained contract lawyers, uninformed or biased judges, and prevent abuses of due process and civil rights while forcing compliance with federal law such as the *Americans with Disabilities Act* and the *Olmstead Act* so that patients are directed to the least restrictive and most helpful living situation consistent with their level of physical and mental functioning.

The ombudsman would also like to see a state wide program where learning could be encouraged and shared among counties. He suggests that counties that are "doing good things" be rewarded and mechanisms be established to share their successes with other counties. I would imagine this to involve some meetings of workers in different counties and workshops to be put on by those counties that are meeting with significant success.

***

Boomers Against Elder Abuse is a Facebook page that tries to increase public awareness of the widespread abuse of senior citizens, primarily through the mechanism of guardianships. It lists nearly 200 cases of guardians abusing their wards and making off with their savings and resources. Because Bill was financially impoverished, the problems with his guardian were not the same kind as those frequently encountered by well-off individuals who have guardians that bilk their estates of all assets while neglecting their clients. For information on those kinds of abuses, see the article by Angela V. Woodhull, PhD entitled "How Fradulent Guardianship/Conservatorship Commences and Continues" (http://www.ejfi.org/Courts/Courts-33.htm). Instead, the problems Bill ran into fall mainly into the realm of violations of *legal* standards for guardianships in the state of Minnesota as specified in *CONSERVATORSHIP AND GUARDIANSHIP IN MINNESOTA*, published by the Minnesota Conference of Chief Judges (Pending, 2003 Amended 2009, 2010). These standards define the law and specify quite clearly what actions are expected of a guardian with respect to a client. The ways in which Bill's guardian failed to live up to these standards are many and some examples will be presented here (sections in italics are quoted from the manual).

There must be cause, or reason, to believe that the person is incapacitated. It is not sufficient to proceed just because a person has a diagnosis which may indicate incapacity. There must be evidence which supports this belief, such as behavior which demonstrates incapacity, and there must be no other less restrictive alternatives available to meet the needs of the person. It must be kept in mind that the individual has the potential and the right to contest any guardianship or conservatorship proceedings.

There was no objective evidence that Bill suffered from any mental incapacity. He was discharged from Anoka Metro Regional Treatment Center and his commitment was rescinded because he did not meet the criteria for being there. The claimed psychiatric maladies used to justify the guardianship were not substantiated and were refuted by Dr. Smart when he discharged Bill and his commitment was rescinded. The stated justification for this guardianship was not updated to reflect Dr. Smart's actions.

There was no evidence of psychosis, hallucinations, delusions or paranoia. There was no evidence to indicate that Bill was ever a danger to himself or others. Bill's inhumane treatment for the three years is sufficient to account for any psychological problems that may have been manifested. There was no evidence that Bill suffered from organic brain dysfunction any more than other persons his age and there may, in fact, be evidence to the contrary that has been suppressed.

There were many other less restrictive alternatives to Bill's placement when he was first discharged from the hospital (or for that matter, when he was initially committed). Bird Brain did not adequately pursue these other alternatives and instead placed him in facilities that could not possibly meet his needs and, in fact, made him worse physically and psychologically.

Bill was denied the right to protest any of his guardianship proceedings and Bird Brain even prevented him from attending a hearing involving his case, presumably on the grounds that there was no money for transportation. In fact, Bill was residing in the same small town where the hearing was held and transportation costs would have been minimal. It is more than likely that she was trying to prevent Bill from contesting whatever she said in court.

The manual states that *the court can grant the guardian or the conservator limited power to exercise authority over the ward or protected person. The guardian or conservator must use this authority*

303

only as is necessary to provide needed care and services. It cannot be used in a manner which limits the ward or protected person's civil rights and restricts his or her personal freedoms. This is to make sure that the decision of a guardian or conservator will not be overly protective or restrictive of the person's rights. Yet Bill's guardian instructed the staff at both Golden Liver and FCC to restrict his liberty, personal freedom and movements without proper authority to do so. She prevented Bill from attending a legal hearing on his case and prevented him from attending medical appointments on at least four different occasions.

Under the heading "ON-GOING RESPONSIBILITIES OF GUARDIANS & CONSERVATORS" the manual states that it is the guardian's job *To maintain a current understanding of the needs of the ward or protected person. This includes maintaining current knowledge of the ward's or protected person's diagnosis, prognosis, treatments, care plan and needs through regular and frequent visits with the ward or protected person as well as frequent contacts with care providers.* But Bird Brain was never able to establish a working relationship with Bill, avoided seeing him and sent the husband of her partner to visit instead. This visitor never announced his position or his function to Bill and at one time he told the client that he was there to "see if you have been a good boy." Such degrading and dehumanizing comments can be considered psychological abuse. Bill did not believe that his guardian had an understanding of his needs or even that she placed any value on them. He did not trust her to act with his best interests in mind and suspected she had deliberately acted to thwart his best interests.

While the manual states, *Respect for the rights maintained by the ward or protected person must remain a primary concern of the guardian or conservator in all matters and in all decisions. The guardian or conservator must exercise his or her powers in a way which allows the ward or protected person as much independence as possible,* Bill's guardian callously disregarded his legal and civil rights and acted to restrict his independence in nearly all decisions she made.

The manual states that, *Upon appointment the guardian or conservator assumes the role of advocate," where an advocate is defined as "a person who speaks in favor of something, someone who makes recommendations. An advocate argues for a cause, defends beliefs, or supports a position. An advocate does these things on behalf of another person.* And further, *In order to fulfill his or her duties the guardian or conservator must become familiar with the ward's or protected person's needs, beliefs and preferences. The guardian or conservator must then make a choice that reflects those beliefs, needs, and preferences. To do this, the guardian or conservator must become informed about what services the ward or protected person is entitled to and which services will meet his or her needs.* But Bird Brain did not advocate on Bill's behalf in any way nor did she respect his needs, beliefs and preferences in any of her choices. She did not advocate with respect to the adequacy of his nursing home or medical care when it was (and had been known to be) inadequate. And she did not act to protect Bill's civil and legal rights, specifically the rights granted under MN 144.651 *Health Care Bill of Rights* and MN 524.5-120 Bill of *Rights for Wards and Protected Persons.*

Before making a decision to change a person's residence the guardian must consider: Are the living arrangements appropriate and the least restrictive? Bill's accommodations at Golden Liver were not suitable for any human being. His "space" was an area not much larger than his bed, separated from his roommate by a curtain. His roommate was given to urinating on the floor and intruding on Mr. Tollefson, looming over his bed in a threatening manner at night. Bill was not allowed to make excursions into the community like other residents. He was not provided with a list of his medications. His nurse practitioner would not show up for appointments. When he had emergency medical issues, they were ignored and he had to make his own arrangements for hospitalization. Needed support services, like bathing and laundry, were usually delayed and only grudgingly available. Clothing was "lost" when sent to the laundry.

At FCC, Bill's condition was allowed to deteriorate so that he went from being able to transfer and get around in his wheelchair to being bedridden. He was forced to sleep on a too short bed for one year, until a state nursing home inspector required that they change it. He was not showered for weeks at a time until intervention by the Ombudsman for Older Minnesotans and then they soon lapsed into their old behavior. When he did finally begin to get showers, he could not wash his hair because of loss of range of motion in his shoulders. The staff would not help him shampoo his head because they were "too busy." He was not provided with a proper sized commode for toileting and the sling for lifting him into place was not appropriate for toileting needs. When he did get a shower, the sling for the Hoyer lift would get wet and then could not be used until it had dried. They did not have a spare sling and did not seek to obtain one. He was surreptitiously administered psychotropic medication that was known to interact adversely with one of his other medications, increasing the likelihood of a seizure. He was often denied transfer to his chair because, he was told, they did not have enough staff. There were no provisions for the ward's social and recreational needs and the only entertainment provided was a TV set.

No plans were being developed by the guardian or his care-givers that would help Bill become able to move to a less restrictive setting. FCC disposed of his wheelchair without asking his consent and without even informing him they had done so. Instead, they gave him a variety of excuses, e. g., that it was in storage in the nursing home, that it had been sent to the place where his other belongings were stored, etc. Bird Brain and her delegates ignored Mr. Tollefson's inquiries regarding his wheelchair. His dentures (valued at $3000) were lost when in the custody of Bird Brain. Her partner's husband told Bill they were put in storage with his other belongings but he would not retrieve them so that Bill could properly chew his food. Later he told Bill that he had brought them with other property from Golden Liver and placed them in his closet. The dentures were not there.

Bird Brain's choices of residences for Bill were inappropriate and were not the least restrictive environments in which he could live at the time of his placement. None of the placements had facilities for aquatic physiotherapy, which was advocated by his discharge psychiatrist at Anoka Metro Regional Treatment Center. The living arrangements made for Bill were not at all like those of his previous lifestyle nor were any attempts made to provide living arrangements that afforded him the minimum amount of independence and self-determination. In fact, the guardian was operating with the bizarre belief that Bill could not live anywhere that did not keep residents in locked confinement.

The manual states, *The guardian promotes the care, comfort, and maintenance of the ward. The ward's attitude towards his or her current situation is known. The guardian is aware of what was the ward's basic, original physical appearance, and psychological and emotional state.* In fact, there was no evidence to indicate that the guardian had done anything to promote the care, comfort and maintenance of Mr. Tollefson other than to place him in inappropriate, understaffed, inadequately functioning nursing homes. She made no attempt to determine Bills basic, original physical appearance, and psychological and emotional state. She actively avoided contact with individuals who had known Bill for over half a century to obtain their perspectives. She was more than indifferent to Bill; she disliked him and did not want to spend any time or effort on his behalf.

When making decisions the guardian or conservator must: take actions and make decisions that encourage and allow the maximum level of independent, or self-reliant, functioning on the part of the ward or protected person, safeguard the decision-making powers of the ward or protected person so that they are not restricted beyond a clearly established need, and make decisions only to the extent necessary to provide needed care and services for the ward or protected person. But Bird Brain did not encourage the maximum level of independent or self-reliant functioning on the part of Bill; in fact, she treated him as if he were totally incompetent in all spheres of his life. She acted more like a jailer than an advocate. At Golden Liver, Bird Brain instructed care-givers to restrict Bill's movements to the grounds, did not allow him to go on shopping trips with other residents, and allowed him no discretion in decision-making. There was no demonstrated need for such restrictions. So too, at FCC Bird Brain restricted Bill's liberty, his ability to participate in his medical care, his ability to visit friends, and his ability to obtain information so he could make an informed decision regarding health insurance coverage. Mr. Tollefson was not allowed a genuine choice regarding any of his nursing home placements.

The guardian is supposed to *get to know the ward or protected person, understand any needs or problems the ward or protected person may have, and be able to ask questions and seek opinions about alternative ways to meet the needs of the ward or protected person.* In contrast, Bird Brain did not bother to get to know Bill to any degree. She was unaware of any of his talents, desires, values, problems or long-term history. She avoided any face-to-face contact with Bill as much as possible and avoided contact with any of his long-term friends. She did not ask questions of him or attempt to enlist his cooperation but only made pronouncements as to what he "must do."

The guardian or conservator is bound by law to: consider the ward's or protected person's reasonable wishes, find the support services that will provide the care that the person requires, and weigh and balance all of the potential benefits or risks to the person. Mr. Tollefson had a reasonable wish, frequently stated to Bird Brain, to go through and sort his property, which she did not allow. He had a reasonable wish to live in his home town but it was not granted. He had needed aquatic physiotherapy to increase his level of physical functioning but it was consistently denied with a resultant deterioration in his level of functioning. Bill had reasonable wishes to be referred to medical specialists for specific medical problems which were denied by his guardian. By placing Bill in inadequately staffed and equipped nursing homes, the guardian exposed him to risks of infection, deterioration in functioning, psychological abuse, and finally death.

Ethical substitute decision making assures: that the ward or protected person is involved and included in community settings and activities whenever reasonably possible; that reasonable efforts have been made to obtain the opinions of the relatives and other involved persons....Substituted judgment means the guardian or conservator makes decisions for the ward or protected person based on how the ward or protected person would have decided if not incapacitated. This standard assumes competence of the ward or protected person prior to incapacity when the ward or protected person would have been able to express an informed choice. This requires that the guardian or conservator knew the person, or is able to find out this information by interviewing people who did know the ward or protected person, before the ward or protected person became incapacitated. But, in fact, Bill was not involved or included in community settings and activities at any of the facilities at which he was placed. Bird Brain made no attempt to facilitate such involvement. Bill's friends of a half century or more and sympathetic relatives were not contacted to obtain their opinions. Therefore, Bird Brain operated with no information about how Bill would have decided if not incapacitated.

Least restrictive alternative means that the guardian or conservator must choose alternatives that are the least likely to interrupt, bother, or interfere with the desires, lifestyle, or preferences of the ward or protected person, and are the most likely alternatives other people in the community would choose if they didn't need a substitute decision-maker, given the level of supervision and protection required for the ward or protected person. Allowing least restrictive alternatives requires: The level of supervision and protection must allow "risk-taking" to the degree that there is no reasonable likelihood that serious harm will happen to the ward or protected person or to others.

The guardian or conservator must participate in planning on behalf of the ward or protected person. The guardian or conservator must consider what services are available under state and federal law. The guardian or conservator must plan for the individual needs of the ward or protected person and assist and represent the ward or protected person. It is the guardian's and conservator's responsibility to determine that services for the ward or protected person are being provided in the least restrictive manner.

As indicated previously, Bird Brain had acted more like a prison guard or jailer than a guardian as described in the present rules. Bill was allowed virtually no freedom while in Golden Liver and his usual life style was totally disrupted. His desires and preferences were ignored and the facility, at the command of Bird Brain, took "no risk" by totally restricting Bill's movements. Bird Brain did not provide for the individual needs of Mr. Tollefson which included the need for aquatic physiotherapy, the need for dental care, the need for vision care, the need for pain management, the need for services of a podiatrist and others. Although Bill was capable of and accustomed to making his own medical appointments, he was denied such self-esteem building participation under the guidance of his guardian.

Informed consent requires that the person giving consent: has the knowledge available to make a reasonable decision; has the capacity or ability to make reasoned decisions based upon information that applies to the situation; and is giving consent voluntarily and without coercion, that is, there is no intimidation or pressure, either obvious or suggested from another person. Although Bill had the knowledge and ability to make reasoned decisions based on information that applied to the situation, he was denied the opportunity to participate in decision making by his guardian. He was intimidated, pressured and humiliated just because he wanted to exercise his own judgment or participate in joint decision-making. In November and December of 2012, Bird Brain would not provide information regarding health insurance options to Mr. Tollefson so that he might study them and help choose the best alternative based on his past experience and what he projected he might need in the future. He had ended up with a less desirable insurance plan two years previously when someone else had made the decision without his input.

Whatever the need may be, the guardian or conservator must always consider the ward's or protected person's wishes. A ward or protected person always has certain rights that must be protected by the guardian or conservator when making decisions. A guardian or conservator may not make decisions that restrict these rights. Bird Brain consistently ignored Bill's rights in all decision-making. If his voice was ever heard at all, it was subsequently ignored.

RIGHTS OF WARDS AND PROTECTED PERSONS: A guardian or conservator has the responsibility to ensure that these rights are not violated. These rights must be reviewed and explained to the ward or protected person in a manner which he or she can best understand. These rights were never explained to Bill by Bird Brain, if she even knew what they were. The specific rights given away by the court were never revealed to Bill by Bird Brain (or by his lawyer or the court, for that matter).

The right to be treated with dignity and respect. Bird Brain did not treat Bill as a person worthy of even minimal esteem or honor. She ignored his phone calls, disregarded his requests and did not deem him worthy of any explanations of her role or her actions.

The right to protection from harm. Bill had been harmed physically by his inadequate medical care and improper placement in inadequate nursing homes while Bird Brain made no effort to ameliorate those harms. Even basic forms of decency were denied such as the need for cleanliness.

The right to receive health care and medical treatment. Bill was denied health care appropriate to his needs. He was refused aquatic physiotherapy, treatment of visual problems (including pressure in the eye), treatment of foot problems and toenail care (his toenails had been cut only once since he arrived), dental care (and they lost his dentures), and treatment for pain.

The right to have personal desires, preferences and opinions given due consideration in decisions made. As indicated many times Bill's desires, preferences and opinion were consistently ignored by Bird Brain in all decisions regarding him.

The right to legal representation. Bill knew he had the right to legal representation and was provided a court-appointed attorney. However, his attorney was no more responsible nor ethical than his guardian. He, too, did not respond to Bill's phone calls, ignored his requests or that of his power of attorney and violated Bill's legal rights. Bird Brain did nothing to assist Bill in getting proper legal representation, as an advocate would do.

A ward is entitled to certain basic protections and rights according to Minnesota Statutes sections 524.5-120:

The right to due consideration of current and previously stated personal desires, medical treatment preferences, religious beliefs, and other preferences and opinions in decisions made by the guardian or conservator;

The right to treatment with dignity and respect;

The right to receive timely and appropriate health care and medical treatment that does not violate known conscientious, religious, or moral beliefs of the ward or protected person;

The right to petition the court to prevent or initiate a change in abode;

The right to care, comfort, social and recreational needs, training, education, habilitation, and rehabilitation care and services, within available resources;

The right to personal privacy;"

The right to petition the court for termination or modification of the guardianship or conservatorship or for other appropriate relief;"

The right to be represented by an attorney in any proceeding or for the purpose of petitioning the court"

Bill's guardian did not advocate to ensure any of these rights for her client and it was clearly her legal responsibility to do so. It was also the Rice County Court's responsibility to oversee her adherence to state law, both with respect to CONSERVATORSHIP AND GUARDIANSHIP IN MINNESOTA and Minnesota Statutes sections 524.5-120, but they did not do so.

Clearly, there needs to be another level of oversight to ensure that both guardian and court do their jobs appropriately. One model is that used by Maricopa County, Arizona in the "Guardian Review Program," which apparently arose because of cut-backs in court personnel. Volunteers act as Court Visitors to help monitor guardianship services in order to ensure quality care and compliance with statutes and court orders. They try to educate guardians about their responsibilities and to educate the public about problems faced by incapacitated persons and the guardianship system. It is not known how well this works, how much training the visitors receive and how much authority they have in bringing about an investigation in particular cases. But, assuming Court Visitors are trained in the laws regarding guardianships and are given the authority to intervene or get someone else to intervene, as well as to educate, the program may have some potential in reducing the kinds of abuse that occurred in Bill's case.

One of the problems is that the ward's voice is not given credibility by either the guardian or the court. Thus, if he or she does not have an ethically-minded and motivated attorney to fight for his rights or relatives that are willing to speak up on his behalf, he has no chance to halt victimization through guardianship abuse. As we saw in Bill's case, his attorney was discharged by the court shortly after a guardian was appointed and he felt no obligation to act on his former client's behalf. A corrective to this might be to have attorneys kept on retainer to represent the client as needed, rather than only after an obstructive, time delaying request for representation is made. The client should be able to just call up his attorney and voice his complaints about his guardian and the attorney should be able to bring the matter to the court for action. Of course this leaves the cost factor open-ended and allows for the client to misuse the system by making inauthentic requests, but some mechanism to control that could probably be devised.

***

The major portion of this book has been concerned with nursing home

311

care of poor persons with disabilities, usually paid for by Medicare and Medicaid for a total of $26 billion per year. That quality of care is a major problem in these nursing facilities is evident from a report from the Department of Health and Human Services, Office of the Inspector General in February of 2014 entitled "Adverse Events in Skilled Nursing Facilities: National Incidence Among Medicare Beneficiaries." The study found that fully *one third* of patients in skilled nursing facilities suffered a medication error, infection or some other kind of injury (e. g., bleeding due to use of blood thinners, blood clots, fluid imbalances and delays to provide care, all of which happened to Bill) during their treatment. Half of these patients had to be readmitted to the hospital, 22 percent of the patients suffered lasting harm and 1.5% died for a cost to Medicare of $208 million during the one month period that the data covered. This extrapolates into an estimated 1538 deaths and 21,777 harmed patients for the population *for one month alone.* Fifty nine percent of the injuries were considered preventable.

All three institutions that Bill was confined to were parts of large for-profit corporations. All of the nursing homes in which Bill was a resident were rated as below average by Medicare. Bill was not in the GLC in St. Paul long enough to really see for himself how bad it was – he was ejected and not allowed to return because he complained that he needed medical treatment for his leg (which he did). I have mentioned how I thought these facilities violated Bill's civil and patient rights but the plain old quality of nursing was poor as well. Looking at the Medicare/Medicaid investigative reports for these facilities gives one an idea of why they got the ratings they did.

Reading the Medicare / Medicaid report on Golden Living Center, St. Louis Park for August 10, 2012, while Bill was a resident, I learned who the four mysterious "suits" were who were visiting with Bill just as he was getting ready for a medical appointment and had to leave before they could finish the interview. They were nursing home inspectors on a routine visit to the facility. The way they seemed to work was to "sample" a certain number of rooms and functions and extrapolate from that how pervasive were the facility's deficiencies.

Their report indicated that GLC St. Louis Park was deficient in housekeeping, maintenance and numerous functions related to running a safe and sanitary facility. They were cited for failure to "ensure resident rooms were kept free of pervading urine odors; the floors, walls, equipment, furniture, and fixtures in resident rooms and toilet rooms were kept clean and in good repair, the resident toilet room faucets and toilet safety frames were kept clean and in good repair in 6 of the 7 facility units."

Strong urine odors were found in the rooms and hallways, stains on wallpaper, peeling remnants of nonskid strips and stains on the floor from the adhesive, creating a surface which couldn't be cleaned adequately. Some toilet safety frames had lime buildup on their metal components. Some sink faucets were loose, leaked continuously and had a buildup of lime on the mouth; some had the chrome worn off the handles. Some toilets ran continuously and floors were sticky. At least one call light did not function. Holes in the walls were found, some patched with unpainted drywall which created a porous and impossible to clean surface and at least one door had a large hole gouged into it. Door frames and walls had heavily peeling and bubbling paint. Floor tiles were loose, missing and chipped, exposing blackish flooring and adhesive, creating an uncleanable surface. (It will be remembered that Bill sustained a cut in his foot from a broken tile in a shower). A scooter had not been cleaned for at least three months and was covered with dust, food splatters and crumbs. A vinyl safety mat on the floor next to a bed was heavily cracked, worn and tattered, which exposed the internal foam and created an uncleanable surface. The door knob was missing from a shared toilet room door and a piece of blue colored tape covered the hole from the other side. Floors had heavy grayish brown colored wax buildup on the edges around the room. Five wheelchairs were stored in a resident's room, creating excessive clutter, but the staff present on the tour did not know why they were stored there. A toilet base seal had a brownish colored stain completely encircling the toilet base and was sealed with uncleanable loose and peeling caulk. The back of the safety frame was soiled with a pinkish colored buildup of debris, similar to mildew and the right plastic handle of the safety frame was cracked. The toilet room had a strong urine smell and the floor was sticky. Dressers had broken drawers and worn away veneers on the top. A wheelchair foot pedal was stored on the floor of a room and heavily soiled with a food like residue, scuffed and uncleanable. A commode, belonging to another resident, was stored behind the door to a room and both side handles were wrapped in a stained heavy coating of white cloth tape, creating an uncleanable surface.

During the tour, staff confirmed the above findings were not new and the maintenance director confirmed that they did not have documentation of any repair requests for the items mentioned above. Review of the facility's undated Master Wheelchair Cleaning Program showed that every wheelchair was supposed to be cleaned monthly during the deep cleaning of that particular resident's room and once a quarter cleaned by deep scrubbing or with a pressure washer. Apparently, from observations of wheelchairs, that policy was not followed. Although the written procedures directed how to clean the resident rooms and toilet rooms, it failed to specify items potentially needing repair or potential problems to be aware of and how to report them. The facility lacked a policy on the frequency of mechanical lift cleaning and lacked a procedure to ensure the mechanical lifts were cleaned between resident use.

The facility was cited for not revising and updating patient care plans to reflect changes in mobility and transfer status or risk for accidental injury. In addition, the facility failed to ensure resident rooms and toilet rooms were free of potential accident hazards such as splintered doors and a loose toilet safety frame (a device used for residents to sit on to use the toilet, providing arms to allow the resident to push up to stand/transfer and stabilize while using the toilet). The seat was unsecured and the arms wobbled approximately six inches to either side, creating an unsteady platform to sit on, to transfer to and from; creating a fall risk.

The facility "failed to ensure food temperatures were consistently checked at the points of service, foods being served to residents were held at required temperatures to prevent the spread of potential food borne illness; resident beverages stored in a refrigerator on the 2 South unit were dated after opening and not expired; the facility kitchen equipment and floors were not kept clean and free of soil, and scoops used for flour and ice were not stored in a manner to prevent the spread of potential food borne illnesses; in addition, the facility failed to ensure foods were not touched after handling of dietary tickets with gloved hands in 2 of 7 resident dining rooms (1 North unit and 2 South unit). These practices had the potential to affect 188 of 193 residents who resided in the facility."

The chemical store room had a large uncovered wheeled garbage cart full of bagged garbage. The floor of the chemical store room was heavily soiled with a sticky, dark black colored liquid and food debris and had multiple foot prints and wheel marks from the garbage cart. The room had a strong garbage odor and a soft, white bread-like substance was present on the clean side of the dish machine where the clean dishes slide out and are stored. A soup bowl had a noodle dried on the outside. The outside of the dish machine was heavily soiled. A staff member said a chemical leak had occurred and the dish machine needed to be cleaned. Flying insects were observed throughout the kitchen as well as mouse traps in the bread storage room.

GLC St. Louis Park was cited for failure to ensure that multi-use blood glucose meters and the community electric razor were sanitized between resident uses to minimize the risk of transmitting potential blood borne or skin borne infections. The facility also failed to ensure toilet plungers were stored in a manner which promoted infection control and minimized exposure to bodily wastes in 2 of 3 shared resident toilet rooms that had uncovered toilet plungers stored next to the toilet. A nurse manager stated the nurses aide staff would need to be re-educated on the proper policy/procedure for cleaning the community razor and stated they were looking for instructions on the use of hand sanitizers and wipes.

The reader may recall that Bill and other residents received a letter from GLC suggesting that the rodent problem was all a result of their doing and required that they be moved from their rooms while they were fumigated. While acknowledging that residents needed to be educated about methods of food storage and the effects of excess clutter, the inspectors cited the facility for failure "to ensure resident rooms, common areas and the kitchen were free from rodents (mice) and flying insects (which included fruit flies). Although the facility had employed a pest control and extermination company since 6/15/12, the facility failed to take internal measures recommended by the pest control company; such as securing external doors to prevent mice from entering the facility, securing loose/stored food items in resident rooms, addressing missing and cracked tiles in resident rooms/facility basement area, and reducing clutter in residents rooms to reduce an infestation of mice and flying insects throughout the facility. This had the potential to affect all of the 193 residents residing in the facility."

While some nurses claimed they had received no complaints about mice, residents said they saw them every day and the administrator said there were five actual mouse sightings reported to her just the day before. One of the people from the pest control company said the staff needed to check garbage cans to make sure they were clean, secure food in sealed plastic bins in resident rooms, and in the kitchen and common areas, clean clutter in resident rooms and other areas in order to decrease the rodent and flying insect problem in the facility. The majority of the fruit flies were found in the back corner behind the elevator where there were loose and broken tiles, water pooling on the floor and in-between the footing and the floor. These were considered the fruit fly breeding areas.

Although the pest control company advised the facility on how to address the mouse infestation with internal methods to prevent entry of mice into the facility and to prevent fruit fly breeding, GLC did not institute the recommendations or provide the pest control staff with consistent facility staff assistance to directly address the mouse and fruit fly infestations in resident rooms and in the kitchen.

In 2011 and 2013 GLC St. Louis Park was cited for some of the same housekeeping and safety deficits as in 2012. In 2011 the facility was cited for failure to ensure that residents with pressure ulcers receive the necessary care and treatment to promote healing and prevent further development of pressure ulcers. A patient with an infected pressure ulcer did not receive a comprehensive assessment of skin risk factors that contributed to promote healing, including seating surfaces pressure reduction, tissue tolerance while seated, and prevention of infections. They did not provide care to reduce the risk of falls for residents reviewed for accidents, and did not ensure a safe environment in the dining rooms.

In 2013 they failed to ensure against misappropriation of resident funds and failure to follow the policy regarding investigation of allegations of such misappropriations. They failed to shower a resident according to her preferences for two showers a week instead of being given a bed bath. They failed to develop a care plan to address a patient's medical condition and did not individualize the plan. They did not provide ADL care as directed in the care plans of two patients. They failed to decrease an anti-psychotic medication as recommended by the pharmacist and the pharmacists failed to report unnecessary medications to the attending physician and director of nursing and ensure these irregularities were acted upon

The facility failed to ensure an insulin vial was labeled with a resident's name and medication rooms were kept in a clean and sanitary manner for 21 of 21 residents who had their medications stored on the refrigerators units. In addition, expired medications were given to two residents.

In the 2013 *Statement of Deficiencies and Plan of Correction* for Faribault Care Center, the Centers for Medicare and Medicaid Services cited the facility for failure to thoroughly investigate and immediately report to the State Department of Health allegations of potential abuse for 2 of 6 residents in the sample who reported allegations of abuse and for failing to protect these residents from potential retaliation during a pending investigation. The allegation of intrusive physical contact between a male nurses aide and a female patient who was considered reliable and had never made a similar allegation, was not reported to the facility administrator and the Director of Nursing (DON) interviewed only one other nurses aide and no other patients about the incident. The DON was unable to recite the facility's policy and procedures regarding protection of residents when allegations of abuse were reported. The possibility that another nurses aide retaliated against the patient who made the allegation by refusing to assist her, rushing her, being rude and abrupt with her was not investigated. The facility was directed to develop policies for prevention of mistreatment, neglect or abuse of patients or theft of their property and to hire only people with no legal history of abusing, neglecting or mistreating residents.

Based on observation and interview, the facility was also cited for failure to accommodate the needs of a resident whose mattress was not long enough. This resident was, of course, our Bill Tollefson. The report did, incorrectly, state that Bill "chose to spend most of the day in bed." Interestingly, the inspector found, using the Brief Interview of Mental Status (BIMS), that Bill was "cognitively intact," something that his guardian and nursing home jailers continued to deny in spite of the evidence to the contrary. The BIMS procedure has the patient recall three words immediately after they are presented and then again after a short time interval. It also assesses knowledge of the year, month and day of the week. A quick rough screening device, it is said to measure attention, orientation and ability to register and recall new information. This probably was the same assessment device used when Bill was at Mayo Clinic that I had wanted to obtain through my request for my power of attorney and health care representative documents from that institution. The guardian appeared to not want me to obtain evidence that contradicted the claimed basis for the guardianship.

The nursing home inspector also found that a Braden Pressure Risk Assessment indicated that Bill was at moderate risk for the development of pressure ulcers. The Braden Scale is a measure of the risk of developing pressure ulcers using a set of six criteria: ability to detect and respond to discomfort or pain related to pressure on parts of the body; skin moisture which can cause the skin to soften and wear away, risking epidermal erosion; lack of activity can promote atrophy of muscles and breakdown of tissue; capability of adjusting body position independently; nutritional status; degree of sliding on beds or chairs which can cause shear and breakdown of cell walls and capillaries. According to the inspector, Bill's sensory perception was "slightly limited, can't always communicate discomfort or the need to be turned. Moisture: skin is occasionally moist requiring an extra linen change approximately every day. Activity: resident is confined to bed, Mobility: very limited, makes occasional slight changes in body or extremity position but unable to make frequent or significant changes in body or extremity position. Friction and shear: problem, requires moderate to maximum assistance in moving, complete lifting without sliding against sheets is impossible, frequently slides down in bed or chair, requiring frequent reposition with maximum assist."

The risk of development of bed sores was very salient with Bill and he frequently complained to and about staff failure to pay attention to these risk factors and his own experience of sweating, itching, and blood spotting from his backside. The facility was required to "Reasonably accommodate the needs and preferences of each resident," but even after his bed was extended and he was provided a new mattress, the problems continued. He was not issued the pressure pad designed to prevent bed sores, he was not issued new bed sheets every day, he continued to sweat and itch, he was not repositioned when he needed to be, and he was not provided with physical therapy to help him become more mobile. In other words, the nursing home staff paid attention only to the fact that the bed they had him sleeping in for over a year was too short; they had no understanding of the overall problem.

FCC was also cited for failure to provide services in accordance with each resident's plan of care, specifically in two wheelchair bound patients who required assistance with toileting. The objective was to have these patients remain clean, dry and have no episodes of skin breakdown. It will be recalled that Bill had many episodes of sitting in his soiled linens waiting for aides to come to clean him up.

Related to this lack of sanitation was another citation for failure of staff to wash their hands after direct contact with resident urinals, bed pans and other contaminated articles for four of four residents during observations of personal care for which hand washing was indicated. Although the facility policy required hand washing as the primary means to prevent the spread of infections, the staff did not obey them. FCC was ordered to have a program that investigates, controls and keeps infection from spreading. This carelessness about sanitation probably was what led to Bill contracting pneumonia. His ulcers also may have been due to lack of sanitation since H.Pylori is transmitted person to person via either the oral-oral or fecal-oral route. According to Wikipedia, "Transmission occurs mainly within families in developed nations yet can also be acquired from the community in developing countries. *H. pylori* may also be transmitted orally by means of fecal matter through the ingestion of waste-tainted water, so a hygienic environment could help decrease the risk of *H. pylori* infection."

FCC was cited for failure to follow care plans related to fall risk by not using bed sensor alarms when appropriate and failure to ensure safe practices when using the Hoyer lift to transfer residents. It was observed that the staff used an improperly hooked sling when transferring one resident resulting in three rib fractures and pain in chest wall, hip and leg. It was found that the facility policy lacked any instructions regarding inspection of the sling accessory devices after it was discovered that staff did not inspect a mesh sling prior to placement around a resident. FCC was ordered to "Make sure that the nursing home area is free from accident hazards and risks and provides supervision to prevent avoidable accidents." It will be remembered that Bill was frequently given "sling excuses" for why they could not move him using the Hoyer lift. In his case, they "solved" their deficit in sling equipment, skills and training by just not moving him whenever they could avoid it, i. e., they didn't allow him to use the commode, skipped showers, and didn't move him into his comfortable electric lift chair.

The facility was ordered to provide housekeeping and maintenance services after it was observed a mildew odor potentially affecting 29 residents was present. A shower was found to have loose trim stained with a mildew type stain and many rooms were observed to have pealing paint and plaster. A door was found to have splintering and rough edges.

An interview with the facility social worker confirmed that the care plan for one resident did not address the resident's anxiety, mood, and behavioral issues even though the patient was receiving psychotropic medication. Non-pharmacological interventions to manage the patient's mood and/or behavioral symptoms was not included. The facility was ordered to "Develop a complete care plan that meets all of a resident's needs, with timetables and actions that can be measured."

There also was identified problems in the use of certain medications. The facility did not ensure that adequate indications for the use and efficacy of PRN psychotropic and pain medications were present. According to the inspecting nurse, "When PRN orders are implemented, nursing staff must monitor the use of such medications to determine: a. The nature of the problem and whether it persists; b. Whether additional evaluation is needed; or c. Whether the medication could be discontinued entirely because the problem is resolved. If a resident uses a PRN medication repeatedly over several days or longer, the nursing staff will discuss with the Physician whether the current medication remains appropriate."Apparently the facility did not follow these rules and it was instructed to "1) Make sure that each resident's drug regimen is free from unnecessary drugs; 2) Each resident's entire drug/medication is managed and monitored to achieve highest well being."

In Bill's case, even after FCC was instructed to make these changes, he was surreptitiously administered psychotropic medications without his awareness or permission and the adverse side-effects of these medications were not monitored or taken into account when deciding whether or not to continue them. He was administered what seemed to be some kind of pain medication that pushed him into a manic state and then was given something else that switched him into a near comatose state shortly thereafter. They continued to give him medications for gout without evaluating whether or not these were actually needed and he was placed on a diabetic diet even though tests that they administered themselves indicated that he was not diabetic. Whether or not he continued to need thyroid medication after he stopped taking amioderone was never assessed; he was just maintained on the drug. So, FCC's inadequacy in drug management was yet another failing that affected Mr. Tollefson. It should be noted here that, nation-wide it is estimated that 15,000 nursing home patients per year die from inappropriately given anti-psychotic drugs, according to FDA drug reviewer David Graham, MD.

Food handling and general maintenance were also sources of citations for FCC. They did not have a regular dietitian but instead shared one with another Deseret facility and a lead staff person had been designated to perform food service management functions but split her day between regular food service duties and management duties. She did not have a certified dietary manager's certificate, nor was she enrolled in a program. The state nursing inspector observed that the facility failed to maintain safe food handling practices, with the potential to affect all residents in the facility. Cross contamination was observed during meal service, open food packages (cake mix, bread crumbs, pasta, and marshmallows) were not stored in sealed containers, and test strips for sanitation fluid testing were unavailable. Kitchen equipment was not maintained in a safe and functional manner: a toaster and blender were not institutional grade and lacked National Sanitation Foundation certification. Ventilation fans weren't working in a soiled utility room with a very strong smell of urine and an inoperable shower fan allowed mildew odors to develop.

Finally and importantly, the facility failed to complete annual performance evaluations for all of their nursing assistants who had been there for over a year. They were ordered to "1) Review the work of each nurse aide every year; and 2) give regular in-service training based upon these reviews." By way of an excuse, the administrator stated that the evaluations had not been completed because there had been three changes in facility ownership in the last year. I think the inspector may have misunderstood that there had been three changes of *administrators*, not ownership, in the last year.

Although Bill would get angry at nurses and nurses aides who would treat him in a derogatory and imperious manner, he knew that the driving force for their unprofessional behavior came from the top. Corporate officers and managers decided on the size and quality of the work force, on the patient density for a particular facility, on how resources were distributed for maintenance and housekeeping as opposed to distributions to stock holders. Bill knew that the staff was being asked to do more than they could possibly do with the resources they were given and their frustration and anger was displaced onto residents. Staff turnover was a good indication of their dissatisfaction with the degree to which they could do their jobs given the constraints imposed by management. There were three different administrators for the FCC facility in one year, at least that many directors of nursing, and who knows how many nurses and nurses aides found better facilities at which to use their skills. Conditions were so bad that one medical clinic that had served them decided to call it quits and another refused to contract with them at all.

Perhaps the profit motive should be removed from nursing home care (or all medical care, for that matter). There are non-profit community nursing homes, such as Northfield Retirement Center (NRC), that seem to be able to provide quality care in a variety of living situations for residents that are dependent on Medicare or Medicaid as well as those who are able to pay. NRC's 30 acre campus includes a fitness center, walking paths, grocery store, cafe, wellness clinic, beauty salon, wifi internet, movie theater, library, lounges, facility TV programing channels, and a large variety of activities for mind, body and spirit. Most important is their values statement, which they seem to take seriously:

"Because we believe our care-receivers and caregivers are people of significant worth, we will:
- provide loving care to all;
- uphold the right of residents to live with honor and dignity;
- provide services without discrimination;
- provide excellent service;
- advocate for the people we serve;
- promote the highest professional standards;
- foster a climate of opportunity for individual growth;
- recognize and respect staff;
- support volunteers and friends;
- be responsible financial stewards."

Perhaps this kind of facility is not possible in large anonymous communities characterized by what the French sociologist Durkheim called "anomie," but only in close-knit small communities with lots of active supporters. Certainly, state operated facilities in Minnesota, although they are non-profit, do not appear to be operated with such dedication as NRC and have many of the same problems as the for-profit nursing homes, e. g., too few and poorly trained staff, lack of resources, lack of oversight. But, for the country as a whole, for-profit nursing homes have one third less staff than do non-profit nursing homes and they have significantly more deficiencies, which translates into more abused and neglected residents.

Assuming that large corporate nursing homes are going to be around for a while (and they are even buying up hospice facilities now because they can turn a good profit with the help of Medicare by taking in non-terminal patients), what can be done to curb their abuses of the elderly and infirm? One thing that might help is more frequent inspections and hefty fines for non-compliance with established standards. Showing up at a nursing home once a year or every two years for an inspection is just not adequate and the nursing homes do not seem to take them seriously. Like Big Pharma, they may treat state imposed fines as just another "cost of doing business" that is less expensive than catching up on deferred maintenance, reducing the number of patients per square foot, hiring well qualified staff and paying them enough so that they do not leave at the first opportunity, or, god forbid, reducing the shareholders return on investment. Of course, more frequent inspections means having more inspectors and that means more money needs to go into that aspect of state government. This, in turn, requires legislators that actually want to solve social and medical problems rather than just promise to cut taxes to garner votes in the next election. And to get those kinds of legislators requires that we have an electorate that is educated in regard to the problems in nursing care. And where does this education come from? Why, from the media doing stories of sufficient length (not sound bites) to actually educate and let people know what they can do about the problem and from activists who spread the word however they can. So, rise up citizens. Join the Boomers Against Elder Abuse or the National Association to Stop Guardianship Abuse. Get off your duffs and vote in some problem-solvers, learn what role you can play in giving our elders a dignified ending to their lives. After all, you are in line to join their ranks, sooner or later.

And what am I to say about all those tax-payer funded agencies that are supposed to prevent or correct injustice and inadequate care? All of the state agencies in Minnesota except for one, the Ombudsman for Elder Minnesotans, were totally unresponsive (even when their mission statements said they handled such problems). The State Department of Health conducted only sham investigations of complaints made to them, ones that were certain to end in the status quo. The governor didn't even feel it necessary to respond at all to a petition pointing to defects in his state's handling of mental patients.

And the feds? They only responded to my HIPAA complaint after an intervention by a senator after a year's delay, and then they investigated the wrong complaint and accepted the word of a gigantic heath care corporation which subsequently made contradictory statements about the person affected by their lack of diligence. And the Department of Justice was so inept that they could not read the first sentence of the first page of an ADA complaint and see that I was one of the complainants. What did they do? I have no idea. I have again asked Senator Tom Udall to intervene to get the feds to say what, if anything, they did with regard to my ADA Complaint. At this writing, they have not responded.

Perhaps I shouldn't expect too much from the Department of Justice. A recent article by the Project on Government Oversight (POGO) indicated that hundreds of federal prosecutors and other Justice Department employees violated rules, laws, or ethical standards relating to their work, according to their own Office of Professional Responsibility (http://www.pogo.org/our-work/reports/2014/hundreds-of-justice-attorneys-violated-standards.html). Of the 650 infractions reviewed from 2002 to 2013, more than 400 were considered "recklessness or intentional misconduct," as opposed to simply errors or cases of poor judgment. There were 48 allegations that attorneys mislead courts, 29 instances of prosecutors failing to provide exculpatory information to defendants and 13 instances where DOJ employees were alleged to have violated constitutional or civil rights.

So what am I to expect if I have to file a request for information from that self-same agency under the Freedom Of Information Act? Probably more of the same.

I must confess that most all of my efforts to achieve some justice for Bill and to keep him from ending up being yet another victim of the gulag did, in fact, fail. The knowledge I gained in so doing is mainly a knowledge of what doesn't work. Consequently, my advise to anyone who finds him/herself in a similar situation is to forget about everything I tried to do, don't count on any government agencies or agents to do anything, forget about getting politicians to help. Document everything as well as you can, and concentrate your efforts on raising enough money to hire a really good attorney that will stand up to the powers that be and work for your interests. That will be an uphill battle, as previously indicated, but it seems to be the only game in town. Then sue the bastards for as much as you can. Threat of financial loss is the only thing they seem to be capable of understanding.

ABOUT THE AUTHOR

Gerald D. Otis was born in Northfield, Minnesota. He graduated from Northfield High School, attended St. Olaf College for two years, worked as a cab driver to save money so that he could graduate from the University of Minnesota in 1961. After completing a clinical internship at the Veterans Administration Hospital in Palo Alto, California he earned his Ph.D. in Psychology from the University of Arizona in 1966. Dr. Otis joined the University of New Mexico School of Medicine where he taught classes, maintained a clinical practice, and headed a research team in a longitudinal study of the career decision making process in medical students and physicians,.

For 10 years after Dr. Otis left the University, he combined a private practice with the design and construction of sculptural furniture and computer programming. During his years as a psychologist he published results of research on incidental learning, interaction of stress and personality, family psychotherapy, physician career choice, psychological type and the Myers-Briggs Type Indicator, post-traumatic stress disorder, and trends in violent death. He has received two awards from the Association for Psychological Type and several awards for his efforts at fine woodworking.

Following 16 years working for the Veterans Administration in southern Oregon, where he specialized in the treatment of post-traumatic stress disorder, Dr. Otis retired from clinical practice and now lives in Las Cruces, New Mexico with his wife Connie. He has authored two books: *Joseph Lee Heywood: His Life and Tragic Death* and *Paroxysm: Love, Murder and Justice in Post Civil War Washington, DC.* He has also edited, with his wife, a collection of poems: *Words of Grace: The Poetry of Grace McCrea Lindahl.*

www.ingramcontent.com/pod-product-compliance
Lightning Source LLC
Chambersburg PA
CBHW051625170526
45167CB00001B/65